THE MEDITERRANEAN DIET
FOR FAMILY

3 Books in 1: All You Need to Know About the Mediterranean Cooking + More Than 350+ Delicious Italian, Spanish, and Greek Style Recipes for Weight Loss and Live Healthy!

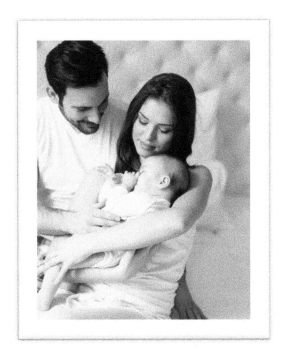

By

Alexander Sandler

TABLE OF CONTENT

PART I—INTRODUCTION

Do you feel like you're always eating and can't get enough of certain foods? Read on...

Many studies have shown that following a low-carb diet allows you to lose weight quickly without having to count every single calorie introduced into your body.

For this reason, you must know the difference between simple and complex carbohydrates.

Like any other macro-nutrient, carbohydrates are needed to provide energy to the body. But which type?

Complex carbohydrates such as brown rice or whole-wheat pasta and whole wheat bread, legumes, oats, many vegetables, potatoes, quinoa provide nutrients to the body and therefore are considered beneficial.

Simple carbohydrates such as white sugar, candy, sweets, and sugary drinks, white flour, and bread do not provide any nutrients to the body. This is why they are also called "empty calories" because they provide nothing but calories.

So the answer is straightforward: you can consume complex carbohydrates, which are widely used in the Mediterranean diet for vegetarians, and you should avoid simple carbohydrates as much as possible.

You will notice that by eating a healthier, more balanced diet that includes plant proteins, fiber, minerals, vitamins, good quality fats

and complex carbohydrates, you will have more energy to carry out your daily activities.

The reason you're always hungry and feel like you can't get enough of certain foods (which is the title of this chapter) is that by eating a lot of high-calorie snacks and simple carbohydrates (the empty-calorie kind), you experience an instant boost but a subsequent crash in your energy level and therefore eat more and gain more weight.

By following the Mediterranean diet for vegetarians, you will notice that your appetite will naturally and automatically stabilize, you will consume fewer calories, and consequently, your weight will also stabilize.

Reducing simple carbohydrates will stabilize your blood sugar levels and allow you to lose weight, eliminate bloating in the abdomen area, and look and feel much healthier.

While many people suggest avoiding fats, avoiding simple carbohydrates can bring more weight loss results. Some fats are, in fact, beneficial, usually fats that come from plant sources such as extra virgin olive oil, nuts, dark chocolate, almonds, avocados, and so on...

A healthy eating program such as the Mediterranean diet provides a viable solution to many diet-related health problems such as obesity, issues related to the metabolic process, inflammation, and heart disease.

When considering any type of diet, remember that food and exercise always go hand in hand. So also make sure to move your body at least 20 minutes a day (4 to 5 days a week).

You could choose a natural, plain yogurt with nuts and honey on top or with berries and oatmeal on top for breakfast.

Remember to read labels. When choosing your products, always avoid those with a long list of ingredients full of artificial elements. If you can buy the organic version, even better.

Another breakfast idea is to have your favorite choice of seasonal fruit with a cup of coffee or tea. If you choose this option, make sure to set the table nicely, cut up the different fruits, and arrange them well on a plate, and you could also sprinkle cinnamon or freshly grated lemon zest.

Don't underestimate the importance of presentation and eating carefully without rushing. It makes a massive difference in terms of satisfaction and not feeling deprived.

If you like oats, you can make oatmeal with berries or nuts on top instead of yogurt, or you could have some type of plant-based milk (like oat, almond, rice, or nut milk) with your favorite choice of natural whole grains.

No matter how you choose to start your day, never skip breakfast and always start with a big glass of water (think of it as a shower, you wouldn't start your day without it, right?).

You can cook brown rice or pasta for lunch and mix it with your favorite choice of veggies.

I like to sauté carrots and zucchini with about 2 to 3 tablespoons of extra virgin olive oil and a clove of garlic and season the veggies with basil and fresh oregano.

Cook the pasta or rice according to the instructions on the package. Once the pasta or rice is cooked, add it to the vegetables, toss and mix well. Your lunch is ready.

Eat pasta or rice for lunch instead of dinner whenever possible because it takes longer to digest. You always want to eat something lighter at dinner.

Another idea for lunch is to make a Mediterranean omelet by simply whisking a couple of eggs with fresh herbs and your favorite choice of vegetables. Cook it well on both sides in a skillet with extra virgin olive oil—season with salt and freshly ground black pepper.

You can easily make a delicious dinner by grilling or cooking different vegetables or mushrooms and seasoning extra virgin olive oil and fresh herbs.

Or you can prepare zucchini and eggplant with fresh tomatoes and black olives, topped with basil, extra virgin olive oil, salt, and pepper.

Another idea for dinner is to prepare a simple dish with legumes and vegetables seasoned with extra virgin olive oil and chili.

You could eat a different variety of raw vegetables with tahini paste (which is a very tasty and delicious paste made with sesame) and a hard-boiled egg or a small piece of parmesan cheese.

These were some ideas; in the next chapter, you will find several Mediterranean and vegetarian recipes to choose from for lunch or dinner.

START TO GET FAMILIAR WITH THE MEDITERRANEAN DIET: SCIENTIFICAL STUDIES AND BENEFITS

In 2013, an article published in the New England Journal of Medicine made headlines in every major newspaper. The report, "Primary Prevention of Cardiovascular Disease with a Mediterranean Diet," detailed a five-year study on the health benefits of eating a Mediterranean diet, especially concerning coronary health and stroke risk.

In this latest clinical study, more than 6,000 people were divided into three groups. The first group of participants followed a Mediterranean diet and were also asked to consume at least one liter of extra virgin olive oil per week. The second group also followed the Mediterranean diet, but they were asked to consume at least 35 grams of healthy nuts per week. Finally, the third group ate a low-fat Western diet. None of the participants were asked to exercise in any particular way, and no-calorie restrictions were imposed on any of the groups. At the end of the study, the results were truly remarkable:

The study also reported that the risk of stroke was similarly reduced. However, it became so evident during the study that those following the Western diet were at a health disadvantage that the research was terminated a year early due to moral and ethical concerns about asking that group to continue.

The results of this study were so dramatic and significant that they attracted international attention. However, this is just one of many studies demonstrating the health benefits of the Mediterranean diet. The scientific and medical communities have praised it for years for its benefits on heart and artery health and kidney function, reducing the risk of stroke, type 2 diabetes, and metabolic syndrome, and even preventing some forms of cancer.

Research supports the many health benefits of the Mediterranean diet

The impact of the Mediterranean diet on heart health is one of its most commonly studied aspects, and there is plenty of research demonstrating its positive effect on coronary and vascular function.

In 2011, for example, researchers at the University of Miami published a study on the cardiovascular benefits of following a Mediterranean diet. The study results showed that consuming fresh fruits and vegetables, whole grains, olive oil, nuts, and fish was an excellent way to improve heart health and decrease the risk of cardiovascular disease.

In 2011, the journal Public Health Nutrition published the results of a study that showed that the high volume of whole grains consumed in the Mediterranean diet made it an effective way to reduce the risk of certain forms of cancer, particularly colorectal cancer.

Then, in 2012, the Department of Internal Medicine and Geriatrics at the University of Palermo published the results of a study that showed that the Mediterranean diet has a positive impact not only on heart health but also on the incidence of diabetes.

And again in 2012, Spanish researchers from the Diabetology, Endocrinology and Nutrition Unit at the Dr. Josep Trueta Hospital in Girona reported that a study of 129 older adults eating a Mediterranean diet with nuts, a Mediterranean diet with olive oil, or a low-fat diet revealed that after two years, both types of Mediterranean diet led to a significant improvement in bone health.

As you can see, the health benefits of the Mediterranean diet have been wholly and extensively studied.

However, much research has shown that the Mediterranean diet may have a much longer list of health benefits beyond the heart. This chapter will look at just a few of the many improvements you can experience on your health when you start the Mediterranean diet.

Additional benefits

Aside from the significant heart and brain benefits, the Mediterranean diet can significantly improve many other key factors in your life. For example, since the Mediterranean diet focuses on eating healthy, exercising, and connecting with others, you can see improvements to your mental health, your physical health, and you'll often feel like you're living a more fulfilling life. Some of the other additional benefits you may experience when you switch to a Mediterranean diet are discussed below.

Longevity

When you eliminate the risk of developing certain conditions such as cardiovascular disease, diabetes, and dementia, you increase your lifespan. But eliminating these health risks is not the only cause of increased longevity with the Mediterranean diet. Increased physical activity and deep social connection also play a significant role in living longer.

Plus Energy

Following a Mediterranean diet focuses on fueling your body. Other diets focus only on filling your body, and this is often done through empty calories. You won't need to rely on sugary drinks, excess caffeine, or sugar-filled energy bars to get you going and keep you moving. You'll feel less weighed down after eating, which means you'll be able to work at higher levels of output.

Clear skin

Healthy skin starts on the inside. When you provide your body with healthy foods, this will radiate through your skin. For example, the antioxidants in extra virgin olive oil are enough to keep your skin young and healthy. But the Mediterranean diet includes several types of fresh fruits and vegetables that are full of antioxidants. These antioxidants help repair damaged cells in the body and promote the growth of healthy cells. Eating a variety of healthy fats also keeps your skin supple and can protect it from premature aging.

Better sleep

Sugar and caffeine can cause significant sleep disturbances. In addition, other foods, such as processed foods, can make it harder to get the right amount of sleep. Your body will want to rest to recover and properly absorb the vitamins and minerals consumed during the day. Your brain will switch into sleep mode with ease because it has received the vitamins it needs to function correctly. When you get the right amount of sleep, you will, in turn, have more energy the next day, and this can also significantly improve your mood. The Mediterranean diet increases the consumption of nutrient-dense foods and avoids excess sugar and processed foods known to cause sleep problems.

In addition, the Mediterranean diet allows you to maintain a healthy weight, reducing your risk of developing sleep disorders such as sleep apnea. Sleep apnea is common in individuals who are overweight and obese. It causes the airway to become blocked, making it difficult to breathe. This results in not getting enough oxygen when you sleep, which can cause you to wake up suddenly and frequently during the night.

Protects against cancer

Many plant-based foods, especially those in the yellow and orange color groups, contain cancer-fighting agents. For example, increasing the antioxidants consumed by eating fresh fruits and vegetables and whole grains can help protect the body's cells from developing cancerous cells. Drinking a glass of red wine also provides cancer-protective compounds.

Maintaining a healthy weight

With the Mediterranean diet, you eat mostly whole, fresh foods. Eating more foods rich in vitamins, minerals, and nutrients is essential to maintaining a healthy weight. The diet is easy to adhere to, and there are no calorie restrictions to follow strictly. This makes it a highly sustainable plan for those who want to lose weight or maintain a healthy weight. Keep in mind. This is not an option to lose weight quickly. However, this lifestyle will allow you to maintain optimal health for years, not just a few months.

THE BENEFITS

Heart health and stroke risk reduction

Heart health is strongly influenced by diet. Maintaining healthy cholesterol levels, blood pressure, blood sugar, and maintaining a healthy weight leads to optimal heart health. Your diet directly affects each of these components. Those who are most at risk are often advised to start on a low-fat diet. A low-fat diet eliminates all fats, including those from oils, nuts, and red meat. Investigations have shown that this diet, which includes healthy fats, is more effective at lowering cardiovascular risks than a standard low-fat diet (This is processed red meat, 2019). This is because the unsaturated fats consumed in the Mediterranean diet lower harmful cholesterol levels and increase good cholesterol levels.

The Mediterranean diet emphasizes the importance of daily activity and stress reduction by enjoying quality time with friends and family. Each of these elements, along with eating more plant-based foods, significantly improves heart health and reduces the risk of many heart-related conditions.

Age-related muscle and bone weakness reduction

Eating a well-balanced diet that provides a wide range of vitamins and minerals is essential for reducing muscle weakness and bone degradation. This is especially important as you age. Accident-related injuries such as tripping, falling, or slipping while walking can cause serious injuries. As you age, this becomes even more of a concern because some simple falls can be fatal. Many accidents occur because of weakening muscle mass and loss of bone density. Women, especially those entering the menopausal stage of their lives, are at greater risk of serious injury from accidental falls because estrogen levels decrease significantly—this decrease in estrogen results in a loss of bone and muscle mass. Reduced estrogen can also cause bone thinning, which over time develops into osteoporosis.

Maintaining healthy bone mass and muscle agility as you age can be a challenge. When you don't get the proper nutrients to promote healthy bones and muscles, you increase your risk of developing osteoporosis. The Mediterranean diet offers an easy way to meet the dietary needs necessary to improve bone and muscle function.

Antioxidants, vitamins C and K, carotenoids, magnesium, potassium, and phytoestrogens are essential minerals and nutrients for optimal musculoskeletal health. Plant-based foods, unsaturated fats, and whole grains help provide the necessary balance of nutrients that keep bones and muscles healthy. Following a Mediterranean diet can improve and reduce bone loss as you age.

Reduces the risk of neurological diseases

Alzheimer's disease

Alzheimer's disease is a form of dementia in which there is significant cognitive decline. Those with Alzheimer's suffer from

- Disorientation
- Memory loss
- Inability to think clearly
- Language problems
- Impaired judgment
- Visual and spatial disorientation

Alzheimer's is a common brain disorder in older adults, age 60 and older, but early signs of Alzheimer's can be present even in adults as young as 30. The condition can progress quickly or slowly, depending on how fast the neurons in the brain begin to die. Although the decline starts in the hippocampus area of the brain, it becomes widespread as it progresses.

Individuals with Alzheimer's show a significant increase in beta-amyloid proteins in the brain and have a much lower level of brain energy. Research has focused on the early identification of people at increased risk for dementia through brain scans and imaging. In one such study, brain scans were conducted on 70 individuals between 30 and 60. Patients did not showed signs of dementia, and 34 of them adhered to a Mediterranean diet while 36 followed a standard Western diet. When brain scans were conducted at the beginning of the study and then two years later. The scans showed that those following the Western diet had a significant loss of brain energy levels and increased beta-amyloid accumulation instead of those on the Mediterranean diet (Mediterranean Diet May Slow Development, 2018). The study highlights how simple lifestyle changes can help reduce the risk of Alzheimer's and other cognitive declines.

This indicates that diet can have an impact on the two leading indicators of Alzheimer's disease development. Just as diet can impact other areas of your health, it can also affect the health of your brain. Cholesterol, blood sugar, and blood vessel health can contribute to your risk of developing Alzheimer's disease. The most common fuel sources for the brain are fresh fruits and vegetables that supply vital vitamins and nutrients. When processed foods, refined grains, and added sugars are consumed too often, this compromises brain function because these foods release toxins into the body. These toxins then cause widespread inflammation, and the brain begins to accumulate plaques that cause cognitive abilities to malfunction (Nutrition and Dementia, 2019).

The Western diet consists of several foods that increase the risk of Alzheimer's, such as processed meat, refined grains such as white bread and pasta, and added sugar. In addition, foods that contain diacetyl, which is a chemical commonly used in the refining process, increase the buildup of beta-amyloid plaques in the brain. Microwave popcorn, margarine, and butter are some of the most frequently consumed foods that contain this harmful chemical. So it's no wonder that Alzheimer's is becoming one of the leading causes of death among Americans.

This diet includes a wide range of foods that have been shown to increase memory and slow cognitive decline. Dark leafy vegetables, fresh berries, extra virgin olive oil, and fresh fish contain vitamins and minerals that can improve brain health. The Mediterranean diet can help you make the necessary diet and lifestyle changes that significantly decrease your risk of Alzheimer's disease.

Parkinson's disease

Parkinson's disease is a slowly progressing neurodegenerative disease that affects dopamine-producing neurons in the brain. Those with Parkinson's disease experience.

- Tremors
- Muscle stiffness
- Balance problems
- Difficulty walking
- Depression
- Sleep problems
- Cognitive disorders

Parkinson's disease is not curable, and the medications and therapies suggested for this condition only help individuals manage symptoms, not slow or stop the progress of the disease. Genetics and environmental factors have been studied to understand better what causes Parkinson's disease to develop. However, while genetics play a factor, exposure to pesticides, herbicides, high cholesterol, low vitamin D levels, and limited physical activity can increase the risk of Parkinson's disease.

Parkinson's disease is also common among individuals who have higher levels of oxidative stress. This damages brain cells and can cause severe cognitive and physical decline. Antioxidants can help reduce the risk of developing Parkinson's disease and repair damaged cells and form stronger brain connections.

The Mediterranean diet encourages the consumption of antioxidant-rich foods such as fresh fruits and vegetables. Eating organic and locally grown fruits and vegetables reduces the risk of exposure to toxins from pesticides and herbicides.

People with Parkinson's are often encouraged to change their diets to include more healthy fats, such as extra virgin olive oil, seeds, nuts, fresh fruits, organic vegetables, and whole grains. This dietary recommendation is the foundation of the Mediterranean diet. Individuals are also encouraged to reduce salt, sugar, and empty calorie foods, which the Mediterranean diet encourages.

Protects against type 2 diabetes

Health professionals recommend the Mediterranean diet for those diagnosed with type 2 or prediabetic diabetes. The combination of healthy foods and regular exercise that the Mediterranean diet promotes are two of the key components in helping individuals manage and even see a remission of symptoms.

Type 2 diabetes develops when your body can no longer produce or properly use the insulin it produces. This causes blood sugar levels to reach dangerous levels. Blood sugar or glucose is what gives your body energy. It provides fuel to your muscles, tissues, and cells so they can function properly. When glucose is released into the bloodstream, it signals the pancreas to start producing insulin so that the cells in your body can adequately absorb the glucose. When you have type 2 diabetes, your pancreas doesn't produce enough insulin. As a result, your cells can't absorb enough, or the insulin isn't used properly, so the glucose stays in your body. A build-up of glucose in the body can cause a long list of health complications. For example, the body can turn to use muscle and fat to get the energy it needs. Blood vessels can also be damaged, which increases the risk of heart attack and stroke.

Those who are at increased risk of developing type 2 diabetes are:
- Individuals who are overweight or obese
- Individuals who have limited physical activity.
- Individuals who have a family history of type 2 diabetes
- Individuals who have insulin resistance
- The most common symptoms of type 2 diabetes include.
- Excessive fatigue
- Frequent numbness in the hands or feet
- Tingling in the hands and feet
- Regular headaches
- Difficulty with vision
- Increased urination
- Unquenchable thirst

Type 2 diabetes can go unnoticed for years. As a result, many individuals are unaware of their condition until a severe health complication arises due to the condition. As a result, those with type 2 diabetes are at increased risk for heart attack, stroke, organ damage, vision loss, hearing loss, and many other health conditions that can reduce the quality of life and shorten lifespan.

What you eat contributes to the production of insulin and the efficiency with which the body can use the insulin produced. Carbohydrates, in particular, are converted into glucose for the body to use as energy. Unfortunately, many individuals eat too many unhealthy carbohydrates, causing the body to be out of balance and blood sugar levels to remain elevated. The most common foods known to increase glucose levels are white bread, pasta, and sugary drinks. The excessive sugar and simple carbohydrates found in these items cause the body to suddenly rise in glucose that the body often cannot handle fast enough.

Carbohydrates themselves are not all bad, and when you choose the right ones, they can help slow down the release of glucose, making it easier for the body to absorb energy. Complex carbohydrates found naturally in many fruits, vegetables, and whole grains are released slowly into the bloodstream. Eating foods rich in fiber also helps slow the release of glucose. Type 2 diabetes has been strongly linked to diet. Diets high in trans fat, sugar, simple carbohydrates, and sodium increase the risk of developing diabetes. Individuals who switch to a Mediterranean diet lower their risk of type 2 diabetes. Those diagnosed as prediabetic, which is often a red flag diagnosis that almost always leads to a diagnosis of type 2 diabetes, may reverse the diagnosis. Those with diabetes will often find that the Mediterranean diet can help them significantly reduce symptoms and take control of their insulin and blood sugar levels.

The Mediterranean diet encourages improvement in both diet and physical activity. These two components are the most important factors that will help you manage your diabetes symptoms and reduce your risk of developing the condition.

HEALTHY LIFESTYLE, NOT ONLY WEIGHT LOSS!

One of the ways to make sure that a diet will help you achieve your weight loss goals is to choose one that allows you to eat a wide variety of delicious foods and doesn't require you to go hungry, go without all of your favorite sweets or buy a lot of expensive and obscure ingredients. This is where the Mediterranean diet stands out. There are no strict rules to follow and no deprivation or need to drive all over town hunting for exotic ingredients or expensive supplements.

DID YOU KNOW? Not only is the Mediterranean diet healthy and delicious, but it can also be a very inexpensive way to lose weight. The emphasis on eating whole (rather than processed) foods in season and buying from farmers' markets means you'll be buying produce at its best flavor and lowest prices. As everyone knows, an apple is cheaper than a strawberry in November, and it tastes better too!

How the Mediterranean diet helps you lose weight

For many people who follow it, the Mediterranean diet leads to weight loss naturally and effortlessly.

While most weight-loss diets focus on counting calories, following a strict menu, weighing and measuring foods, or undertaking a rigorous exercise program, the Mediterranean diet focuses on enjoying a wide variety of healthy foods and taking the time to savor meals and share them with others. It is a joyful and healthy way to eat.

By eliminating processed and fast foods from your diet, which are loaded with unhealthy fats, sugar, and chemicals, you can significantly decrease your calorie intake by eating more food. In addition, without counting calories or fat grams, you can trade unhealthy, "empty" foods for those that promote good health and support the loss of stored fat.

For years, the low-fat diet has been promoted as the only authentic way to lose weight, but we now know this is not true. Instead, a low-fat diet very often results in weight gain and can be unhealthy.

A research hospital in Switzerland recently looked at six separate studies comparing the Mediterranean diet and a low-fat diet. People who followed the Mediterranean diet for the studies experienced more significant weight loss, lower body fat percentages, lower blood pressure, and better blood sugar levels than those on the low-fat diet.

Because it also includes a wide variety of healthy, fresh foods, the Mediterranean diet provides a healthy amount of fiber and "good" fats, both of which support weight loss by helping you feel full. A high-fiber diet also slows the rate at which sugar is absorbed into the bloodstream, which controls both blood sugar and insulin levels. Too much insulin in the bloodstream blocks fat loss, as insulin triggers fat storage. Fiber from whole grains, fruits, and vegetables also improves digestion, which can be an essential factor in weight loss. Many of the antioxidants found in fresh fruits and vegetables, such as lutein in apples, have also promoted weight loss. Overall, the Mediterranean diet allows people to lose weight naturally and healthily, without starving themselves or eliminating food groups. Not only will you be able to lose weight on a diet. You'll have fun while doing it.

Breakfast

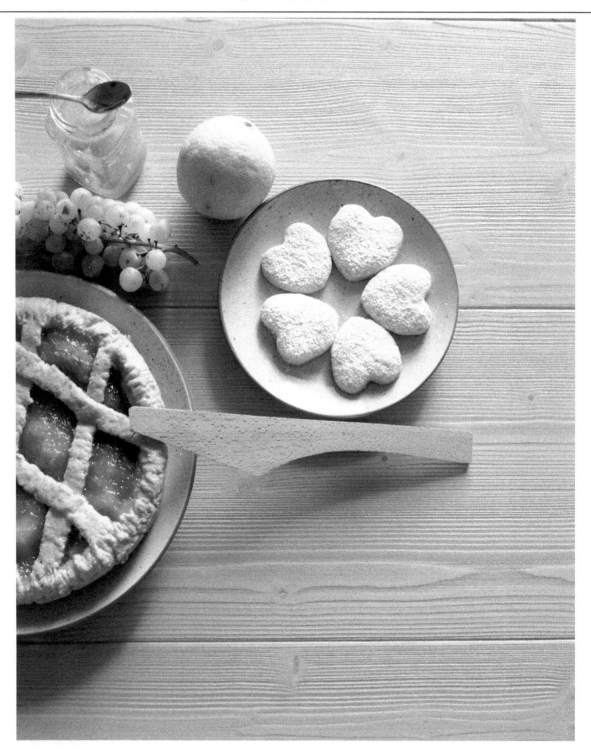

1) CARROT OATMEAL BREAKFAST

Cooking Time: 10 Minutes   **Servings:** 2

Ingredients:

- ✓ 1 cup steel-cut oats
- ✓ 1/2 cup raisins
- ✓ 1/2 tsp ground nutmeg
- ✓ 1/2 tsp ground cinnamon
- ✓ 2 carrots, grated
- ✓ 2 cups of water
- ✓ 2 cups unsweetened almond milk
- ✓ 1 tbsp honey

Directions:

- ❖ Spray instant pot from inside with cooking spray.
- ❖ Add all ingredients into the instant pot and stir well.
- ❖ Seal pot with lid and cook on high for 10 minutes.
- ❖ Once done, release pressure using quick release. Remove lid.
- ❖ Stir and serve.

Nutrition: Calories: 3;Fat: 6.6 g;Carbohydrates: 73.8 g;Sugar: 33.7 g;Protein: 8.1 g;Cholesterol: 0 mg

2) ARBORIO RICE RUM-RAISIN PUDDING

Cooking Time: 4 Hours   **Servings:** 2

Ingredients:

- ✓ ¾ cup Arborio rice
- ✓ 1 can evaporated milk
- ✓ ½ cup raisins
- ✓ ¼ tsp nutmeg, grated
- ✓ 1½ cups water
- ✓ 1/3 cup sugar
- ✓ ¼ cup dark rum
- ✓ sea salt or plain salt

Directions:

- ❖ Start by mixing rum and raisins in a bowl and set aside.
- ❖ Then, heat the evaporated milk and water in a saucepan and then simmer.
- ❖ Now, add sugar and stir until dissolved.
- ❖ Finally, convert this milk mixture into a slow cooker and stir in rice and salt. Cook on low heat for hours.
- ❖ Now, stir in the raisin mixture and nutmeg and let sit for 10 minutes.
- ❖ Serve warm.

Nutrition: Calories: 3, Total Fat: 10.1g, Saturated Fat: 5.9, Cholesterol: 36 mg, Sodium: 161 mg, Total Carbohydrate: 131.5 g, Dietary Fiber: 3.3 g, Total Sugars: 54.8 g, Protein: 14.4 g, Vitamin D: 0 mcg, Calcium: 372 mg, Iron: 2 mg, Potassium: 712 mg

3) MEDITERRANEAN-STYLE QUINOA WITH FETA EGG MUFFINS

Cooking Time: 30 Minutes   **Servings:** 12

Ingredients:

- ✓ 8 eggs
- ✓ 1 cup cooked quinoa
- ✓ 1 cup crumbled feta cheese
- ✓ 1/4 tsp salt
- ✓ 2 cups baby spinach finely chopped
- ✓ 1/2 cup finely chopped onion
- ✓ 1 cup chopped or sliced tomatoes, cherry or grape tomatoes
- ✓ 1/2 cup chopped and pitted Kalamata olives
- ✓ 1 tbsp chopped fresh oregano
- ✓ 2 tsp high oleic sunflower oil plus optional extra for greasing muffin tins

Directions:

- ❖ Pre-heat oven to 350 degrees F
- ❖ Prepare 1silicone muffin holders on a baking sheet, or grease a 12-cup muffin tin with oil, set aside
- ❖ In a skillet over medium heat, add the vegetable oil and onions, sauté for 2 minutes
- ❖ Add tomatoes, sauté for another minute, then add spinach and sauté until wilted, about 1 minute
- ❖ Remove from heat and stir in olives and oregano, set aside
- ❖ Place the eggs in a blender or mixing bowl and blend or mix until well combined
- ❖ Pour the eggs in to a mixing bowl (if you used a blender) then add quinoa, feta cheese, veggie mixture, and salt, and stir until well combined
- ❖ Pour mixture in to silicone cups or greased muffin tins, dividing equally, and bake for 30 minutes, or until eggs have set and muffins are a light golden brown
- ❖ Allow to cool completely
- ❖ Distribute among the containers, store in fridge for 2-3 days

- ❖ To Serve: Heat in the microwave for 30 seconds or until slightly heated through
- ❖ Recipe Notes: Muffins can also be eaten cold. For the quinoa, I recommend making a large batch \'7b2 cups water per each cup of dry, rinsed quinoa\'7d and saving the extra for leftovers.

Nutrition: Calories:1Total Carbohydrates: 5g;Total Fat: 7g;Protein: 6g

4) GREEK YOGURT BLUEBERRY PANCAKES

Cooking Time: 15 Minutes   **Servings:** 6

Ingredients:

- ✓ 1 1/4 cup all-purpose flour
- ✓ 2 tsp baking powder
- ✓ 1 tsp baking soda
- ✓ 1/4 tsp salt
- ✓ 1/4 cup sugar
- ✓ 3 eggs
- ✓ 3 tbsp vegan butter unsalted, melted
- ✓ 1/2 cup milk
- ✓ 1 1/2 cups Greek yogurt plain, non-fat
- ✓ 1/2 cup blueberries optional
- ✓ Toppings:
- ✓ Greek yogurt
- ✓ Mixed berries – blueberries, raspberries and blackberries

Directions:

- ❖ In a large bowl, whisk together the flour, salt, baking powder and baking soda
- ❖ In a separate bowl, whisk together butter, sugar, eggs, Greek yogurt, and milk until the mixture is smooth
- ❖ Then add in the Greek yogurt mixture from step to the dry mixture in step 1, mix to combine, allow the patter to sit for 20 minutes to get a smooth texture – if using blueberries fold them into the pancake batter
- ❖ Heat the pancake griddle, spray with non-stick butter spray or just brush with butter
- ❖ Pour the batter, in 1/4 cupful's, onto the griddle
- ❖ Cook until the bubbles on top burst and create small holes, lift up the corners of the pancake to see if they're golden browned on the bottom
- ❖ With a wide spatula, flip the pancake and cook on the other side until lightly browned
- ❖ Distribute the pancakes in among the storage containers, store in the fridge for 3 day or in the freezer for 2 months
- ❖ To Serve: Reheat microwave for 1 minute (until 80% heated through) or on the stove top, drizzle warm syrup on top, scoop of Greek yogurt, and mixed berries (including blueberries, raspberries, blackberries)

Nutrition: Calories:258;Total Carbohydrates: 33g;Total Fat: 8g;Protein: 11g

5) BREAKFAST VEGETABLE BOWL

Cooking Time: 5 Minutes   **Servings:** 2

Ingredients:

- ✓ Breakfast Bowl:
- ✓ 1 ½ cups cooked quinoa
- ✓ 1 lb asparagus[1], cut into bite-sized pieces, ends trimmed and discarded
- ✓ 1 tbsp avocado oil or olive oil
- ✓ 3 cups shredded kale leaves
- ✓ 1 batch lemony dressing
- ✓ 3 cups shredded, uncooked Brussels sprouts
- ✓ 1 avocado, peeled, pitted and thinly-sliced
- ✓ 4 eggs, cooked to your preference (optional)
- ✓ Garnishes:
- ✓ Toasted sesame seeds
- ✓ Crushed red pepper
- ✓ Sunflower seeds
- ✓ Sliced almonds
- ✓ Hummus
- ✓ Lemon Dressing:
- ✓ 2 tsp Dijon mustard
- ✓ 1 garlic clove, minced
- ✓ 2 tbsp avocado oil or olive oil
- ✓ 2 tbsp freshly-squeezed lemon juice
- ✓ Salt, to taste
- ✓ Freshly-cracked black pepper, to taste

Directions:

- ❖ In a large sauté pan over medium-high heat, add the oil
- ❖ Once heated, add the asparagus and sauté for 4-5 minutes, stirring occasionally, until tender. Remove from heat and set side
- ❖ Add the Brussels sprouts, quinoa, and cooked asparagus, and toss until combined
- ❖ Distribute among the container, store in fridge for 2-3 days
- ❖ To serve: In a large, mixing bowl combine the kale and lemony dressing. Use your fingers to massage the dressing into the kale for 2-3 minutes, or until the leaves are dark and softened, set aside. In a small mixing bowl, combine the avocado, lemon juice, dijon mustard, garlic clove, salt, and pepper. Assemble the bowls by smearing a spoonful of hummus along the side of each bowl, then portion the kale salad evenly between the four bowls. Top with the avocado slices, egg, and your desired garnishes
- ❖ Recipe Note: Feel free to sub the asparagus with your favorite vegetable(s), sautéing or roasting them until cooked

Nutrition: Calories:632;Carbs: 52g;Total Fat: 39g;Protein: 24g

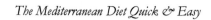

6) BREAKFAST EGG-ARTICHOKE CASSEROLE

Cooking Time: 30 To 35 Minutes   **Servings: 8**

Ingredients:

- ✓ 14 ounces artichoke hearts, if using canned remember to drain them
- ✓ 16 eggs
- ✓ 1 cup shredded cheddar cheese
- ✓ 10 ounces chopped spinach, if frozen make sure it is thawed and well-drained
- ✓ 1 clove of minced garlic
- ✓ ½ cup ricotta cheese
- ✓ ½ cup parmesan cheese
- ✓ ½ tsp crushed red pepper
- ✓ 1 tsp sea salt
- ✓ ½ tsp dried thyme
- ✓ ¼ cup onion, shaved
- ✓ ¼ cup milk

Directions:

- ❖ Grease a 9 x -inch baking pan or place a piece of parchment paper inside of it.
- ❖ Turn the temperature on your oven to 350 degrees Fahrenheit.
- ❖ Crack the eggs into a bowl and whisk them well.
- ❖ Pour in the milk and whisk the two ingredients together.
- ❖ Squeeze any excess moisture from the spinach with a paper towel.
- ❖ Toss the spinach and leafless artichoke hearts into the bowl. Stir until well combined.
- ❖ Add the cheddar cheese, minced garlic, parmesan cheese, red pepper, sea salt, thyme, and onion into the bowl. Mix until all the ingredients are fully incorporated.
- ❖ Pour the eggs into the baking pan.
- ❖ Add the ricotta cheese in even dollops before placing the casserole in the oven.
- ❖ Set your timer for 30 minutes, but watch the casserole carefully after about 20 minutes. Once the eggs stop jiggling and are cooked, remove the meal from the oven. Let the casserole cool down a bit and enjoy!

Nutrition: calories: 302, fats: 18 grams, carbohydrates: grams, protein: 22 grams.

7) CAULIFLOWER RICE BOWL BREAKFAST

Cooking Time: 12 Minutes   **Servings: 6**

Ingredients:

- ✓ 1 cup cauliflower rice
- ✓ 1/2 tsp red pepper flakes
- ✓ 1 1/2 tsp curry powder
- ✓ 1/2 tbsp ginger, grated
- ✓ 1 cup vegetable stock
- ✓ 4 tomatoes, chopped
- ✓ 3 cups broccoli, chopped
- ✓ Pepper
- ✓ Salt

Directions:

- ❖ Spray instant pot from inside with cooking spray.
- ❖ Add all ingredients into the instant pot and stir well.
- ❖ Seal pot with lid and cook on high for 12 minutes.
- ❖ Once done, allow to release pressure naturally for 10 minutes then release remaining using quick release. Remove lid.
- ❖ Stir and serve.

Nutrition: Calories: 44;Fat: 0.8 g;Carbohydrates: 8.2 g;Sugar: 3.8 g;Protein: 2.8 g;Cholesterol: 0 mg

8) CUCUMBER-DILL SAVORY YOGURT

Cooking Time: 10 Minutes   **Servings: 4**

Ingredients:

- ✓ 2 cups low-fat (2%) plain Greek yogurt
- ✓ 4 tsp minced shallot
- ✓ 4 tsp freshly squeezed lemon juice
- ✓ ¼ cup chopped fresh dill
- ✓ 2 tsp olive oil
- ✓ ¼ tsp kosher salt
- ✓ Pinch freshly ground black pepper
- ✓ 2 cups chopped Persian cucumbers (about 4 medium cucumbers)

Directions:

- ❖ Combine the yogurt, shallot, lemon juice, dill, oil, salt, and pepper in a large bowl. Taste the mixture and add another pinch of salt if needed.
- ❖ Scoop ½ cup of yogurt into each of 4 containers. Place ½ cup of chopped cucumbers in each of 4 separate small containers or resealable sandwich bags.
- ❖ STORAGE: Store covered containers in the refrigerator for up to 5 days.

Nutrition: Total calories: 127; Total fat: 5g; Saturated fat: 2g; Sodium: 200mg; Carbohydrates: 9g; Fiber: 2g; Protein: 11g

9) SPICE CRANBERRY TEA

Cooking Time: 18 Minutes   **Servings:** 2

Ingredients:

- ✓ 1-ounce cranberries
- ✓ ½ lemon, juice, and zest
- ✓ 1 cinnamon stick
- ✓ 2 teabags
- ✓ ½ inch ginger, peeled and grated
- ✓ raw honey to taste
- ✓ 3 cups water

Directions:

- ❖ Start by adding all the Ingredients: except honey into a pot or saucepan.
- ❖ Bring to a boil and then simmer for about 115 minutes.
- ❖ Strain and serve the tea.
- ❖ Add honey or any other sweetener of your preference.
- ❖ Enjoy.

Nutrition: Calories: 38, Total Fat: 0.3g, Saturated Fat: 0.1, Cholesterol: 0 mg, Sodium: 2 mg, Total Carbohydrate: 10 g, Dietary Fiber: 4.9 g, Total Sugars: 1.1 g, Protein: 0.7 g, Vitamin D: 0 mcg, Calcium: 77 mg, Iron: 1 mg, Potassium: 110 mg

10) ZUCCHINI PUDDING

Cooking Time: 10 Minutes   **Servings:** 4

Ingredients:

- ✓ 2 cups zucchini, grated
- ✓ 1/2 tsp ground cardamom
- ✓ 1/4 cup swerve
- ✓ 5 oz half and half
- ✓ 5 oz unsweetened almond milk
- ✓ Pinch of salt

Directions:

- ❖ Spray instant pot from inside with cooking spray.
- ❖ Add all ingredients into the instant pot and stir well.
- ❖ Seal pot with lid and cook on high for 10 minutes.
- ❖ Once done, allow to release pressure naturally for 10 minutes then release remaining using quick release. Remove lid.
- ❖ Stir well and serve.

Nutrition: Calories: ;Fat: 4.7 g;Carbohydrates: 18.9 g;Sugar: 16 g;Protein: 1.9 g;Cholesterol: 13 mg

11) MEDITERRANEAN-STYLE BREAKFAST BURRITO

Cooking Time: 20 Minutes   **Servings:** 6

Ingredients:

- ✓ 9 eggs
- ✓ 3 tbsp chopped sun-dried tomatoes
- ✓ 6 tortillas that are 10 inches
- ✓ 2 cups baby spinach
- ✓ ½ cup feta cheese
- ✓ ¾ cups of canned refried beans
- ✓ 3 tbsp sliced black olives Salsa, sour cream, or any other toppings you desire

Directions:

- ❖ Wash and dry your spinach.
- ❖ Grease a medium frying pan with oil or nonstick cooking spray.
- ❖ Add the eggs into the pan and cook for about 5 minutes. Make sure you stir the eggs well, so they become scrambled.
- ❖ Combine the black olives, spinach, and sun-dried tomatoes with the eggs. Stir until the ingredients are fully incorporated.
- ❖ Add the feta cheese and then set the lid on the pan so the cheese will melt quickly.
- ❖ Spoon a bit of egg mixture into the tortilla.
- ❖ Wrap the tortillas tightly.
- ❖ Wash your pan or get a new skillet. Remember to grease the pan.
- ❖ Set each tortilla into the pan and cook each side for a couple of minutes. Once they are lightly brown, remove them from the pan and allow the burritos to cool on a serving plate. Top with your favorite condiments and enjoy!
- ❖ To store the burritos, wrap them in aluminum foil and

place them in the fridge. They can be stored for up to two days.

Nutrition: calories: 252, fats: grams, carbohydrates: 21 grams, protein: 14 grams

12) DRY FRUIT HEALTHY PORRIDGE

Cooking Time: 8 Hours   **Servings: 6**

Ingredients:

- ✓ 2 cups steel-cut oats
- ✓ 1/8 tsp ground nutmeg
- ✓ 1 tsp vanilla
- ✓ 1 1/2 tsp cinnamon
- ✓ 1/2 cup dry apricots, chopped
- ✓ 1/2 cup dry cranberries, chopped
- ✓ 1/2 cup dates, chopped
- ✓ 1/2 cup raisins
- ✓ 8 cups of water
- ✓ Pinch of salt

Directions:

- ❖ Spray instant pot from inside with cooking spray.
- ❖ Add all ingredients into the instant pot and stir well.
- ❖ Seal the pot with a lid and select slow cook mode and cook on low for 8 hours.
- ❖ Stir well and serve.

Nutrition: Calories: 196;Fat: 2 g;Carbohydrates: 42 g;Sugar: 18.4 g;Protein: 4.g;Cholesterol: 0 mg

13) SCRAMBLED EGGS PESTO

Cooking Time: 10 Minutes   **Servings: 2**

Ingredients:

- ✓ 5 eggs
- ✓ 2 tbsp butter
- ✓ 2 tbsp pesto
- ✓ 4 tbsp milk
- ✓ salt to taste
- ✓ pepper to taste

Directions:

- ❖ Beat the eggs into a bowl and add salt and pepper as per your taste.
- ❖ Then, heat a pan and add the butter, then the eggs, stirring continuously.
- ❖ While stirring continuously, add the pesto.
- ❖ Switch off the heat and quickly add the creamed milk and mix it well with eggs.
- ❖ Serve hot.

Nutrition: Calories: 342, Total Fat: 29.8g, Saturated Fat: 12.3, Cholesterol: 44mg, Sodium: 345 mg, Total Carbohydrate: 3.4g, Dietary Fiber: 0.3 g, Total Sugars: 3.2 g, Protein: 16.8 g, Vitamin D: 47 mcg, Calcium: 148 mg, Iron: 2 mg, Potassium: 168 mg

14) SWEET POTATOES AND SPICED MAPLE YOGURT WITH WALNUTS BREAKFAST

Cooking Time: 45 Minutes   **Servings: 4**

Ingredients:

- ✓ 4 red garnet sweet potatoes, about 6 inches long and 2 inches in diameter
- ✓ 2 cups low-fat (2%) plain Greek yogurt
- ✓ ¼ tsp pumpkin pie spice
- ✓ 1 tbsp pure maple syrup
- ✓ ½ cup walnut pieces

Directions:

- ❖ Preheat the oven to 425°F. Line a sheet pan with a silicone baking mat or parchment paper.
- ❖ Prick the sweet potatoes in multiple places with a fork and place on the sheet pan. Bake until tender when pricked with a paring knife, 40 to 45 minutes.
- ❖ While the potatoes are baking, mix the yogurt, pumpkin pie spice, and maple syrup until well combined in a medium bowl.
- ❖ When the potatoes are cool, slice the skin down the middle vertically to open up each potato. If you'd like to eat the sweet potatoes warm, place 1 potato in each of containers and ½ cup of spiced yogurt plus 2 tbsp of walnut pieces in each of 4 other containers. If you want to eat the potatoes cold, place ½ cup of yogurt and 2 tbsp of walnuts directly on top of each of the 4 potatoes in the 4 containers.
- ❖ STORAGE: Store covered containers in the refrigerator for up to days.

Nutrition: Total calories: 350; Total fat: 13g; Saturated fat: 3g; Sodium: 72mg; Carbohydrates: 4; Fiber: 5g; Protein: 16g

15) BLUEBERRY PEACH OATMEAL

Cooking Time: 4 Hours   **Servings: 4**

Ingredients:

- ✓ 1 cup steel-cut oats
- ✓ 1/2 cup blueberries
- ✓ 3 1/2 cups unsweetened almond milk
- ✓ 7 oz can peach
- ✓ Pinch of salt

Directions:

- ❖ Spray instant pot from inside with cooking spray.
- ❖ Add all ingredients into the instant pot and stir well.
- ❖ Seal the pot with a lid and select slow cook mode and cook on low for 4 hours.
- ❖ Stir well and serve.

Nutrition: 1;Fat: 4.5 g;Carbohydrates: 25.4 g;Sugar: 8.6 g;Protein: 3.9 g;Cholesterol: 0 mg

16) Scrambled Eggs Mediterranean-Style

Cooking Time: 10 Minutes   **Servings: 2**

Ingredients:

- ✓ 1 tbsp oil
- ✓ 1 yellow pepper, diced
- ✓ 2 spring onions, sliced
- ✓ 8 cherry tomatoes, quartered
- ✓ 2 tbsp sliced black olives
- ✓ 1 tbsp capers
- ✓ 4 eggs
- ✓ 1/4 tsp dried oregano
- ✓ Black pepper
- ✓ Topping:
- ✓ Fresh parsley, to serve

Directions:

- ❖ In a frying pan over medium heat, add the oil
- ❖ Once heated, add the diced pepper and chopped spring onions, cook for a few minutes, until slightly soft
- ❖ Add in the quartered tomatoes, olives and capers, and cook for 1 more minute
- ❖ Crack the eggs into the pan, immediately scramble with a spoon or spatula
- ❖ Sprinkle with oregano and plenty of black pepper, and stir until the eggs are fully cooked
- ❖ Distribute the eggs evenly into the containers, store in the fridge for 2-3 days
- ❖ To Serve: Reheat in the microwave for 30 seconds or in a toaster oven until warmed through

Nutrition: Calories:249;Carbs: 13g;Total Fat: 17g;Protein: 14g

17) MEDITERRANEAN-STYLE VEGGIE QUICHE

Cooking Time: 55 Minutes   **Servings:** 8

Ingredients:

- 1/2 cup sundried tomatoes - dry or in olive oil*
- Boiling water
- 1 prepared pie crust
- 2 tbsp vegan butter
- 1 onion, diced
- 2 cloves garlic, minced
- 1 red pepper, diced
- 1/4 cup sliced Kalamata olives
- 1 tsp dried oregano
- 1 tsp dried parsley
- 1/3 cup crumbled feta cheese
- 4 large eggs
- 1 1/4 cup milk
- 2 cups fresh spinach or 1/2 cup frozen spinach, thawed and squeezed dry
- Salt, to taste
- Pepper, to taste
- 1 cup shredded cheddar cheese, divided

Directions:

- If you're using dry sundried tomatoes - In a measure cup, add the sundried tomatoes and pour the boiling water over until just covered, allow to sit for 5 minutes or until the tomatoes are soft. The drain and chop tomatoes, set aside
- Preheat oven to 375 degrees F
- Fit a 9-inch pie plate with the prepared pie crust, then flute edges, and set aside
- In a skillet over medium high heat, melt the butter
- Add in the onion and garlic, and cook until fragrant and tender, about 3 minutes
- Add in the red pepper, cook for an additional 3 minutes, or until the peppers are just tender
- Add in the spinach, olives, oregano, and parsley, cook until the spinach is wilted (if you're using fresh) or heated through (if you're using frozen), about 5 minutes
- Remove the pan from heat, stir in the feta cheese and tomatoes, spoon the mixture into the prepared pie crust, spreading out evenly, set aside
- In a medium-sized mixing bowl, whisk together the eggs, 1/2 cup of the cheddar cheese, milk, salt, and pepper
- Pour this egg and cheese mixture evenly over the spinach mixture in the pie crust
- Sprinkle top with the remaining cheddar cheese
- Bake for 50-55 minutes, or until the crust is golden brown and the egg is set
- Allow to cool completely before slicing
- Wrap the slices in plastic wrap and then aluminum foil and place in the freezer.
- To Serve: Remove the aluminum foil and plastic wrap, and microwave for 2 minutes, then allow to rest for 30 seconds, enjoy!
- Recipe Notes: You'll find two types of sundried tomatoes available in your local grocery store—dry ones and ones packed in olive oil. Both will work for this recipe.
- If you decide to use dry ones, follow the directions in the recipe to reconstitute them. If you're using oil-packed sundried tomatoes, skip the first step and just remove them from the oil, chop them, and continue with the recipe.
- Season carefully! Between the feta, cheddar, and olives, this recipe is naturally salty.

Nutrition: Calories:239;Carbs: ;Total Fat: 15g;Protein: 7g

18) PUDDING WITH CHIA

Cooking Time: 15 Minutes   **Servings: 2**

Ingredients:

✓ ½ cup chia seeds
✓ 2 cups milk
✓ 1 tbsp honey

Directions:

❖ Combine and mix the chia seeds, milk, and honey in a bowl.
❖ Put the mixture in the freezer and let it set.
❖ Take the pudding out of the freezer only when you see that the pudding has thickened.
❖ Serve chilled.

Nutrition: Calories: 429, Total Fat: 22.4g, Saturated Fat: 4.9, Cholesterol: 20 mg, Sodium: 124 mg, Total Carbohydrate: 44.g, Dietary Fiber: 19.5 g, Total Sugars: 19.6 g, Protein: 17.4 g, Vitamin D: 1 mcg, Calcium: 648 mg, Iron: 4 mg, Potassium: 376 mg

19) RICE BOWLS FOR BREAKFAST

Cooking Time: 8 Minutes   **Servings: 4**

Ingredients:

✓ 1 cup of brown rice
✓ 1 tsp ground cinnamon
✓ 1/4 cup almonds, sliced
✓ 2 tbsp sunflower seeds
✓ 1/4 cup pecans, chopped
✓ 1/4 cup walnuts, chopped
✓ 2 cup unsweetened almond milk
✓ Pinch of salt

Directions:

❖ Spray instant pot from inside with cooking spray.
❖ Add all ingredients into the instant pot and stir well.
❖ Seal pot with lid and cook on high for 8 minutes.
❖ Once done, allow to release pressure naturally for 5 minutes then release remaining using quick release. Remove lid.
❖ Stir well and serve.

Nutrition: Calories: 291;Fat: 12 g;Carbohydrates: 40.1 g;Sugar: 0.4 g;Protein: 7.g;Cholesterol: 0 mg

20) TAHINI EGG SALAD AND PITA

Cooking Time: 12 Minutes   **Servings: 4**

Ingredients:

✓ 4 large eggs
✓ ¼ cup freshly chopped dill
✓ 1 tbsp plus 1 tsp unsalted tahini
✓ 2 tsp freshly squeezed lemon juice
✓ ⅛ tsp kosher salt
✓ 4 whole-wheat pitas, quartered

Directions:

❖ Place the eggs in a saucepan and cover with water. Bring the water to a boil. As soon as the water starts to boil, place a lid on the pan and turn the heat off. Set a timer for minutes.
❖ When the timer goes off, drain the hot water and run cold water over the eggs to cool.
❖ When the eggs are cool, peel them, place the yolks in a medium bowl, and mash them with a fork. Then chop the egg whites.
❖ Add the chopped egg whites, dill, tahini, lemon juice (to taste), and salt to the bowl, and mix to combine.
❖ Place a heaping ⅓ cup of egg salad in each of 4 containers. Place the pita in 4 separate containers or resealable bags so that the bread does not get soggy.
❖ STORAGE: Store covered containers in the refrigerator for up to 5 days.

Nutrition: Total calories: 242; Total fat: 10g; Saturated fat: 2g; Sodium: 300mg; Carbohydrates: 29g; Fiber: 5g; Protein: 13g

21) MANGO STRAWBERRY- GREEN SMOOTHIE

Cooking Time: 10 Minutes **Servings:** 2

Ingredients:

- ✓ 1½ cups low-fat (2%) milk
- ✓ 2 cups packed baby spinach leaves
- ✓ ½ cup sliced Persian or English cucumber, skin on
- ✓ ⅔ cup frozen strawberries
- ✓ ⅔ cup frozen mango chunks
- ✓ 1 medium very ripe banana, sliced (about ⅔ cup)
- ✓ ½ small avocado
- ✓ 1 tsp honey

Directions:

- ❖ Place the milk, spinach, cucumber, strawberries, mango, banana, and avocado in a blender.
- ❖ Blend until smooth and taste. If the smoothie isn't sweet enough, add the honey.
- ❖ Distribute the smoothie between 2 to-go cups.
- ❖ STORAGE: Store smoothie cups in the refrigerator for up to 3 days.

Nutrition: Total calories: 261; Total fat: 8g; Saturated fat: 2g; Sodium: 146mg; Carbohydrates: 40g; Fiber: ; Protein: 11g

22) ALMOND-CHOCOLATE BANANA BREAD

Cooking Time: 25 Minutes **Servings:** 4

Ingredients:

- ✓ Cooking spray or oil to grease the pan
- ✓ 1 cup almond meal
- ✓ 2 large eggs
- ✓ 2 very ripe bananas, mashed
- ✓ 1 tbsp plus 2 tsp maple syrup
- ✓ ½ tsp vanilla extract
- ✓ ½ tsp baking powder
- ✓ ¼ tsp ground cardamom
- ✓ ⅓ cup dark chocolate chips, very roughly chopped

Directions:

- ❖ Preheat the oven to 350°F and spray an 8-inch cake pan or baking dish with cooking spray or rub with oil.
- ❖ Combine all the ingredients in a large mixing bowl. Then pour the mixture into the prepared pan.
- ❖ Place the pan in the oven and bake for 25 minutes. The edges should be browned, and a paring knife should come out clean when the banana bread is pierced.
- ❖ When cool, slice into wedges and place 1 wedge in each of 4 containers.
- ❖ STORAGE: Store covered containers at room temperature for up to 2 days, refrigerate for up to 7 days, or freeze for up to 3 months.

Nutrition: Total calories: 3; Total fat: 23g; Saturated fat: 6g; Sodium: 105mg; Carbohydrates: 37g; Fiber: 6g; Protein: 10g

23) EGG WHITE SANDWICH MEDITERRANEAN-STYLE BREAKFAST

Cooking Time: 30 Minutes **Servings:** 1

Ingredients:

- ✓ 1 tsp vegan butter
- ✓ ¼ cup egg whites
- ✓ 1 tsp chopped fresh herbs such as parsley, basil, rosemary
- ✓ 1 whole grain seeded ciabatta roll
- ✓ 1 tbsp pesto
- ✓ 1-2 slices muenster cheese (or other cheese such as provolone, Monterey Jack, etc.)
- ✓ About ½ cup roasted tomatoes
- ✓ Salt, to taste
- ✓ Pepper, to taste
- ✓ Roasted Tomatoes:
- ✓ 10 oz grape tomatoes
- ✓ 1 tbsp extra virgin olive oil
- ✓ Kosher salt, to taste
- ✓ Coarse black pepper, to taste

Directions:

- ❖ In a small nonstick skillet over medium heat, melt the vegan butter
- ❖ Pour in egg whites, season with salt and pepper, sprinkle with fresh herbs, cook for 3-4 minutes or until egg is done, flip once
- ❖ In the meantime, toast the ciabatta bread in toaster
- ❖ Once done, spread both halves with pesto
- ❖ Place the egg on the bottom half of sandwich roll, folding if necessary, top with cheese, add the roasted tomatoes and top half of roll sandwich
- ❖ To make the roasted tomatoes: Preheat oven to 400 degrees F. Slice tomatoes in half lengthwise. Then place them onto a baking sheet and drizzle with the olive oil, toss to coat. Season with salt and pepper and roast in oven for about 20 minutes, until the skin appears wrinkled

Nutrition: Calories:458;Total Carbohydrates: 51g;Total Fat: 0g;Protein: 21g

24) APRICOT-STRAWBERRY SMOOTHIE

Cooking Time: 15 Minutes   **Servings:** 2

Ingredients:

- ✓ 1 cup strawberries, frozen
- ✓ ¾ cup almond milk, unsweetened
- ✓ 2 apricots, pitted and sliced

Directions:

- ❖ Put all the Ingredients: into the blender.
- ❖ Blend them for a minute or until you reach desired foamy texture.
- ❖ Serve the smoothie.
- ❖ Enjoy.

Nutrition: Calories: 247, Total Fat: 21.9 g, Saturated Fat: 19 g, Cholesterol: 0 mg, Sodium: 1mg, Total Carbohydrate: 14.4 g, Dietary Fiber: 4.1 g, Total Sugars: 9.7 g, Protein: 3 g, Vitamin D: 0 mcg, Calcium: 30 mg, Iron: 2 mg, Potassium: 438 mg

25) BREAKFAST BARS WITH APPLE QUINOA

Cooking Time: 40 Minutes   **Servings:** 12

Ingredients:

- ✓ 2 eggs
- ✓ 1 apple peeled and chopped into ½ inch chunks
- ✓ 1 cup unsweetened apple sauce
- ✓ 1 ½ cups cooked & cooled quinoa
- ✓ 1 ½ cups rolled oats
- ✓ 1/4 cup peanut butter
- ✓ 1 tsp vanilla
- ✓ 1/2 tsp cinnamon
- ✓ 1/4 cup coconut oil
- ✓ ½ tsp baking powder

Directions:

- ❖ Heat oven to 350 degrees F
- ❖ Spray an 8x8 inch baking dish with oil, set aside
- ❖ In a large bowl, stir together the apple sauce, cinnamon, coconut oil, peanut butter, vanilla and eggs
- ❖ Add in the cooked quinoa, rolled oats and baking powder, mix until completely incorporated
- ❖ Fold in the apple chunks
- ❖ Spread the mixture into the prepared baking dish, spreading it to each corner
- ❖ Bake for 40 minutes, or until a toothpick comes out clean
- ❖ Allow to cool before slicing
- ❖ Wrap the bars individually in plastic wrap. Store in an airtight container or baggie in the freezer for up to a month.
- ❖ To serve: Warm up in the oven at 350 F for 5 minutes or microwave for up to 30 seconds

Nutrition: (1 bar): Calories:230;Total Fat: 10g;Total Carbs: 31g;Protein: 7g

26) KALE, PEPPER, AND CHICKPEA SHAKSHUKA

Cooking Time: 35 Minutes   **Servings: 5**

Ingredients:

- ✓ 1 tbsp olive oil
- ✓ 1 small red onion, thinly sliced
- ✓ 1 red bell pepper, thinly sliced
- ✓ 1 green bell pepper, thinly sliced
- ✓ 1 bunch kale, stemmed and roughly chopped
- ✓ ½ cup packed cilantro leaves, chopped
- ✓ ½ tsp kosher salt
- ✓ 1 tsp smoked paprika
- ✓ 1 (14.5-ounce) can diced tomatoes
- ✓ 1 (14-ounce) can low-sodium chickpeas, drained and rinsed
- ✓ ⅔ cup water
- ✓ 5 eggs
- ✓ 2½ whole-wheat pitas (optional)

Directions:

- ❖ Preheat the oven to 375°F.
- ❖ Heat the oil in an oven-safe 1inch skillet over medium-high heat. Once the oil is shimmering, add the onions and red and green bell peppers. Sauté for 5 minutes, then cover, leaving the lid slightly ajar. Cook for 5 more minutes, then add the kale and cover, leaving the lid slightly ajar. Cook for 10 more minutes, stirring occasionally.
- ❖ Add the cilantro, salt, paprika, tomatoes, chickpeas, and water, and stir to combine.
- ❖ Make 5 wells in the mixture. Break an egg into a small bowl and pour it into a well. Repeat with the remaining eggs.
- ❖ Place the pan in the oven and bake until the egg whites are opaque and the eggs still jiggle a little when the pan is shaken, about 12 to 1minutes, but start checking at 8 minutes.
- ❖ When the shakshuka is cool, scoop about 1¼ cups of veggies into each of 5 containers, along with 1 egg each. If using, place ½ pita in each of 5 resealable bags.
- ❖ STORAGE: Store covered containers in the refrigerator for up to 5 days.

Nutrition: Total calories: 244; Total fat: 9g; Saturated fat: 2g; Sodium: 529mg; Carbohydrates: 29g; Fiber: ; Protein: 14g

27) BROCCOLI ROSEMARY CAULIFLOWER MASH

Cooking Time: 12 Minutes   **Servings: 3**

Ingredients:

- ✓ 2 cups broccoli, chopped
- ✓ 1 lb cauliflower, cut into florets
- ✓ 1 tsp dried rosemary
- ✓ 1/4 cup olive oil
- ✓ 1 tsp garlic, minced
- ✓ Salt

Directions:

- ❖ Add broccoli and cauliflower into the instant pot. Pour enough water into the pot to cover broccoli and cauliflower.
- ❖ Seal pot with lid and cook on high for 1minutes.
- ❖ Once done, allow to release pressure naturally. Remove lid.
- ❖ Drain broccoli and cauliflower well and clean the instant pot.
- ❖ Add oil into the pot and set the pot on sauté mode.
- ❖ Add broccoli, cauliflower, rosemary, garlic, and salt and cook for 10 minutes.
- ❖ Mash the broccoli and cauliflower mixture using a potato masher until smooth.
- ❖ Serve and enjoy.

Nutrition: Calories: 205;Fat: 17.2 g;Carbohydrates: 12.6 g;Sugar: 4.7 g;Protein: 4.8 g;Cholesterol: 0 mg

28) APPLE, PUMPKIN, AND GREEK YOGURT MUFFINS

Cooking Time: 20 Minutes   **Servings: 12**

Ingredients:

- ✓ Cooking spray to grease baking liners
- ✓ 2 cups whole-wheat flour
- ✓ 1 tsp aluminum-free baking powder (see tip)
- ✓ 1 tsp baking soda
- ✓ ⅛ tsp kosher salt
- ✓ 2 tsp ground cinnamon
- ✓ ½ tsp ground ginger
- ✓ ½ tsp ground allspice
- ✓ ⅔ cup pure maple syrup
- ✓ 1 cup low-fat (2%) plain Greek yogurt
- ✓ 1 cup 100% canned pumpkin
- ✓ 1 large egg
- ✓ ¼ cup extra-virgin olive oil
- ✓ 1½ cups chopped green apple (leave peel on)
- ✓ ½ cup walnut pieces

Directions:

- ❖ Preheat the oven to 400°F and line a muffin tin with baking liners. Spray the liners lightly with cooking spray.
- ❖ In a large bowl, whisk together the flour, baking powder, baking soda, salt, cinnamon, ginger, and allspice.
- ❖ In a medium bowl, combine the maple syrup, yogurt, pumpkin, egg, olive oil, chopped apple, and walnuts.
- ❖ Pour the wet ingredients into the dry ingredients and combine just until blended. Do not overmix.
- ❖ Scoop about ¼ cup of batter into each muffin liner and bake for 20 minutes, or until the tops look browned and a paring knife comes out clean when inserted. Remove the muffins from the tin to cool.
- ❖ STORAGE: Store covered containers at room temperature for up to 4 days. To freeze the muffins for up to 3 months, wrap them in foil and place in an airtight resealable bag.

Nutrition: Total calories: 221; Total fat: 9g; Saturated fat: 1g; Sodium: 18g; Carbohydrates: 32g; Fiber: 4g; Protein: 6g

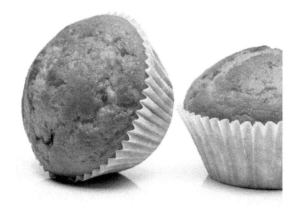

Lunch and Dinner

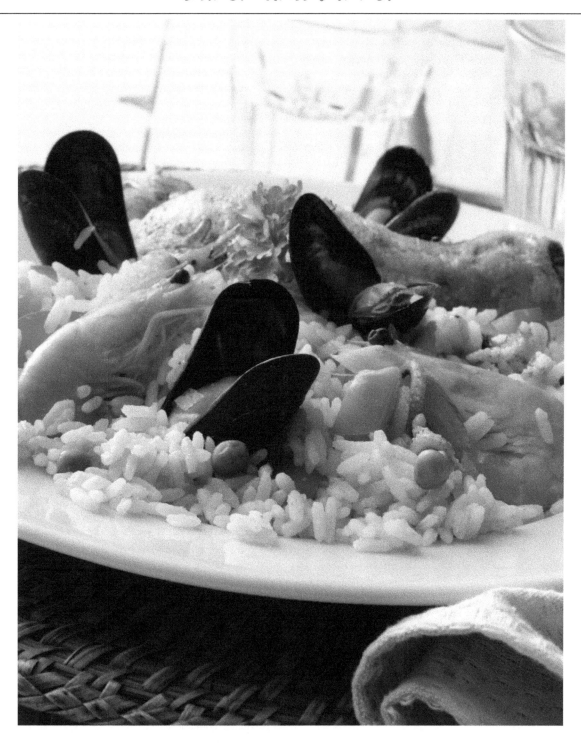

29) TYPICAL CREAMY SHRIMP-STUFFED PORTOBELLO MUSHROOMS

Cooking Time: 40 Minutes   **Servings:** 3

Ingredients:

- ✓ 1 tsp olive oil, plus 2 tbsp
- ✓ 6 portobello mushrooms, caps and stems separated and stems chopped
- ✓ 2 tsp chopped garlic
- ✓ 10 ounces uncooked peeled, deveined shrimp, thawed if frozen, roughly chopped
- ✓ 1 (14.5-ounce) can no-salt-added diced tomatoes
- ✓ 1 (14.5-ounce) can no-salt-added diced tomatoes
- ✓ 4 tbsp roughly chopped fresh basil
- ✓ ½ cup mascarpone cheese
- ✓ ¼ cup panko bread crumbs
- ✓ 4 tbsp grated Parmesan, divided
- ✓ ¼ tsp kosher salt
- ✓ 6 ounces broccoli florets, finely chopped (about 2 cups)

Directions:

- ❖ Preheat the oven to 350°F. Line a sheet pan with a silicone baking mat or parchment paper. Rub 1 tsp of oil over the bottom (stem side) of the mushroom caps and place on the lined sheet pan, stem-side up.
- ❖ Heat the remaining 2 tbsp of oil in a 12-inch skillet on medium-high heat. Once the oil is shimmering, add the chopped mushroom stems and broccoli, and sauté for 2 to minutes. Add the garlic and shrimp, and continue cooking for 2 more minutes. Add the tomatoes, basil, mascarpone, bread crumbs, 3 tbsp of Parmesan, and the salt. Stir to combine and turn the heat off.
- ❖ With the mushroom cap openings facing up, mound slightly less than 1 cup of filling into each mushroom. Top each with ½ tsp of the remaining Parmesan cheese. Bake the mushrooms for 35 minutes. Place 2 mushroom caps in each of 3 containers.
- ❖ STORAGE: Store covered containers in the refrigerator for up to 4 days.

Nutrition: Total calories: 47 Total fat: 31g; Saturated fat: 10g; Sodium: 526mg; Carbohydrates: 26g; Fiber: 7g; Protein: 26g

30) EASY ROSEMARY EDAMAME, ZUCCHINI, AND SUN-DRIED TOMATOES WITH GARLIC-CHIVE QUINOA

Cooking Time: 15 Minutes   **Servings:** 4

Ingredients:

- ✓ FOR THE GARLIC-CHIVE QUINOA
- ✓ 1 tsp olive oil
- ✓ 1 tsp chopped garlic
- ✓ ⅔ cup quinoa
- ✓ 1⅓ cups water
- ✓ ¼ tsp kosher salt
- ✓ 1 (¾-ounce) package fresh chives, chopped
- ✓ FOR THE ROSEMARY EDAMAME, ZUCCHINI, AND SUN-DRIED TOMATOES
- ✓ 1 tsp oil from sun-dried tomato jar
- ✓ 2 medium zucchini, cut in half lengthwise and sliced into half-moons (about 3 cups)
- ✓ 1 (12-ounce) package frozen shelled edamame, thawed (2 cups)
- ✓ ½ cup julienne-sliced sun-dried tomatoes in olive oil, drained
- ✓ ¼ tsp dried rosemary
- ✓ ⅛ tsp kosher salt

Directions:

- ❖ TO MAKE THE GARLIC-CHIVE QUINOA
- ❖ Heat the oil over medium heat in a saucepan. Once the oil is shimmering, add the garlic and cook for 1 minute, stirring often so it doesn't burn.
- ❖ Add the quinoa and stir a few times. Add the water and salt and turn the heat up to high. Once the water is boiling, cover the pan and turn the heat down to low. Simmer the quinoa for 15 minutes, or until the water is absorbed.
- ❖ Stir in the chives and fluff the quinoa with a fork.
- ❖ Place ½ cup quinoa in each of 4 containers.
- ❖ TO MAKE THE ROSEMARY EDAMAME, ZUCCHINI, AND SUN-DRIED TOMATOES
- ❖ Heat the oil in a 12-inch skillet over medium-high heat. Once the oil is shimmering, add the zucchini and cook for 2 minutes.
- ❖ Add the edamame, sun-dried tomatoes, rosemary, and salt, and cook for another 6 minutes, or until the zucchini is crisp-tender.
- ❖ Spoon 1 cup of the edamame mixture into each of the 4 quinoa containers.
- ❖ STORAGE: Store covered containers in the refrigerator for up to 5 days.

Nutrition: Total calories: 312; Total fat: ; Saturated fat: 1g; Sodium: 389mg; Carbohydrates: 39g; Fiber: 9g; Protein: 15g

31) SPECIAL CHERRY, VANILLA, AND ALMOND OVERNIGHT OATS

Cooking Time: 10 Minutes   **Servings:** 5

Ingredients:

- ✓ 1⅔ cups rolled oats
- ✓ 3⅓ cups unsweetened vanilla almond milk
- ✓ 5 tbsp plain, unsalted almond butter
- ✓ 2 tsp vanilla extract
- ✓ 1 tbsp plus 2 tsp pure maple syrup
- ✓ 3 tbsp chia seeds
- ✓ ½ cup plus 2 tbsp sliced almonds
- ✓ 1⅔ cups frozen sweet cherries

Directions:

- ❖ In a large bowl, mix the oats, almond milk, almond butter, vanilla, maple syrup, and chia seeds until well combined.
- ❖ Spoon ¾ cup of the oat mixture into each of 5 containers.
- ❖ Top each serving with 2 tbsp of almonds and ⅓ cup of cherries.
- ❖ STORAGE: Store covered containers in the refrigerator for up to 5 days. Overnight oats can be eaten cold or warmed up in the microwave.

Nutrition: Total calories: 373; Total fat: 20g; Saturated fat: 1g; Sodium: 121mg; Carbohydrates: 40g; Fiber: 11g; Protein: 13g

32) EASY ROTISSERIE CHICKEN, BABY KALE, FENNEL, AND GREEN APPLE SALAD

Cooking Time: 15 Minutes   **Servings:** 3

Ingredients:

- ✓ 1 tsp olive oil
- ✓ 1 tsp chopped garlic
- ✓ ⅔ cup quinoa
- ✓ 1⅓ cups water
- ✓ 1 cooked rotisserie chicken, meat removed and shredded (about 9 ounces)
- ✓ 1 fennel bulb, core and fronds removed, thinly sliced (about 2 cups)
- ✓ 1 small green apple, julienned (about 1½ cups)
- ✓ 8 tbsp Honey-Lemon Vinaigrette, divided
- ✓ 1 (5-ounce) package baby kale
- ✓ 6 tbsp walnut pieces

Directions:

- ❖ Heat the oil over medium heat in a saucepan. Once the oil is shimmering, add the garlic and cook for minute, stirring often so that it doesn't burn.
- ❖ Add the quinoa and stir a few times. Add the water and turn the heat up to high. Once the water is boiling, cover the pan and turn the heat down to low. Simmer the quinoa for 15 minutes, or until the water is absorbed. Cool.
- ❖ Place the chicken, fennel, apple, and cooled quinoa in a large bowl. Add 2 tbsp of the vinaigrette to the bowl and mix to combine.
- ❖ Divide the baby kale, chicken mixture, and walnuts among 3 containers. Pour 2 tbsp of the remaining vinaigrette into each of 3 sauce containers.
- ❖ STORAGE: Store covered containers in the refrigerator for up to days.

Nutrition: Total calories: 9; Total fat: 39g; Saturated fat: 6g; Sodium: 727mg; Carbohydrates: 49g; Fiber: 8g; Protein: 29g

33) ZA'ATAR SALMON ROAST WITH PEPPERS AND SWEET POTATOES

Cooking Time: 25 Minutes   **Servings: 4**

Ingredients:

- ✓ FOR THE VEGGIES
- ✓ 2 large red bell peppers, cut into ½-inch strips
- ✓ 1 pound sweet potatoes, peeled and cut into 1-inch chunks
- ✓ 1 tbsp olive oil
- ✓ ¼ tsp kosher salt
- ✓ FOR THE SALMON
- ✓ 2¾ tsp sesame seeds

- ✓ 2¾ tsp dried thyme leaves
- ✓ 2¾ tsp sumac
- ✓ 1 pound skinless, boneless salmon fillet, divided into 4 pieces
- ✓ ⅛ tsp kosher salt
- ✓ 1 tsp olive oil
- ✓ 2 tsp freshly squeezed lemon juice

Directions:

- ❖ TO MAKE THE VEGGIES
- ❖ Preheat the oven to 4°F.
- ❖ Place silicone baking mats or parchment paper on two sheet pans.
- ❖ On the first pan, place the peppers and sweet potatoes. Pour the oil and sprinkle the salt over both and toss to coat. Spread everything out in an even layer. Place the sheet pan in the oven and set a timer for 10 minutes.
- ❖ TO MAKE THE SALMON
- ❖ Mix the sesame seeds, thyme, and sumac together in a small bowl to make the za'atar spice mix.
- ❖ Place the salmon fillets on the second sheet pan. Sprinkle the salt evenly across the fillets. Spread ¼ tsp of oil and ½ tsp of lemon juice over each piece of salmon.
- ❖ Pat 2 tsp of the za'atar spice mix over each piece of salmon.
- ❖ When the veggie timer goes off, place the salmon in the oven with the veggies and bake for 10 minutes for salmon that is ½ inch thick and for 15 minutes for salmon that is 1 inch thick. The veggies should be done when the salmon is done cooking.
- ❖ Place one quarter of the veggies and 1 piece of salmon in each of 4 separate containers.
- ❖ STORAGE:Store covered containers in the refrigerator for up to 4 days.

Nutrition: Total calories: 295; Total fat: 10g; Saturated fat: 2g; Sodium: 249mg; Carbohydrates: 29g; Fiber: 6g; Protein: 25g

34) ITALIAN EGG CAPRESE BREAKFAST CUPS

Cooking Time: 17 minutes   **Servings: 12**

Ingredients:

- ✓ 1/2 tsp garlic powder
- ✓ 4 tbsp basil sliced
- ✓ 12 mozzarella balls
- ✓ 3 cups spinach
- ✓ 12 large eggs

- ✓ 1.25 cups chopped tomatoes
- ✓ 1/2 tsp black pepper
- ✓ 3/4 tsp salt
- ✓ 1-2 tbsp Parmesan cheese grated
- ✓ balsamic vinegar as required

Directions:

- ❖ In greased muffin cups, make a layer of spinach at the bottom.
- ❖ Arrange tomatoes, mozzarella, and basil above the spinach layer.
- ❖ In a mixing bowl, mix salt, cheese, black pepper, garlic powder, and eggs.
- ❖ Add the egg/cheese mixture in layered muffin cups.
- ❖ Place the muffin cups for 20 minutes in a preheated oven at 350 degrees.
- ❖ Drizzle balsamic vinegar and serve.

Nutrition: Calories: 141 kcal Fat: 10 g Protein: 11 g Carbs: 1 g Fiber: 1.8 g

35) MEDITERRANEAN-STYLE MINI FRITTATAS

Cooking Time: 25 minutes   **Servings:** 12

Ingredients:

- ✓ ¼ cup crumbled feta cheese
- ✓ 1 tsp olive oil
- ✓ 1 cup chopped mushrooms
- ✓ 1 cup sliced zucchini
- ✓ 1/3 cup diced red onion
- ✓ ¼ cup chopped Kalamata olives
- ✓ 2 cups spinach
- ✓ ½ tsp dried oregano
- ✓ ½ cup fat-free milk
- ✓ Six eggs
- ✓ Black pepper to taste

Directions:

- ❖ Sauté mushrooms, zucchini, and onions for about two minutes in heated oil in a skillet over medium flame.
- ❖ Mix spinach in the mushroom mixture after lowering the flame. Add oregano and olives.
- ❖ Cook for two more minutes with occasional stirring. When spinach is done, remove the cooking skillet and set aside.
- ❖ Mix pepper, eggs, cheese, milk, and sautéed veggies in a bowl.
- ❖ In an oil muffin pan, pour egg/veggies mixture.
- ❖ Bake in a preheated oven at 350 degrees for 20 minutes and serve.

Nutrition: Calories: 128 kcal Fat: 8 g Protein: 9 g Carbs: 4 g Fiber: 1 g

36) NAPOLI CAPRESE AVOCADO TOAST

Preparation Time: **Cooking Time:** 10 minutes   **Servings:** 1

Ingredients:

- ✓ Two avocados
- ✓ ¼ cup chopped basil leaves
- ✓ 2 tsp lemon juice
- ✓ 4 oz sliced mozzarella
- ✓ Sea salt to taste
- ✓ Four toasted slices of bread
- ✓ Black pepper to taste
- ✓ 1 cup halved grape tomatoes
- ✓ Balsamic glaze for drizzling

Directions:

- ❖ In a bowl, add sliced avocados, salt, lemon juice, and pepper and mix well.
- ❖ Over medium flame, lightly toast the bread.
- ❖ Using a knife, spread avocados mixture over bread slices.
- ❖ Sprinkle salt, basil, cheese, pepper, balsamic glaze, and tomatoes.
- ❖ Serve and enjoy it.

Nutrition: Calories: 338 kcal Fat: 20.4 g Protein: 12.8 g Carbs: 25.8 g Fiber: 9.2 g

37) SPECIAL ASPARAGUS AND MUSHROOM FRITTATA WITH GOAT CHEESE

Preparation Time: **Cooking Time:** 8 minutes   **Servings:** 4

Ingredients:

- ✓ 2 tbsp goat cheese
- ✓ Two eggs
- ✓ 1pinch of kosher salt
- ✓ 1 tsp of milk
- ✓ 1 tbsp butter
- ✓ Five trimmed asparagus spears
- ✓ Three sliced brown mushrooms
- ✓ 1 tbsp chopped green onion

Directions:

- ❖ In a pan, cook mushrooms over medium flame for about three minutes.
- ❖ Stir in asparagus and cook for two more minutes.
- ❖ In a bowl, add one tsp of water, eggs, and salt and mix well.
- ❖ Add the egg mixture to the mushroom mixture, followed by a drizzling of goat cheese and green onions.
- ❖ Let them cook well until the egg mixture is properly formed.
- ❖ Shift the pan to the preheated oven and bake for three minutes.
- ❖ Drizzle cheese and serve.

Nutrition: Calories: 331 kcal Fat: 26 g Protein: 20 g Carbs: 7 g Fiber: 2 g

38) TASTY TAHINI BANANA SHAKES

Preparation Time: 5 minutes | **Cooking Time:** 0 minute | **Servings:** 3

Ingredients:

- ¼ cup ice, crushed
- 1 ½ cups almond milk
- ¼ cup tahini
- 4 Medjool dates
- Two sliced bananas
- One pinch of ground cinnamon

Directions:

- Blend all the ingredients in the blender to obtain a creamy and smooth mixture.
- Pour mixture in cups and serve after sprinkling cinnamon over the top.

Nutrition: Calories: 299 kcal Fat: 12.4 g Protein: 5.7 g Carbs: 47.7 g Fiber: 5.6 g

39) EASY SHAKSHUKA

Preparation Time: 15 minutes | **Cooking Time:** 20 minutes | **Servings:** 6

Ingredients:

- 1 tsp ground cumin
- 2 tbsp olive oil
- One chopped red bell pepper
- Six eggs
- ¼ tsp salt
- Three minced cloves garlic
- Ground black pepper to taste
- 2 tbsp tomato paste
- ½ tsp smoked paprika
- ¼ tsp red pepper flakes
- 2 tbsp chopped cilantro for garnish
- ½ cup feta cheese
- One chopped yellow onion
- 28 oz fire-roasted tomatoes, crushed
- Crusty bread for serving

Directions:

- Heat oil in a skillet over medium flame and cook bell pepper, onions, and salt in it for six minutes with constant stirring.
- After six minutes, stir in tomato paste, red pepper flakes, cumin, garlic, and paprika. Cook for another two minutes.
- Add crushed tomatoes and cilantro to the onion mixture. Let it simmer.
- Reduce the flame and simmer for five minutes.
- Use salt and pepper to adjust the flavor.
- Crack eggs in small well made at different areas using a spoon. Pour tomato mixture over eggs to help them cook while staying intact.
- Bake the skillet in a preheated oven at 375 degrees for 12 minutes.
- Garnish with cilantro, flakes, and cheese and serve.

Nutrition: Calories: 216 kcal Fat: 12.8 g Protein: 11.2 g Carbs: 16.6 g Fiber: 4.4 g

40) EASY GREEN JUICE

Preparation Time: 15 minutes | **Cooking Time:** 0 minute | **Servings:** 2

Ingredients:

- 5 oz kale
- 1 tsp crushed ginger
- One apple
- Five trimmed celery stalks
- ½ English cucumber
- 1 oz parsley

Directions:

- Blend all the ingredients in the blender and pour into serving cups.

Nutrition: Calories: 92 kcal Fat: 0.8 g Protein: 2.8 g Carbs: 21 g Fiber: 6.2 g

41) GREEK-STYLE CHICKEN GYRO SALAD

Preparation Time: 15 minutes   **Cooking Time:** 7 minutes   **Servings:** 4

Ingredients:

- ✓ Chicken
- ✓ 3 tsp dried oregano
- ✓ 2 tbsp olive oil
- ✓ 1 tbsp red wine vinegar
- ✓ 1.25 lb boneless chicken breasts
- ✓ 1 tsp ground black pepper
- ✓ 1 tbsp lemon juice
- ✓ 1 tsp Kosher salt
- ✓ Salad
- ✓ 1 cup diced English cucumber
- ✓ 6 cups lettuce

- ✓ 1 cup feta cheese diced
- ✓ 1 cup diced tomatoes
- ✓ 1/2 cup diced red onions
- ✓ 1 cup crushed pita chips
- ✓ Tzatziki Sauce
- ✓ 1 tbsp white wine vinegar
- ✓ 3/4 tsp Kosher salt
- ✓ 8 oz Greek yogurt
- ✓ One minced clove garlic
- ✓ 2/3 cup grated English cucumber
- ✓ 1 tbsp lemon juice
- ✓ 3/4 tsp ground black pepper
- ✓ 2 tsp dried dill weed
- ✓ One pinch of sugar

Directions:

- ❖ Heat oil in a skillet and add chicken, salt, oregano, and black pepper. Cook for five minutes over medium flame.
- ❖ Reduce the flame to low and add lemon juice and vinegar and simmer for five minutes.
- ❖ Continue cooking until the chicken is done. Now, the chicken is ready and set aside.
- ❖ Combine tomatoes, pita chips, chicken, lettuce, cucumber, and onions. Mix and set aside. The salad is ready.
- ❖ In another bowl, whisk yogurt, cucumber, garlic, lemon juice, vinegar, dill, salt, pepper, and sugar. Mix well. The sauce is ready.
- ❖ Now, pour the sauce over the salad and serve with cooked chicken.

Nutrition: Calories: 737 kcal Fat: 29 g Protein: 64 g Carbs: 54 g Fiber: 6 g

42) TUSCAN-STYLE TUNA AND WHITE BEAN SALAD

Preparation Time: 5 minutes   **Cooking Time:** 0 minute   **Servings:** 2

Ingredients:

- ✓ 2 tbsp extra virgin olive oil
- ✓ 15 oz cannellini beans
- ✓ 4 cups spinach
- ✓ 5 oz white albacore
- ✓ 1/4 cup sliced olives
- ✓ 1/2 cup diced cherry tomatoes

- ✓ One sliced red onion
- ✓ 1/2 lemon
- ✓ Kosher salt to taste
- ✓ 1/4 cup feta cheese
- ✓ Black pepper to taste

Directions:

- ❖ Combine white beans, olives, lemon juice, arugula, onions, tuna, olive oil, and tomatoes in a mixing bowl.
- ❖ Sprinkle pepper and salt and feta cheese and serve.

Nutrition: Calories: 436 kcal Fat: 22 g Protein: 30 g Carbs: 39 g Fiber: 12 g

43) MEDITERRANEAN-STYLE OUTRAGEOUS HERBACEOUS CHICKPEA SALAD

Preparation Time: 20 minutes   **Cooking Time:** 20 minutes   **Servings:** 4

Ingredients:

- ✓ 1/2 cup chopped celery with leaves
- ✓ 30 oz chickpeas
- ✓ 1.5 cups chopped parsley
- ✓ 1/2 cup chopped onion
- ✓ 3 tbsp olive oil

- ✓ 3 tbsp lemon juice
- ✓ Two minced cloves garlic
- ✓ 1/2 tsp kosher salt
- ✓ One chopped red bell pepper
- ✓ 1/2 tsp black pepper

Directions:

- ❖ Combine bell pepper, onion, chickpeas, celery, and parsley in a mixing bowl.
- ❖ In another bowl. Mix olive oil, garlic, salt, lemon juice, and pepper.
- ❖ Pour olive oil mixture over chickpeas mixture and mix well and serve.

Nutrition: Calories: 474 kcal Fat: 16 g Protein: 20 g Carbs: 65 g Fiber: 18 g

44) EASY AVOCADO CAPRESE SALAD

Preparation Time: 5 minutes   **Cooking Time:** 0 minute   **Servings:** 1

Ingredients:

- ✓ 1 cup sliced cherry tomatoes
- ✓ 1/4 cup basil leaves
- ✓ 1/2 cup mozzarella cheese balls
- ✓ ½ avocado

- ✓ 2 tsp extra virgin olive oil
- ✓ Salt to taste
- ✓ 2 tsp balsamic vinegar
- ✓ Black pepper to taste

Directions:

- ❖ In a bowl, combine cheese, tomatoes, avocado, olive oil, salt, basil, vinegar, and black pepper.
- ❖ Mix well and serve.

Nutrition: Calories: 456 kcal Fat: 37 g Protein: 17 g Carbs: 20 g Fiber: 9 g

45) CENTRE ITALY CITRUS SHRIMP AND AVOCADO SALAD

Preparation Time: 5 minutes   **Cooking Time:** 10 minutes   **Servings:** 3

Ingredients:

- ✓ 1 tbsp olive oil
- ✓ 1/2 cup lemon juice
- ✓ 1 cup of orange juice
- ✓ 1/2 tsp stone house seasoning
- ✓ 3 lb shrimp
- ✓ 2 tbsp chopped parsley
- ✓ 8 cups salad greens
- ✓ 1/2 cup citrus vinaigrette
- ✓ 1/2 sliced red onion
- ✓ One sliced avocado

Directions:

- ❖ In a bowl, mix orange juice, stone house seasoning, oil, and lemon juice.
- ❖ Transfer the bowl mixture to the heated skillet. Cook for five minutes over medium flame.
- ❖ Stir in shrimps and cook for five more minutes.
- ❖ Sprinkle parsley and set aside. Citrus shrimps are ready.
- ❖ Prepare the Citrus Vinaigrette Dressing as per the instruction given on the package.
- ❖ In a bowl, whisk citrus vinaigrette until it emulsified. Mix salad greens, avocado, shrimps, and onion in a citrus vinaigrette. Serve and enjoy it.

Nutrition: Calories: 430 kcal Fat: 21 g Protein: 48 g Carbs: 12 g Fiber: 3 g

46) SIMPLE COUSCOUS WITH SUNDRIED TOMATO AND FETA

Preparation Time: 12 minutes   **Cooking Time:**   **Servings:** 6

Ingredients:

- ✓ 1.25 cups dried couscous
- ✓ 1 tsp powdered vegetable stock
- ✓ 1.25 cups boiled water
- ✓ One chopped garlic clove
- ✓ 14 oz chickpeas
- ✓ 1 tsp coriander powder
- ✓ ½ cup chopped coriander
- ✓ One chopped onion
- ✓ ½ cup chopped parsley
- ✓ 7 oz sun-dried tomato
- ✓ One lemon zest
- ✓ 4 oz arugula lettuce
- ✓ Black pepper
- ✓ 5 tbsp lemon juice
- ✓ 2 oz feta cheese
- ✓ ½ tsp black pepper
- ✓ Salt to taste

Directions:

- ❖ In a bowl, combine garlic, chickpeas, stock powder, couscous, and coriander.
- ❖ Add hot water to the bowl and mix well. Cover the bowl and keep it aside for about five minutes.
- ❖ Add sun-dried tomatoes, lemon juice, coriander, rocket, pepper, parsley, salt, onions, and lemon zest and toss well.
- ❖ Sprinkle feta cheese and serve.

Nutrition: Calories: 260 kcal Fat: 9.2 g Protein: 10 g Carbs: 39 g Fiber: 5.8 g

47) ORIGINAL GARLICKY SWISS CHARD AND CHICKPEAS

Preparation Time: 10 minutes   **Cooking Time:** 10 minutes   **Servings:** 4

Ingredients:

- ✓ 1 cup chopped sundried tomatoes
- ✓ 1 tbsp olive oil Two minced garlic cloves One sliced shallot Two bunches of chopped Swiss chard
- ✓ 15 oz chickpeas One lemon
- ✓ 1/4 cup vegetable broth

Directions:

- ❖ Cook shallot in heated oil over medium flame until they turned translucent.
- ❖ After shallots are translucent, stir in garlic and cook for three minutes.
- ❖ Mix chard and broth and cover, and let it simmer for a few minutes.
- ❖ Add lemon juice, sundried tomatoes, lemon zest, and chickpeas and mix to combine. Cook for three minutes.
- ❖ Serve and enjoy.

Nutrition: Calories: 519 kcal Fat: 9 g Protein: 14 g Carbs: 87 g Fiber: 10 g

48) EASY ARUGULA SALAD WITH PESTO SHRIMP, PARMESAN, AND WHITE BEANS

Preparation Time: 35 minutes   **Cooking Time:** 15 minutes   **Servings: 3**

Ingredients:

- 4 tbsp olive oil
- 1/2 lb raw shrimp Two minced cloves garlic
- 1/4 tsp ground black pepper
- 1/4 tsp salt
- One pinch of red pepper flakes
- 1/4 cup pesto Genovese 2 cups cherry tomatoes
- 8 cups Arugula
- 1/8 cup grated parmesan cheese
- 1/2 lemon
- 1/2 cup white beans

Directions:

- In a mixing bowl, add salt, chili flakes, olive oil, shrimp, and black pepper. Mix well and keep it aside for 30 minutes for enhanced flavor.
- Heat olive oil in a skillet over a high flame. Cook shrimps in oil, two minutes from each side.
- Lower the flame and stir in tomatoes and garlic. Cook for five more minutes with occasional stirring.
- Shift cooked shrimps' mixture in a bowl and mix with pesto.
- In a bowl, mix olive oil, arugula, and lemon juice. Add cheese, tomatoes, salt, beans, and black pepper. Mix well.
- Serve arugula mixture with cooked shrimps.

Nutrition: Calories: 276 kcal Fat: 6.7 g Protein: 30 g Carbs: 23.3 g Fiber: 5.5 g

49) CANTALOUPE AND MOZZARELLA CAPRESE SALAD

Preparation Time: 10 minutes   **Cooking Time:** 0 minute   **Servings: 8**

Ingredients:

- 1 tbsp white wine vinegar sliced cantaloupes
- Eight shredded prosciutto
- 8 oz mozzarella balls
- ¼ cup chopped basil leaves tbsp extra-virgin olive oil
- ¼ cup chopped mint leaves
- Salt to taste
- 1.5 tbsp honey
- Black pepper to taste

Directions:

- Take cantaloupe balls out of cantaloupe using melon baller and place in a bowl.
- Add mozzarella cheese ball, prosciutto, basil, and mint leaves. Mix well.
- In another bowl, mix honey, vinegar, and olive oil. Pour the dressing over a cantaloupe mixture and mix well.
- Serve and enjoy it.

Nutrition: Calories: 232 kcal Fat: 15 g Protein: 10 g Carbs: 17 g Fiber: 2 g

50) SIMPLE ARUGULA SALAD

Preparation Time: 5 minutes   **Cooking Time:** 0 minute   **Servings: 2**

Ingredients:

- 4 cups arugula tbsp olive oil
- 1/2 tsp kosher salt tbsp lemon juice
- 1/2 tsp black pepper
- 1/4 cup grated parmesan cheese
- 1 tsp honey

Directions:

- Combine honey, black pepper, parmesan cheese, olive oil, salt, arugula, and lemon juice. Toss to coat well.
- Serve and enjoy.

Nutrition: Calories: 203 kcal Fat: 18 g Protein: 6 g Carbs: 6 g Fiber: 1 g

51) MEDITERRANEAN-STYLE QUINOA SALAD

Preparation Time: 15 minutes   **Cooking Time:** 0 minute   **Servings: 4**

Ingredients:

- 1.5 cups dry quinoa
- 1/2 tsp kosher salt
- 1/2 cup extra virgin olive oil
- 1 tbsp balsamic vinegar minced garlic cloves
- 1/2 tsp minced basil
- 1/2 tsp crushed thyme
- Black pepper to taste cups arugula
- 15 oz garbanzo
- One package salad savors for toppings

Directions:

- In a pot, add water, salt, and quinoa. Cook until quinoa is done. Drain and set aside.
- Whisk garlic, pepper, thyme, olive oil, salt, basil, and vinegar in a bowl. The dressing is ready. Keep it aside.
- In a big sized bowl, combine salad savor content, arugula, quinoa, and beans.
- Pour dressing over the arugula mixture and serve after sprinkling basil over it.

Nutrition: Calories: 583 kcal Fat: 33 g Protein: 15 g Carbs: 58 g Fiber: 10 g

52) GREEK-STYLE PASTA SALAD WITH CUCUMBER AND ARTICHOKE HEARTS

Preparation Time: 5 minutes　　**Cooking Time:** 0 minute　　**Servings:** 10

Ingredients:

- ½ cup olive oil
- Four minced garlic cloves
- 1/4 cup white balsamic vinegar tbsp oregano
- 1 cup crumbled feta cheese
- 1 tsp ground pepper
- 15 oz sliced artichoke hearts
- 1 lb pasta noodles cooked

- ✓ 12 oz roasted and chopped red bell peppers
- ✓ One sliced English cucumber
- ✓ 8 oz sliced Kalamata olives
- ✓ ¼ sliced red onion
- ✓ 1/3 cup chopped basil leaves
- ✓ 1 tsp kosher salt

Directions:

- ❖ Combine vinegar, oregano, salt, olive oil, garlic, and black pepper in a bowl and mix well. Set aside.
- ❖ In a big sized bowl, combine olives, onions, cheese, artichoke hearts, cooked pasta, cucumber and bell peppers,
- ❖ Drizzle dressing over the artichoke hearts mixture and toss to coat. Garnish with feta cheese and basil and serve after half an hour.

Nutrition: Calories: 415.43 kcal Fat: 23.15 g Protein: 9.54 g Carbs: 42.54 g Fiber: 4.46 g

53) SPECIAL QUINOA AND KALE PROTEIN POWER SALAD

Preparation Time: 5 minutes　　**Cooking Time:** 15 minutes　　**Servings:** 5

Ingredients:

- ✓ One sliced zucchini
- ✓ ½ tbsp extra virgin olive oil
- ✓ ¼ tsp turmeric
- ✓ ¼ tsp cumin
- ✓ ¼ tsp paprika tsp minced garlic,

- ✓ One pinch of red pepper flakes
- ✓ ½ cup cooked quinoa
- ✓ Salt to taste
- ✓ 1 cup drained chickpeas
- ✓ 1 cup chopped curly kale

Directions:

- ❖ In a bowl, whisk chili flakes, cumin, paprika, salt, olive oil, garlic, and turmeric. Keep it aside.
- ❖ Toast quinoa for one minute in olive oil.
- ❖ Cook toasted quinoa following the instructions given over the package. Set aside.
- ❖ Sauté garlic, kale, chickpeas, and zucchini in heated olive oil in the same skillet used to toast quinoa.
- ❖ Cook for a few minutes until the mixture starts to sweat. Sprinkle salt and remove skillet from flame.
- ❖ In a bowl, combine veggies mixture and quinoa and leave for 10 minutes.
- ❖ In a skillet, sauté spices in oil for two minutes and add in veggies mixture.
- ❖ Serve and enjoy.

Nutrition: Calories: 106 kcal Fat: 3 g Protein: 5 g Carbs: 16 g Fiber: 4 g

54) ITALIAN ANTIPASTO SALAD PLATTER

Preparation Time: 20 minutes　　**Cooking Time:** 0 minute　　**Servings:** 4

Ingredients:

- ✓ ½ chopped red bell pepper
- ✓ One chopped garlic clove
- ✓ 12 sliced black olive
- ✓ ¼ cup olive oil
- ✓ 2 tbsp balsamic vinegar
- ✓ 1 tbsp chopped basil
- ✓ Black pepper to taste

- ✓ 6 oz artichoke hearts
- ✓ 5 oz Italian blend
- ✓ Salt to taste
- ✓ 1 cup broccoli florets
- ✓ ½ cup sliced onion
- ✓ Eight strawberry tomatoes 3 oz salami dried 4 oz mozzarella cheese

Directions:

- ❖ In a mixing bowl, mix salt, vinegar, olive oil, black pepper, garlic, and basil. The dressing is ready.
- ❖ Whisk vinaigrette and salad blend in a bowl.
- ❖ Transfer the salad blend mixture to a platter and organize all the leftover ingredients on the platter and serve.

Nutrition: Calories: 351 kcal Fat: 25.9 g Protein: 16.2 g Carbs: 14.8 g Fiber: 3.8 g

55) WHOLE WHEAT GREEK-STYLE PASTA SALAD

Preparation Time: 15 minutes   **Cooking Time:** 0 minute   **Servings:** 6

Ingredients:

- ✓ 1 lb rotini pasta
- ✓ One chopped cucumber
- ✓ 1 cup sliced cherry tomatoes
- ✓ One chopped yellow capsicum
- ✓ 1 cup chopped Kalamata olives
- ✓ One diced red onion 2 tbsp chopped dill
- ✓ ½ cup feta cheese
- ✓ Salt to taste
- ✓ Black pepper to taste
- ✓ Dressing
- ✓ 2 minced garlic cloves
- ✓ ¼ cup olive oil
- ✓ 3 tbsp red wine vinegar
- ✓ ½ lemon juice
- ✓ Salt to taste
- ✓ ½ tsp oregano
- ✓ Black pepper to taste

Directions:

- ❖ Bring water to boil in a pot. Stir in salt and cook pasta in it until it is done.
- ❖ Strain pasta and set aside.
- ❖ Mix Olive oil, vinegar, salt, lemon juice, oregano, pepper, and garlic in a bowl. The dressing is ready.
- ❖ Combine cooked pasta, cucumber, olives, feta cheese, onions, bell pepper, tomatoes, and dill in a salad serving bowl.
- ❖ Drizzle dressing over the mixture and toss to coat.
- ❖ Serve and enjoy it.

Nutrition: Calories: 437 kcal Fat: 16 g Protein: 14 g Carbs: 64 g Fiber: 2 g

56) POMODORO AND HEARTS OF PALM SALAD

Preparation Time: 15 minutes   **Cooking Time:** 0 minute   **Servings:** 4

Ingredients:

- ✓ 14 oz sliced hearts of palm, diced avocados tbsp lime juice cup sliced grape tomatoes
- ✓ 1/4 cup sliced green onion
- ✓ 1/2 cup chopped cilantro
- ✓ Salt to taste

Directions:

- ❖ In a bowl, combine drained and sliced palm hearts, lime juice, tomatoes, avocados, and onions.
- ❖ Mix salt to adjust the taste.
- ❖ Sprinkle cilantro to enhance the taste and serve.

Nutrition: Calories: 199 kcal Fat: 15 g Protein: 5 g Carbs: 15 g Fiber: 10 g

57) GREEK QUINOA TABBOULEH WITH CHICKPEAS

Preparation Time: 20 minutes   **Cooking Time:** 15 minutes   **Servings:** 8

Ingredients:

- ✓ 1 cup quinoa
- ✓ 2 cups of water
- ✓ 1.5 cups chickpeas cooked cups sliced cherry tomatoes cups slicing cucumber
- ✓ 3/4 cups chopped parsley
- ✓ 2/3 cups chopped onions Tbsp chopped mint
- ✓ Ground Pepper to taste
- ✓ Dressing
- ✓ 1/3 cups olive oil lemon zest tbsp lemon juice
- ✓ 1.5 tsp minced garlic
- ✓ ¾ tsp salt

Directions:

- ❖ In a bowl, mix lemon juice, salt, oil, lemon zest, and garlic. The dressing is ready.
- ❖ In a deep pot, add two cups of water, a pinch of salt, and quinoa. Let it boil.
- ❖ When the water starts boiling, lower the flame to low and cover. Let it simmer for about 15 minutes.
- ❖ Strain quinoa and set aside to cool down.
- ❖ In a bowl, combine onions, cucumbers, mint, tomatoes, cooked quinoa, parsley, black pepper, and chickpeas.
- ❖ Add dressing in quinoa mixture and mix well.
- ❖ Adjust flavor using black pepper and salt and serve.

Nutrition: Calories: 206 kcal Fat: 12 g Protein: 5 g Carbs: 22 g Fiber: 3 g

58) GREEK-STYLE AVOCADO SALAD

Preparation Time: 20 minutes   **Cooking Time:** 0 minute   **Servings: 8**

Ingredients:

- ✓ Two sliced English cucumbers
- ✓ 1.5 lb chopped tomatoes
- ✓ 1/4 sliced red onion 1/2 cups sliced Kalamata olives
- ✓ 1/4 cup chopped parsleysliced avocados
- ✓ 1 cup feta cheese

- ✓ 1/2 cup extra virgin olive oil
- ✓ 1/2 cup red wine vinegar minced garlic cloves
- ✓ 1 tbsp oregano
- ✓ 2 tsp sugar
- ✓ 1 tsp kosher salt
- ✓ 1 tsp ground black pepper

Directions:

- ❖ Mix tomatoes, parsley, onions, cucumbers, avocado, and olives. Set aside.
- ❖ Whisk vinegar, sugar, olive oil, salt, oregano, garlic, and pepper in a jar. Close the lid and shake to get the emulsified mixture. You can add salt, black pepper, and sugar to adjust the taste according to you. The dressing is ready.
- ❖ Transfer the dressing to the salad bowl and toss well.
- ❖ Garnish with feta cheese and serve.

Nutrition: Calories: 323 kcal Fat: 29 g Protein: 5 g Carbs: 14 g Fiber: 6 g

59) WINTER COUSCOUS SALAD

Preparation Time: 10 minutes   **Cooking Time:** 25 minutes   **Servings: 8**

Ingredients:

- ✓ Salad
- ✓ 1.5 cups dry pearl couscous
- ✓ 2 lb cubed butternut squash
- ✓ 1/2 cup dried cranberries
- ✓ 1/2 chopped red onion
- ✓ sliced fennel bulb
- ✓ tbsp olive oil bunch sliced kale
- ✓ 1/2 cup chopped pecans

- ✓ Dressing
- ✓ 2 tbsp apple cider vinegar
- ✓ 1/3 cup olive oil
- ✓ 2 tbsp honey tbsp Dijon mustard
- ✓ 1 tbsp lemon juice
- ✓ Kosher salt to taste tbsp orange juice
- ✓ Black pepper to taste

Directions:

- ❖ Put fennel, onions, and butternut squash over a baking tray lined with a parchment sheet.
- ❖ Sprinkle salt, olive oil, and black pepper over butternut squash.
- ❖ Bake in a preheated oven at 400 degrees for 30 minutes.
- ❖ Cook couscous by following the instructions given on the package.
- ❖ Mix mustard, olive oil, juice, vinegar, honey, salt, and black pepper in a jar and shake until the mixture emulsifies. The dressing is ready.
- ❖ In a bowl, combine baked veggies, kale, pecans, couscous, and cranberries. Pour dressing over the mixture and toss well.
- ❖ Serve and enjoy it.

Nutrition: Calories: 266 kcal Fat: 21 g Protein: 4 g Carbs: 18 g Fiber: 3 g

60) ITALIAN SLOW COOKER CHICKEN CACCIATORA

Preparation Time: 15 minutes   **Cooking Time:** 240 minutes   **Servings: 5**

Ingredients:

- ✓ Three chopped garlic cloves
- ✓ 1.5 tbsp olive oil
- ✓ 1.25 tbsp balsamic vinegar
- ✓ 1 tsp kosher salt
- ✓ 1/2 tsp black pepper
- ✓ 2 tsp Italian seasoning

- ✓ 28 oz crushed tomatoes
- ✓ 2 lb boneless chicken breastschopped yellow onion
- ✓ One chopped green bell pepper
- ✓ 8 oz sliced cremini mushrooms

Directions:

- ❖ Rub the chicken with salt and black pepper and cook in heated oil in a skillet over a high flame for five minutes from both sides.
- ❖ Shift the chicken to the slow cooker.
- ❖ Sauté onions in heated oil for three minutes in a skillet over medium flame.
- ❖ Stir in vinegar and garlic and cook for one more minute.
- ❖ Shift the garlic mixture to the slow cooker.
- ❖ Add mushrooms, tomatoes, Italian seasoning, and bell pepper and mix.
- ❖ Cover the cooker and cook on low flame for four hours.
- ❖ After chicken is done, sprinkle salt, vinegar, and pepper and serve with rice or whatever you like.

Nutrition: Calories: 228 kcal Fat: 8 g Protein: 32 g Carbs: 10 g Fiber: 3 g

61) GREEK-STYLE BAKED COD WITH LEMON AND GARLIC

Preparation Time: 10 minutes   **Cooking Time:** 12 minutes   **Servings:** 4

Ingredients:

- ✓ Five minced garlic cloves 1.5 lb Cod fillet
- ✓ ¼ cup chopped parsley
- ✓ Lemon Juice Mixture
- ✓ 5 tbsp Olive oil
- ✓ 5 tbsp lemon juice
- ✓ 2 tbsp butter

- ✓ Coating
- ✓ 1/3 cup all-purpose flour
- ✓ ¾ tsp salt
- ✓ ¾ tsp paprika 1 tsp coriander
- ✓ ¾ tsp cumin
- ✓ ½ tsp black pepper

Directions:

- ❖ In a medium-sized bowl, combine olive oil, butter, and lemon juice and keep it aside.
- ❖ Whisk flour, salt, spices, and pepper in a bowl and keep it aside.
- ❖ Coat fish with lemon mixture followed by coating with flour mixture.
- ❖ Sauté coated fish in heated olive oil in a skillet over medium flame for two minutes from each side.
- ❖ Mix garlic into lemon juice and pour over sautéed fish.
- ❖ Bake in a preheated oven at 400 degrees for almost 10 minutes.
- ❖ Drizzle parsley and serve with your favorite salad or rice.

Nutrition: Calories: 312 kcal Fat: 18.4 g Protein: 23.1 g Carbs: 16.1 g Fiber: 14 g

62) EASY ONE-PAN BAKED HALIBUT AND VEGETABLES

Preparation Time: 10 minutes   **Cooking Time:** 15 minutes   **Servings:** 6

Ingredients:

- ✓ For the Sauce:
- ✓ Zest of two lemons tsp dried oregano
- ✓ ½ tsp black pepper
- ✓ 1 cup Olive oil
- ✓ 4 tbsp lemon juice
- ✓ 1 tsp seasoned salt tbsp minced garlic tsp dill
- ✓ ¾ tsp coriander

- ✓ For the Fish
- ✓ sliced yellow onion
- ✓ 1 lb green beans lb sliced halibut fillet
- ✓ 1 lb cherry tomatoes

Directions:

- ❖ Whisk olive oil, onions, oregano, salt, dill, pepper, tomatoes, lemon zest, green beans, juice, coriander, and garlic in a bowl.
- ❖ Spread vegetable mixture over one side of the baking tray.
- ❖ Coat halibut fillets with the sauce and place them on a baking tray.
- ❖ Pour the leftover sauce over the vegetable mixture and fillets.
- ❖ Bake in a preheated oven at 425 degrees for 15 minutes.

Nutrition: Calories: 390 kcal Fat: 31.3 g Protein: 17.5 g Carbs: 8.8 g Fiber: 4.1 g

63) AFRICAN MOROCCAN FISH

Preparation Time: 10 minutes   **Cooking Time:** 30 minutes   **Servings: 6**

Ingredients:

- ✓ Olive oil as required
- ✓ 2 tbsp tomato paste
- ✓ Eight minced garlic cloves
- ✓ Two diced tomatoes
- ✓ ½ tsp cumin
- ✓ 15 oz chickpeas sliced red pepper cup water

- ✓ Kosher salt to taste
- ✓ Handful of cilantros
- ✓ Black pepper to taste
- ✓ 1.5 lb cod fillet pieces
- ✓ 1.5 tsp allspice mixture
- ✓ ¾ tsp paprika
- ✓ 1 tbsp lemon juice
- ✓ ½ sliced lemon

Directions:

- ❖ Sauté garlic in heated oil for one minute.
- ❖ Stir in bell pepper and diced tomatoes and tomato paste and cook for five minutes over medium flame with constant stirring.
- ❖ Mix garlic, salt, chickpeas, cilantro, pepper, water, and half tsp of allspice mixture. Let it boil and reduce the flame and simmer for 20 minutes.
- ❖ Whisk leftover allspice mixture, paprika, salt, cumin, and pepper in a bowl.
- ❖ Rub fish with spice mixture and oil.
- ❖ Place fish and fish mixture in a pan, followed by a cooked chickpea mixture, lemon slices, and juice.
- ❖ Let it cook for 15 minutes over low flame.
- ❖ Sprinkle cilantro and serve.
- ❖ Sprinkle spice mixture over the fish

Nutrition: Calories: 463 kcal Fat: 5.7 g Protein: 23.7 g Carbs: 67.2 g Fiber: 2.3 g

64) ITALIAN-STYLE BAKED CHICKEN

Preparation Time: 10 minutes   **Cooking Time:** 18 minutes   **Servings: 6**

Ingredients:

- ✓ 2 lb boneless chicken breast
- ✓ Pepper to taste tsp thyme
- ✓ One sliced red onion tsp dry oregano
- ✓ 1 tsp sweet paprika tbsp olive oil minced garlic cloves

- ✓ 1 tbsp of lemon juice halved Campari tomatoes
- ✓ Salt to taste
- ✓ Handful chopped parsley for garnishing
- ✓ Basil leaves as required for garnishing

Directions:

- ❖ Flatten the chicken pieces suing meat mallet in a zip lock bag.
- ❖ Rub chicken pieces with black pepper and salt and add them to the bowl. Add lemon juice, garlic, oil, and spices and mix well to fully coat the chicken.
- ❖ Place onions in an oiled baking tray followed by chicken and tomatoes.
- ❖ Bake in a preheated oven at 425 degrees for 10 minutes while covering the tray with foil.
- ❖ After ten minutes, uncover and bake again for eight more minutes.
- ❖ Serve after sprinkle parsley over the baked chicken.

Nutrition: Calories: 290 kcal Fat: 11.5 g Protein: 35.9 g Carbs: 11 g Fiber: 0.8 g

65) EASY LEMON GARLIC SALMON

Preparation Time: 10 minutes   **Cooking Time:** 18 minutes   **Servings: 6**

Ingredients:

- ✓ Salmon
- ✓ 2 lb salmon fillet
- ✓ 2 tbsp parsley for garnishing
- ✓ Olive oil
- ✓ Kosher salt
- ✓ ½ sliced lemon
- ✓ Lemon-Garlic Sauce
- ✓ Zest of one lemon
- ✓ 3 tbsp olive oil
- ✓ 3 tbsp of lemon juice
- ✓ Five chopped garlic cloves tsp sweet paprika tsp dry oregano
- ✓ ½ tsp black pepper

Directions:

- ❖ In a bowl, whisk olive oil, pepper, garlic, lemon zest and juice, oregano, and paprika in a mixing bowl and set aside. The lemon garlic sauce is ready.
- ❖ Brush baking tray with oil lined with foil paper.
- ❖ Place seasoned (with salt) salmon on a baking tray and pour the sauce over the salmon.
- ❖ Bake in a preheated oven at 375 degrees for 20 minutes.
- ❖ Broil baked salmon for three minutes and serve after garnishing.

Nutrition: Calories: 338 kcal Fat: 25.8 g Protein: 33.1 g Carbs: 11.8 g Fiber: 3 g

66) SHEET PAN CHICKEN AND VEGETABLES

Preparation Time: 15 minutes   **Cooking Time:** 45 minutes   **Servings: 6**

Ingredients:

- ✓ 2 lb red potatoes
- ✓ 2 tbsp olive oil
- ✓ One chopped onion
- ✓ Three minced garlic cloves
- ✓ 1 tsp powdered rosemary
- ✓ .25 tsp salt
- ✓ 3/4 tsp pepper
- ✓ Six chicken thighs
- ✓ 1/2 tsp paprika
- ✓ 6 cups baby spinach

Directions:

- ❖ Mix onion, rosemary, potatoes, oil, salt, garlic, and pepper in a bowl. Shift the potato mixture into a baking tray sprayed with oil.
- ❖ Combine salt, pepper, paprika, and rosemary in another bowl and sprinkle over chicken. Place chicken pieces over potato mixture and bake in a preheated oven at 425 degrees for 35 minutes.
- ❖ Take chicken out of oven and place in serving dish. Put spinach over veggies and bake for another ten minutes. Transfer cooked veggies over chicken and serve.

Nutrition: Calories: 357 kcal Fat: 14 g Protein: 28 g Carbs: 28 g Fiber: 4 g

67) SICILIAN FISH STEW

Preparation Time: 10 minutes   **Cooking Time:** 35 minutes   **Servings: 6**

Ingredients:

- ✓ Olive oil
- ✓ Two chopped celery ribs chopped yellow onion
- ✓ Salt to taste
- ✓ Four minced garlic cloves tbsp toasted pine nuts
- ✓ Black pepper to taste
- ✓ ½ tsp dried thyme
- ✓ ¾ cup dry white wine
- ✓ One pinch of red pepper flakes
- ✓ 28 oz plum tomatoes
- ✓ Tomato juice
- ✓ ¼ cup golden raisins cups vegetable broth
- ✓ 2 tbsp capers
- ✓ ½ cup chopped parsley leaves
- ✓ 2 lb sliced skinless bass fillet
- ✓ Italian bread for serving

Directions:

- ❖ Sauté onions and celery, black pepper, and salt in a Dutch oven over medium flame with constant stirring for four minutes.
- ❖ Add flakes, thyme, and garlic, and cook for one minute.
- ❖ Mix tomato juice and white wine and let it simmer.
- ❖ When the liquid is concentrated to half, add capers, tomatoes, raisins, and stock.
- ❖ Cook for 20 more minutes.
- ❖ Rub fish with pepper and salt and add in cooking solution and mix well. Let it simmer for five minutes.
- ❖ Remove from the flame and let it cool for five minutes while the oven is covered.
- ❖ Sprinkle parsley and pine nuts and serve.

Nutrition: Calories: 320 kcal Fat:11.6 g Protein: 31.2 g Carbs: 19.8 g Fiber: 2.8 g

68) GREEK CHICKEN SOUVLAKI

Preparation Time: 45 minutes **Cooking Time:** 40 minutes **Servings: 4**

Ingredients:

- ✓ Margination
- ✓ 12 boneless chicken thighs
- ✓ 4 tbsp olive oil tsp dried mint tsp dried oregano
- ✓ 1 tsp ground cumin
- ✓ 1 tsp sweet paprika crushed garlic cloves
- ✓ 1 tsp coriander
- ✓ ½ tsp ground cinnamon
- ✓ 1 tbsp lemon juice
- ✓ Zest of one lemon
- ✓ Wedges cut slices of one lemon slices

- ✓ Pitta wraps
- ✓ 250 g white bread flour tsp caster sugar
- ✓ 7 g dried yeast tsp olive oil
- ✓ Tzatziki sauce
- ✓ crushed garlic clove
- ✓ ½ chopped cucumber small bunch of chopped mint leaves
- ✓ 200 g Greek yogurt
- ✓ 1 tbsp lemon juice
- ✓ To serve
- ✓ Four chopped tomatoes One lettuce
- ✓ One sliced red onion

Directions:

- ❖ In a large mixing bowl, add chicken and black pepper, salt, and all the ingredients mentioned in the marination list. Toss to coat well. Leave it overnight for better results in the refrigerator.
- ❖ Whisk flour, sugar, salt, and yeast in a bowl. Pour 2 tsp oil and warm water about 150 ml and mix to form a dough. Knead the dough for ten minutes.
- ❖ Cover the bowl and set aside for 60 minutes.
- ❖ Make four portions of the raised dough, roll them into circles, and set aside 20 more minutes. The dough for pita bread is ready.
- ❖ In a bowl, mix all the ingredients of the Tzatziki sauce and set aside. The Tzatziki sauce is ready.
- ❖ Thread chicken pieces on skewers separately, place the skewers over the top of roasting tin, place overheated grill, and cook the chicken for 20 minutes while brushing with oil. When chicken is done, set aside.
- ❖ Brush the flattened pita bread with oil and place in a heated pan. Cook for three minutes, and when it turned golden from the underside, then flip and cook the other side for three more minutes. When the bread is fully cooked, cover it and keep it warm until further use.
- ❖ Make kebabs out of grilled chicken and place in pita bread followed by tomato, onion, lettuce, lemon slices, and drizzle Tzatziki sauce and serve.

Nutrition: Calories: 707 kcal Fat: 34 g Protein: 46 g Carbs: 52 g Fiber: 4 g

69) EASY GRILLED SWORDFISH

Preparation Time: 15 minutes **Cooking Time:** 8 minutes **Servings: 4**

Ingredients:

- ✓ Ten garlic cloves
- ✓ 2 tbsp lemon juice
- ✓ 1/3 cup olive oil 2 tsp coriander
- ✓ 1 tsp Spanish paprika
- ✓ ¾ tsp cumin

- ✓ ¾ tsp salt
- ✓ Four swordfish steaks
- ✓ ½ tsp black pepper
- ✓ Crushed red pepper to taste

Directions:

- ❖ Blend olive oil, pepper, garlic, salt, and lemon juice in a blender to obtain a smooth mixture.
- ❖ Coat swordfish with the garlic blended mixture and keep it aside for 15 minutes.
- ❖ Heat grill on high flame. Place fish and cook for five minutes from each side.
- ❖ Sprinkle lemon juice and flakes and serve.

Nutrition: Calories: 398 kcal Fat: 30.7 g Protein: 28.4 g Carbs: 3.1 g Fiber: 0.6 g

70) GREEK-STYLE SHRIMP WITH TOMATOES AND FETA

Preparation Time: 10 minutes   **Cooking Time:** 40 minutes   **Servings:** 4

Ingredients:

- ✓ 4 tbsp olive oil
- ✓ 3/4 cup chopped shallots
- ✓ Four chopped garlic cloves
- ✓ 28 oz diced tomatoes 1 tsp salt
- ✓ 1/4 tsp pepper 2 tsp cumin
- ✓ 1/2 tsp crushed pepper flakes
- ✓ 1 tbsp honey
- ✓ 1.5 lb shrimp
- ✓ 6 oz feta cheese
- ✓ 3/4 tsp dried oregano 2 tbsp chopped mint

Directions:

- ❖ Cook garlic and shallots in heated oil in a skillet over low flame for eight minutes.
- ❖ Stir in salt, cumin, honey, tomatoes, tomato juices, flakes, and pepper.
- ❖ Let the sauce boil and cook for 20 minutes with occasional stirring.
- ❖ Remove from flame and add shrimps in the sauce. Sprinkle feta cheese and oregano.
- ❖ Bake in a preheated oven at 400 degrees for 15 minutes.
- ❖ Shift the shrimp pan to broil and broil for two minutes.
- ❖ Garnish with mint and serve.

Nutrition: Calories: 431 kcal Fat: 25 g Protein: 32 g Carbs: 21 g Fiber: 5 g

71) SIMPLE SALMON KABOBS

Preparation Time: 10 minutes   **Cooking Time:** 8 minutes   **Servings:** 6

Ingredients:

- ✓ 1.5 lb sliced Salmon fillet
- ✓ One sliced red onion
- ✓ One sliced zucchini
- ✓ Kosher salt to taste
- ✓ Black pepper to taste
- ✓ Marinade
- ✓ 1/3 cup Olive Oil
- ✓ Zest of one lemon 2 tbsp lemon juice minced garlic cloves
- ✓ 1 tsp chili pepper 2 tsp dry oregano
- ✓ 2 tsp chopped thyme leaves
- ✓ 1 tsp cumin
- ✓ ½ tsp coriander

Directions:

- ❖ Mix all the ingredients of margination in a bowl.
- ❖ In another bowl, add pepper, onions, salt, salmon, and zucchini and mix well.
- ❖ Add marinade and mix well. Set aside for 20 minutes.
- ❖ Thread onions, salmon, and zucchini in skewers.
- ❖ Place skewers overheated grill, cover them, and grill for eight minutes.
- ❖ When salmons are ready, serve and enjoy it.

Nutrition: Calories: 267 kcal Fat: 11 g Protein: 35 g Carbs: 7 g Fiber: 3 g

72) ORIGINAL SAUTÉED SHRIMP AND ZUCCHINI

Preparation Time: 8 minutes   **Cooking Time:** 7 minutes   **Servings:** 3

Ingredients:

- ✓ lb shrimp
- ✓ 1 tsp salt Two zucchinis 2 tbsp chopped garlic
- ✓ 1 tbsp butter
- ✓ Black pepper to taste 1.5 tbsp lemon juice
- ✓ 2 tbsp chopped parsley
- ✓ Olive oil as required

Directions:

- ❖ Add salt, shrimps, and pepper in a bowl. Mix them well.
- ❖ Cook shrimps in heated oil over medium flame for two minutes from each side. Shift cooked shrimps in a plate.
- ❖ Cook zucchini in heated oil in the same pan for two minutes, then sprinkle pepper and salt.
- ❖ Transfer shrimps to the pan and mix. Add garlic and sauté for two minutes.
- ❖ Add butter and cook to melt it.
- ❖ When shrimps, garlic, and zucchini are cooked, add lemon juice and mix well.
- ❖ Drizzle parsley and serve.

Nutrition: Calories: 216 kcal Fat: 6 g Protein: 33 g Carbs: 6 g Fiber: 1 g

73) EASY SHRIMP PASTA WITH ROASTED RED PEPPERS AND ARTICHOKES

Preparation Time: 10 minutes   **Cooking Time:** 25 minutes   **Servings: 8**

Ingredients:

- ✓ 12 oz farfalle pasta
- ✓ 1/4 cup butter
- ✓ 1.5 lb shrimp
- ✓ Three chopped garlic cloves
- ✓ 1 cup sliced artichoke hearts
- ✓ 12 oz roasted and chopped red bell peppers
- ✓ 1/2 cup dry white wine
- ✓ 1/4 cup basil
- ✓ 1/2 cup whipping cream
- ✓ 3 tbsp drained capers
- ✓ 1 tsp grated lemon peel
- ✓ 3/4 cup feta cheese
- ✓ 2 tbsp lemon juice
- ✓ 2 oz toasted pine nuts

Directions:

- ❖ Boil water in a pot and cook pasta in it.
- ❖ Drain pasta and set aside.
- ❖ Melt butter in a skillet over medium flame. Sauté garlic and cook for one minute.
- ❖ Stir in shrimps and cook for about two minutes.
- ❖ Mix artichokes, capers, bell pepper, and wine. Let it boil.
- ❖ Lower the flame and let it simmer for two minutes with occasional stirring.
- ❖ Add whipping cream, lemon juice, and lemon zest.
- ❖ Let it boil for five minutes.
- ❖ Transfer the cooked shrimps over pasta and mix well.
- ❖ Spread cheese, basil, and nuts and serve.

Nutrition: Calories: 627 kcal Fat: 24 g Protein: 38 g Carbs: 58 g Fiber: 3 g

74) QUICK 30 MINUTES CAPRESE CHICKEN

Preparation Time: 10 minutes   **Cooking Time:** 20 minutes   **Servings: 4**

Ingredients:

- ✓ Two boneless chicken breasts
- ✓ Black pepper to taste
- ✓ 1 tbsp butter
- ✓ 1 tbsp extra virgin olive oil
- ✓ 6 oz Pesto
- ✓ Eight chopped tomatoes
- ✓ Six grated mozzarella cheese
- ✓ Balsamic glaze as needed
- ✓ Kosher salt to taste
- ✓ Basil as required

Directions:

- ❖ Mix salt, sliced chicken, and pepper in a bowl. Set aside for ten minutes.
- ❖ Melt butter in a skillet over medium flame.
- ❖ Cook chicken pieces in melted butter for five minutes from both sides.
- ❖ Remove from the flame. Sprinkle pesto and place mozzarella cheese and tomatoes over chicken pieces.
- ❖ Bake in a preheated oven at 400 degrees for 12 minutes.
- ❖ Garnish with balsamic glaze and serve.

Nutrition: Calories: 232 kcal Fat: 15 g Protein: 18 g Carbs: 5 g Fiber: 1 g

75) SPECIAL GRILLED LEMON CHICKEN SKEWERS

Preparation Time: 10 minutes   **Cooking Time:** 10 minutes   **Servings: 6**

Ingredients:

- ✓ Two boneless chicken breasts
- ✓ Seven green onions
- ✓ Four minced garlic cloves
- ✓ Three lemons
- ✓ 1 tbsp dried oregano
- ✓ 1 tsp kosher salt
- ✓ 1/4 cup olive oil
- ✓ 1/2 tsp black pepper

Directions:

- ❖ Whisk salt, lemon juice, olive oil, garlic, lemon zest, black pepper, oregano, and sliced chicken pieces in a bowl. Set aside for four hours.
- ❖ Thread chicken, onions, and lemon slices onto the skewer.
- ❖ Grill chicken skewers for 15 minutes on preheated grill over medium flames with often turning.
- ❖ Serve when chicken is fully cooked.

Nutrition: Calories: 142 kcal Fat: 1 g Protein: 16 g Carbs: 3 g Fiber: 1 g

76) TASTY SAUTÉED CHICKEN WITH OLIVES CAPERS AND LEMONS

Preparation Time: 5 minutes **Cooking Time:** 30 minutes **Servings: 4**

Ingredients:

- ✓ Six boneless chicken thighs
- ✓ Two sliced lemons
- ✓ One minced garlic clove minced
- ✓ 2/4 cup extra virgin olive oil
- ✓ 2 tbsp all-purpose flour
- ✓ 2 tbsp butter
- ✓ 1 cup chicken broth kosher salt to taste
- ✓ 3/4 cup Sicilian green olives
- ✓ 2 tbsp parsley
- ✓ 1/4 cup capers
- ✓ Black pepper to taste

Directions:

- ❖ Add salt, chicken, and pepper in a bowl and toss well. Set aside for 15 minutes.
- ❖ Cook lemon slices (half of them) in heated olive oil over medium flame for five minutes from both sides.
- ❖ Shift the cooked brown lemon slices on the plate.
- ❖ Coat chicken pieces with rice flour and cook in heated olive oil in the skillet for seven minutes from both sides. Transfer the cooked chicken to the plate.
- ❖ Sauté garlic in heated oil in the same pan for about half a minute. Stir in olives, chicken broth, lemons, and capers. Cook over high flame for few minutes.
- ❖ When half of the broth is left, add parsley and butter. Cook for one minute.
- ❖ Add salt and pepper to adjust the taste and serve.

Nutrition: Calories: 595 kcal Fat: 34 g Protein: 51 g Carbs: 5.5 g Fiber: 9 g

77) DELICIOUS AMARETTO COOKIES

Preparation Time: 4 minutes **Cooking Time:** 30 minutes **Servings: 30 cookies**

Ingredients:

- ✓ 1 tsp almond extract
- ✓ 2.5 cup almond flour
- ✓ Three egg whites ½ cup fine sugar
- ✓ 1/2 tsp vanilla extract

Directions:

- ❖ Preheat the oven to 300°F, lined with parchment paper.
- ❖ In a blender, pulse together all the flour and the sugar. Add the vanilla and almond powder and pump for a couple of seconds. Add the eggs to a bowl, and complete the process until the dough is soft.
- ❖ Put the spoonsful of the dough on the parchment of the paper-lined baking sheet and the sugar dust.
- ❖ Bake at 300°F for 24-30 minutes before serving. Cool completely before serving.

Nutrition: Calories: 62 kcal Fat:3 g Protein:1 g Carbs: 7 g Fiber: g

78) FUDGY BLACK BEAN BROWNIES

Preparation Time: 5 minutes **Cooking Time:** 40 minutes **Servings: 16**

Ingredients:

- ✓ 15-oz black beans
- ✓ 3 tbsp oil
- ✓ 1/4 tsp salt
- ✓ Three eggs
- ✓ 1 tsp vanilla
- ✓ 2/3 cup sugar
- ✓ 1/4 cup cocoa powder
- ✓ 1/2 tsp baking powder
- ✓ 1/2 cup chocolate chips

Directions:

- ❖ Preheat oven to 350 o F (176 o C). Put black beans in pestle and mortar and make a paste. In a mixing bowl, mix all the bean vanilla puree, oil, and eggs.
- ❖ In the mixing bowl, add cocoa powder, baking powder, sugar, coffee, and salt. Stir chocolate chips and add dry mixture to wet ingredients.
- ❖ Bake the batter in oil sprayed pan for 30 to 40 min, till it is seen cooked and the middle doesn't twirl much as you shake the pan.

79) EASY BLUEBERRY PANCAKES

Preparation Time: 10 minutes **Cooking Time:** 15 minutes **Servings: 6**

Ingredients:

- ✓ 15-oz black beans
- ✓ 1/4 tsp salt
- ✓ Three flavorless oil
- ✓ Three eggs
- ✓ 1 tsp vanilla
- ✓ 2/3 cup sugar
- ✓ 1/4 cup cocoa powder
- ✓ 1/2 tsp baking powder
- ✓ 1/2 cup chocolate chips

Directions:

- ❖ In a bowl, mix all flour, salt, baking powder, and sugar. In another bowl, beat egg and milk. Add milk and egg into the flour mixture. Mix it and fold it with blueberries. Set down for one h.
- ❖ Heat a pan over medium-high heat. Pour the batter onto the griddle. Turn its both sides brown to eat.

Nutrition: Calories: 117 kcal Fat: 5.3 g Protein:3 g Carbs: 16 g Fiber: 1.4 g

80) SWEET BLUEBERRY AND BANANA PROTEIN BREAD

Preparation Time: 10 minutes **Cooking Time:** 40 minutes **Servings: 8 people**

Ingredients:

- ✓ 1 cup Blueberries
- ✓ 2 Egg
- ✓ 1 tsp Cinnamon
- ✓ 2 Banana
- ✓ 1 tsp Vanilla Extract
- ✓ 2 tsp Baking Powder

Directions:

- ❖ Preheat oven to 350 degrees.
- ❖ In a mixing bowl, mix almond flour, baking powder, cinnamon, and protein powder.
- ❖ In a large bowl, mix applesauce, eggs, yogurt, and vanilla with mashed banana. Add it into dry ingredients with Â 0.5 of the blueberries. Put the other Â1/2of of the blueberries into the lower layer; now put the bread on top. Bake at 350 degrees till the toothpick comes out clean from the center.

Nutrition: Calories:139 kcal Fat:5.13 g Protein: 10.04 g Carbs:14.94 g Fiber: 2.24 g

81) ORIGINAL BOYSENBERRY AND APPLE COBBLER

Preparation Time: 10 minutes **Cooking Time:** 40 minutes **Servings: 4**

Ingredients:

- ✓ 1/2 cup flour
- ✓ Two sliced apples
- ✓ 1/2 cup sugar
- ✓ 1/2 cup oats
- ✓ 1/2 tsp Pepper
- ✓ 50 g molten butter
- ✓ 1/2 cup milk
- ✓ One can boysenberries

Directions:

- ❖ Preheat oven to 180°C for baking.
- ❖ Mix oats flour, bakers, and sugar blend. Add it in milk and butter and mix them all.
- ❖ Place apples on a baking tray, remove 1/2 the boysenberries' liquid, then mix it well with the apples.
- ❖ Pour the batter and bake in the oven for 30-40 min until it is golden colored or cooked.
- ❖ Serve with ice cream or cream or both!

Nutrition: Calories: 360 kcal Fat:12 g Protein: 5 g Carbs:62 g Fiber: 5g

82) SPECIAL PEACH UPSIDE-DOWN PUDDING

Preparation Time: 25 minutes **Cooking Time:** 45 minutes **Servings: 8**

Ingredients:

- ✓ 1/4 cup butter
- ✓ 1/2 cup milk
- ✓ 1.5 cup peeled peaches
- ✓ 1/2 cup brown sugar
- ✓ 1.25 cup all-purpose flour
- ✓ 1/4 tsp salt
- ✓ 1.25 tsp baking powder
- ✓ 1/2 cup butter
- ✓ One large egg
- ✓ 3/4 cup granulated sugar
- ✓ 1 tsp vanilla

Directions:

- ❖ Place 0.25 cup butter in baking pan. Heat in a 350° oven for 5 minutes till the butter is melted. Remove it from the oven. Add some brown sugar while stirring till the sugar is completely dissolved. Place sugar paste uniformly in the pan. Apply peach pieces over brown sugar mixture.

- ❖ In a large bowl, mix the flour, baking powder, and salt. In a large bowl, beat 0.5 cup butter with a beater on medium to high speed for 30 seconds. Beat in granulated sugar. Put egg and vanilla in it while beating. Now add the flour and milk to the already beaten butter mixture by beating on low speed for every addition. Place batter properly over the peaches in the pan.

- ❖ Bake it until a toothpick in the middle comes out clean. Cool it around 5 min. Shift it onto a large serving platter. Cool it further & serve hot.

Nutrition: Calories:372 kcal Fat:18 g Protein:4 g Carbs: 49 g Fiber: 1 g

83) EASY MUESLI MUFFINS

Preparation Time: 10 minutes **Cooking Time:** 25 minutes **Servings: 7**

Ingredients:

- ✓ 100 g flour
- ✓ 2 tsp baking powder
- ✓ 50 g plain flour
- ✓ 1/2 tsp cinnamon
- ✓ One pinch salt
- ✓ Two eggs
- ✓ 100 g muesli
- ✓ 35 g milk
- ✓ 100 g butter
- ✓ 100 g panela sugar
- ✓ 100 ml of milk
- ✓ 1 tsp vanilla extract

Directions:

- ❖ Preheat the oven to 400 degrees. Take the butter and melt it in a pan.

- ❖ Now mix the dry ingredients. A large bowl adds the two flours, baking powder, ground cinnamon, muesli, orange zest, sugar, salt, and chocolate chips.

- ❖ Mix the wet ingredients with dry. In another bowl, add the milk, eggs, and vanilla. Beat the eggs with the milk by using a fork. Now add the cooled butter and mix it again.

- ❖ Load the muffin cases with more muesli. Cover the cases with the batter mixture using a cake spoon. You want them to be half to two-thirds complete. You will plan to measure each muffin to ensure the same amount. Any of them would weigh around 90g. Taking a couple more of your chosen muesli. Delete the dried fruit from the (placing it back in your cereal container). Spread the oats, seeds, and nuts over the top of the raw muffins.

- ❖ Bake it for 25 min. You have to change the direction of the tray every 18 min. Allow the muffins to rest on a cooling rack.

Nutrition: Calories: 380 kcal Fat:20 g Protein:7 g Carbs: 45 g Fiber: 2 g

84) TASTY ORANGE AND BERRY SELF-SAUCING PUDDING

Preparation Time: 10 minutes   **Cooking Time:** 10 minutes   **Servings:** 04

Ingredients:

- ✓ 125 g berries
- ✓ Oil spray
- ✓ ½ cup flour
- ✓ 30 g Reduced fat oil

- ✓ 1/4 cup Skim milk
- ✓ 1/4 cup Brown sugar
- ✓ ½ tsp Orange rind
- ✓ 1/4 cup Orange juice

Directions:

- ❖ Spray oil in four 0.75 -cup microwave-safe trays with oil. Distribute 1/2the berries in 4 dishes.
- ❖ Put spread in a medium microwave-safe till it is melted.
- ❖ Add flour and milk to melted spread while stirring. Add rind & 1/2 the sugar and mix it well. Fold it in the leftover berries and dress with remaining sugar.
- ❖ Add juice and 1/3 cup (80ml) boiling water in a jug. Slowly pour the juice into the dishes. Microwave it on (75% power) for 5–6 min. Set down for 5 minutes before serving.

Nutrition: Calories: 280 kcal Fat:8 g Protein:5 g Carbs: 44 g Fiber: 3.7g

85) ITALIAN PANFORTE

Preparation Time: 20 minutes   **Cooking Time:** 40 minutes   **Servings: 20 slices**

Ingredients:

- ✓ 3/4 cup roasted almonds
- ✓ 1.5 cup candied fruit
- ✓ 3/4 tsp nutmeg
- ✓ 3/4 whole hazelnuts roasted
- ✓ 3 tbsp honey
- ✓ 1 cup granulated sugar

- ✓ 1 tbsp water
- ✓ 1 cup flour
- ✓ 3/4 tsp coriander powder
- ✓ 1 tsp cinnamon
- ✓ 3/4 tsp ground cloves
- ✓ 1 tbsp icing sugar

Directions:

- ❖ Preheat oven to 300 degrees. Spray the cake pan with oil.
- ❖ In a mixing bowl, mix the nuts and candied fruit. In a medium skillet, whisk the flour and flavors.
- ❖ In a small pan, mix honey, water, and sugar, heat on medium flame with continuous stirring till the mixture starts to boil, lower the slow heat boiling for 2-3 min.
- ❖ Add the honey mixture to the nut mixture and mix them. Add the flour mixture and quickly stir.
- ❖ Put the batter into the prepared cake pan and with wet hands. Dust the top with a tbsp of icing sugar before baking. Bake it for 35 to 40 min.
- ❖ Let the cake cool for 10 to 15 min. Place it on a cake stand and make it cool and dust with icing sugar. Took a piece with a sharp knife and enjoyed it!

Nutrition: Calories: 196 kcal Fat:5 g Protein:3 g Carbs: 36 g Fiber: 2 g

86) ORIGINAL PEAR AND CRUMBLE

Preparation Time: 10 minutes   **Cooking Time:** 45 minutes   **Servings:** 6

Ingredients:

- ✓ Crumble topping
- ✓ 200 g flour
- ✓ 100 g ground almonds
- ✓ 100 g butter
- ✓ 75 g caster sugar

- ✓ Fruit filling
- ✓ 500 g plums
- ✓ 1 tsp corn flour
- ✓ Two pears
- ✓ 3 tbsp caster sugar

Directions:

- ❖ Preheat the oven to 18 degrees.
- ❖ Put 200-gram flour, 100-gram butter,100-gram ground almonds, and 75-gram caster sugar into a food processor and blitz till the batter look a lot like crumbs. On the other hand, spread the butter into the flour until the mixture looks like uneven breadcrumbs.Add the almonds and sugar and set it down.
- ❖ To make the filling
- ❖ Rinse 500g plums, cut into quarters dumping the stones, and place in a narrow baking tray. Peel, core, and thickly slice two pears add to the dish. Season with 1 tsp corn flour and 3 tbsp caster sugar and mix it.
- ❖ To complete
- ❖ Place the fruit level in the dish and dress over the crushed topping. Put the dish on a baking sheet and bake until golden.

Nutrition: Calories: 480 kcal Fat:22 g Protein:8 g Carbs: 66 g Fiber: 6 g

87) SIMPLE WARM FRUIT DESSERT

Preparation Time: 10 minutes   **Cooking Time:** 60 minutes   **Servings:** 6

Ingredients:

- ✓ Three sliced Apples
- ✓ ½ tsp Lemon juiced
- ✓ Three cored & sliced pears
- ✓ 1 tsp Ground Cinnamon
- ✓ ½ tbsp Orange Zest

- ✓ 2 Cup Grapes
- ✓ 1/4 tsp Ground Nutmeg
- ✓ 2 cup cranberries
- ✓ 1 Orange Juiced
- ✓ 1/3 cup Maple Syrup
- ✓ 2 tbsp Coconut Oil

Directions:

- ❖ Preheat the oven to 300 degrees and spray it with coconut oil.
- ❖ Mix apples and pears in a bowl. Add lemon zest, cinnamon, nutmeg, and toss the fruits with a spoon to coat with the juice.
- ❖ Shift the fruits in the baking dish & add in grapes and cranberries.
- ❖ In a mixing bowl, whisk fresh orange zest, Apple syrup, and coconut oil. Put the dressing over the fruits.
- ❖ Bake it in the oven for one hour. Once the fruits are done, remove them from the oven and let them cool at room temperature.
- ❖ Season with some cinnamon and serve.

Nutrition: Calories: 258 kcal Fat: 5 g Protein:1 g Carbs:57 g Fiber:8 g

88) FROZEN BANANA ICE-CREAM

Preparation Time: 3 minutes   **Cooking Time:** 0 minute   **Servings:** 1

Ingredients:

- ✓ 2 tbsp peanut butter
- ✓ Two frozen bananas

- ✓ 5 tbsp almond milk

Directions:

- ❖ In a blender, mix the bananas and the milk.
- ❖ Once they are partly chopped up, add in the nut butter.

Nutrition: Calories: 125 kcal Fat: 0.4 g Protein:1.3 g Carbs:26.9 g Fiber: 3.1 g

89) MUSHROOM AND SPINACH OMELETTE

Preparation Time: 15 minutes   **Cooking Time:** 15 minutes   **Servings:** 2

Ingredients:

- ✓ One egg
- ✓ 1 cup spinach
- ✓ 1 tbsp shredded Parmesan cheese
- ✓ Three egg whites
- ✓ 1 tbsp grated Cheddar cheese
- ✓ ⅛ tsp red pepper flakes
- ✓ 1/4 tsp salt
- ✓ ⅛ tsp garlic powder
- ✓ ⅛ tsp black pepper
- ✓ ⅛ tsp nutmeg
- ✓ ½ tsp olive oil
- ✓ 1/4 cup green onion
- ✓ ½ cup sliced mushrooms
- ✓ 2 tbsp red bell pepper
- ✓ ½ cup tomato

Directions:

- ❖ Beat egg and egg whites in a bowl. Mix in cheese, salt, flakes, garlic, nutmeg, and pepper.
- ❖ Heat oil in skillet; cook and stir mushrooms, onion, and pepper for 5 min. Put spinach in a skillet and cook. Add the egg and tomato mixture in it and keep cooking till it sets on top. Once done, cut into pieces, and serve instantly.

Nutrition: Calories: 114.4 kcal Fat:5.1 g Protein: 12.5 g Carbs: 5.7 g Fiber: 1.8 g

90) TASTY RASPBERRY STRAWBERRY SMOOTHIE

Preparation Time: 10 minutes   **Cooking Time:** 10 minutes   **Servings:** 1

Ingredients:

- ✓ 1 tbsp honey
- ✓ 1 cup hulled fresh strawberries
- ✓ ½ cup milk
- ✓ ½ cup raspberries
- ✓ ½ cup vanilla yogurt
- ✓ 1 tsp vanilla extract

Directions:

- ❖ Put all the ingredients in a blender and blend until a smooth consistency is attained.

Nutrition: Calories: 317.7 kcal Fat: 4.7 g Protein: 11.7 g Carbs: 58.6 g Fiber: 7.1 g

91) ENGLISH PORRIDGE (OATMEAL)

Preparation Time: 2 minutes   **Cooking Time:** 2 minutes   **Servings:** 1

Ingredients:

- ✓ Base Recipe
- ✓ ½ cup oats
- ✓ 1/2cup water
- ✓ 1/2cup milk
- ✓ 1 Pinch salt
- ✓ Maple Brown Sugar
- ✓ 1 tsp sugar
- ✓ 2 tbsp chopped pecans
- ✓ 1 tsp maple syrup
- ✓ 1/8 tsp cinnamon
- ✓ Banana Nut
- ✓ ½ banana sliced
- ✓ 1 tbsp flaxseed
- ✓ 2 tbsp walnuts
- ✓ 1/8 tsp cinnamon
- ✓ Strawberry & Cream
- ✓ 1/2cup strawberries
- ✓ 2 tsp honey
- ✓ 1 tbsp half and half
- ✓ 1/8 tsp vanilla extract
- ✓ Chocolate Peanut Butter
- ✓ 2 tsp cocoa powder
- ✓ 2 tsp chocolate chips
- ✓ 1 tbsp peanut butter
- ✓ 1 tsp roasted peanuts

Directions:

- ❖ Microwave Instructions
- ❖ Place all the ingredients heat in the microwave on high for 2 minutes. Then add 15-sec increments until the oatmeal is puffed and softened.
- ❖ Stovetop Instructions
- ❖ Bring the water and milk to a boil in a pan. Lower the heat & pour in the oats. Cook it while stirring, till the oats are soft and have absorbed most of the liquid.Turn off the stove and let it for 2 to 3 min.
- ❖ Assembly
- ❖ Stir in the toppings and let rest for a few minutes to cool. Serve warm.

Nutrition: Calories: 227 kcal Fat:6 g Protein: 9 g Carbs: 33 g Fiber: 4 g

92) MOROCCAN FATTOUSH SALAD

Preparation Time: 20 minutes   **Cooking Time:** 20 minutes   **Servings:** 6

Ingredients:

- ✓ Two loaves of pita bread
- ✓ • ½ tsp sumac
- ✓ • Olive Oil
- ✓ • Salt and pepper
- ✓ • One chopped English cucumber
- ✓ • One chopped lettuce
- ✓ • Five chopped Roma tomatoes

- ✓ Five radishes
- ✓ • Five chopped green onions
- ✓ • 2 cup parsley leaves
- ✓ Lime-vinaigrette
- ✓ • 1/4 tsp cinnamon
- ✓ • 1 tsp lime juice
- ✓ • Salt and pepper
- ✓ • 1/3 cup Virgin Olive Oil
- ✓ • 1 tsp sumac
- ✓ • 1/4 tsp allspice

Directions:

- ❖ Toast the bread in the oven. Heat olive oil and fry until browned. Add salt, pepper, and 1/2tsp of sumac. Turn off heat & place pita chips on paper towels to drain.
- ❖ In a mixing bowl, mix the chopped lettuce, cucumber, tomatoes, green onions with the sliced radish and parsley.
- ❖ For seasoning, whisk the lemon or lime juice, olive oil, and spices in a small bowl.
- ❖ Sprinkle the salad & toss lightly. Finally, add the pita chips and more sumac if you like. Shifts to small serving bowls or plates. Enjoy!

Nutrition: Calories: 345 kcal Fat:20.4 g Protein: 9.1 g Carbs:39.8 g Fiber: 1 g

93) CALABRIA CICORIA E FAGIOLI

Preparation Time: **Cooking Time:**   **Servings:** 6

Ingredients:

- ✓ 200 g dried cannellini beans
- ✓ • 6 tbsp olive oil
- ✓ • 400 g curly endive

- ✓ Four garlic cloves
- ✓ • 600 ml of water
- ✓ • Two red chilies
- ✓ • Salt and pepper to taste

Directions:

- ❖ Put the dried beans to soak for 12 h (they increase in size). Drain them and boil for two h in fresh unsalted water. Salt at the end of the cooking time. If using canned beans, drain them from their liquid and rinse them before use. Rinse the endive and cut it up into short lengths.
- ❖ Heat the olive oil, fry the garlic without browning, and then add the endive and chilies. Keeping the heat high, stir-fry for a minute or two, coating the endive with the oil, then add the drained cannellini beans, some salt, and the water. Bring to the boil, cover the pan, and lower the heat. Cook until the endive is soft and most of the liquid has been absorbed.

Nutrition: Calories:225 kcal Fat: 21 g Protein: 3 g Carbs: 6 g Fiber:1 g

94) CAMPANIA POACHED EGGS CAPRESE

Preparation Time: 10 minutes   **Cooking Time:** 10 minutes   **Servings:** 2

Ingredients:

- ✓ 4 tsp pesto
- ✓ • 1 tbsp white vinegar
- ✓ • Four eggs
- ✓ • 2 tsp salt

- ✓ 2 English muffins
- ✓ • salt to taste
- ✓ • One tomato sliced
- ✓ • Four slices of mozzarella cheese

Directions:

- ❖ Fill 2 to 3 inches of a pan with water and boil over a high flame. Lower the heat, add the vinegar, 2 tsp of salt in it, and let it simmer.
- ❖ Put a cheese slice and a slice of tomato on every English muffin half and put in a toaster oven for 5 min or till the cheese melts and the English muffin is well toasted.
- ❖ Break an egg in a bowl and add in the water one by one. Let the eggs cook for 2.5 to 3 minutes or until the yolks have solidified and the egg whites are firm. Take the eggs out of the water and put them on a kitchen towel to absorb excess water.
- ❖ For assembling, first put an egg on top of every muffin, add a tsp of pesto sauce on the egg, and scatter the salt.

Nutrition: Calories: 482.1 kcal Fat: g Protein: 33.3 g Carbs: 31.7 g Fiber:1.2 g

95) GREEK EGGS AND GREENS BREAKFAST DISH

Preparation Time: 10 minutes   **Cooking Time:** 10 minutes   **Servings: 2**

Ingredients:

- ✓ 1 tbsp olive oil
- ✓ • salt to taste
- ✓ • 2 cup chopped rainbow chard
- ✓ • ½ cup arugula
- ✓ 1 cup spinach
- ✓ • Two cloves garlic
- ✓ • ½ cup grated Cheddar cheese
- ✓ • Four eggs
- ✓ • black pepper to taste

Directions:

❖ Heat oil over moderate pressure. Sauté the chard, spinach, and arugula until soft, around three minutes. Add garlic, continue cooking until aromatic, approx. Two min.

❖ In a cup, combine the eggs and the cheese; dump into the mixture of the chard. Heat and cook for 5 - 6 minutes. Season to taste with salt and pepper.

Nutrition: Calories:332.5 kcal Fat: 26.2 g Protein: 21 g Carbs:4.2 g Fiber: 1 g

96) ITALIAN BREAKFAST PITA PIZZA

Preparation Time: 25 minutes   **Cooking Time:** 30 minutes   **Servings: 2**

Ingredients:

- ✓ Four slices of bacon
- ✓ 2 tbsp olive oil
- ✓ 1/4 onion
- ✓ Four eggs
- ✓ Two pita bread rounds
- ✓ 2 tbsp pesto
- ✓ ½ tomato
- ✓ One avocado
- ✓ ½ cup slashed spinach
- ✓ 1/4 cup mushrooms
- ✓ ½ cup grated Cheddar cheese

Directions:

❖ Heat the oven to 350 ° F (175° C).

❖ In a medium saucepan, put the bacon and cook over medium-high heat, rotating periodically, when browned uniformly, around ten minutes. Cook the onion in the same skillet till smooth. Put it aside. In the skillet, melt the olive oil. Add the eggs and cook, stirring regularly, for 3 to 5 minutes.

❖ Add the pita bread to the cake pan. Cover with bacon, fried eggs, onions, mushrooms, and spinach; sprinkle the pesto over through the pita. Dress over the toppings of Cheddar cheese.

❖ Bake it in the preheated oven for10 min. Serve with avocado pieces.

Nutrition: Calories: 873.2 kcal Fat: 62 g Protein: 36.8 g Carbs:43.5 g Fiber: 9.5 g

97) NAPOLI CAPRESE ON TOAST

Preparation Time: 15 minutes   **Cooking Time:** 5 minutes   **Servings: 14**

Ingredients:

- ✓ 14 slices bread
- ✓ 1 lb mozzarella cheese
- ✓ Two cloves garlic
- ✓ 1/3 cup basil leaves
- ✓ 3 tbsp olive oil
- ✓ Three tomatoes
- ✓ salt to taste
- ✓ black pepper to taste

Directions:

❖ Baked the bread slices and spread the garlic on one side of each piece. Put a slice of mozzarella cheese, 1 to 2 basil leaves, and a slice of tomato on each piece of toast. Sprinkle with olive oil, spray salt, and black pepper.

Nutrition: Calories: 203.5 kcal Fat: 10 g Protein: 10.5 g Carbs: 16.5 g Fiber: 1.1 g

98) TUSCAN EGGS FLORENTINE

Preparation Time: 10 minutes   **Cooking Time:** 10 minutes   **Servings: 3**

Ingredients:

- ✓ 2 tbsp butter
- ✓ Two cloves garlic
- ✓ 3 tbsp cream cheese
- ✓ ½ cup mushroom
- ✓ ½ fresh spinach
- ✓ Salt to taste
- ✓ Six eggs
- ✓ Black pepper to taste

Directions:

❖ Put the butter in a non-stick skillet; heat and mix the mushrooms and garlic till the garlic is flavorsome for about 1 min. Add spinach to the mushroom paste and cook until spinach is softened for 2 - 3 mins,

❖ Mix the mushroom-spinach mixer; add salt and pepper. Cook, with mixing, until the eggs are stiff; turn. Pour with cream cheese over the egg mixture and cook before cream cheese started melting just over five minutes.

Nutrition: Calories: 278.9 kcal Fat: 22.9 g Protein:15.7 g Carbs: 4.1 g Fiber:22.9

99) SPECIAL QUINOA BREAKFAST CEREAL

Preparation Time: 5 minutes   **Cooking Time:** 16 minutes   **Servings: 4**

Ingredients:

- ✓ ½ cup almonds
- ✓ 1 tsp cinnamon
- ✓ 2 cups of water
- ✓ 1/3 cup seeds
- ✓ ½ cup apricots
- ✓ ½ tsp nutmeg
- ✓ 1 cup quinoa

Directions:

- ❖ Combine water and quinoa in a medium saucepan and continue cooking. Lower the heat and boil when much of the water has been drained for 8–12 minutes. Whisk in apricots, almonds, linseeds, cinnamon, and nutmeg; simmer till the quinoa is soft.

Nutrition: Calories: 349.9 kcal Fat:15.1 g Protein: 11.8 g Carbs: 44.5 g Fiber: 9.3 g

100)   SIMPLE ZUCCHINI WITH EGG

Preparation Time: 5 minutes   **Cooking Time:** 15 minutes   **Servings: 2**

Ingredients:

- ✓ Two zucchinis
- ✓ Black pepper to taste
- ✓ Two eggs
- ✓ 1 tsp water
- ✓ 1.5 tbsp olive oil
- ✓ salt to taste

Directions:

- ❖ Heat the oil in a saucepan over medium heat; sauté the zucchini until soft, around 10 minutes. Season with salt and black pepper.
- ❖ Add the eggs with a fork in a bowl; add more water and mix until uniformly mixed. Spill the eggs over the zucchini; continue cooking until the eggs are boiled and rubbery for almost 5 minutes. Dress it with salt and black pepper.

Nutrition: Calories: 21.7 kcal Fat: 15.7 g Protein: 10.2 g Carbs: 11.2 g Fiber: 3.6 g

101)   MEDITERRANEAN BAKED EGGS IN AVOCADO

Preparation Time: 10 minutes   **Cooking Time:** 15 minutes   **Servings: 2**

Ingredients:

- ✓ One avocado
- ✓ 2 tsp chives
- ✓ One pinch parsley
- ✓ One pinch of salt and black pepper
- ✓ Two eggs
- ✓ Two slice bacon

Directions:

- ❖ Preheat the oven to 425 degrees.
- ❖ Break the eggs in a tub, willing to maintain the yolks preserved.
- ❖ Assemble the avocado halves in the baking bowl, rest them on the side. Slowly spoon one egg yolk in the avocado opening. Keep spooning the white egg into the hole till it is finished. Do the same with leftover egg yolk, egg white, and avocado. Dress with chives, parsley, sea salt, and pepper for each of the avocados.
- ❖ Gently put the baking dish in the preheated oven and cook for about 15 min well before the eggs are cooked. Sprinkle with bacon over the avocado.

Nutrition: Calories: 280.3 kcal Fat:23.5 g Protein: 11.3 g Carbs:9.3 g Fiber:6.9 g

102) **TASTY SCRUMPTIOUS BREAKFAST SALAD**

Preparation Time: 35 minutes   **Cooking Time:** 5 minutes   **Servings: 4**

Ingredients:

- ✓ Five eggs
- ✓ Two avocados
- ✓ One head romaine lettuce
- ✓ Two tomatoes
- ✓ Four clementine
- ✓ 1-pint strawberries

- ✓ One onion
- ✓ One cucumber
- ✓ One apple
- ✓ One peeled mango
- ✓ One nectarine
- ✓ 1/4 cup vinaigrette

Directions:

- ❖ Boil eggs in a pan. Turn off the flame. Let the eggs rest in hot water for 15 min.
- ❖ Cover spinach, avocados, tomatoes, strawberries, clementine, cabbage, peach, apple, nectarine, and cucumber in a large mixing bowl or on an individual platter. Sprinkle the vinaigrette at the tip.
- ❖ Take eggs from hot water; cool in ice water. Peel it and chop it. Spread the eggs over the salad.

Nutrition: Calories: 447.5 kcal Fat: 24.2 g Protein:13.4 g Carbs: 53.7 g Fiber: 15.6 g

103) **GENOVESE SOCCA (FARINATA)**

Preparation Time: 10 minutes   **Cooking Time:** 20 minutes   **Servings: 4**

Ingredients:

- ✓ 1 cup chickpea flour
- ✓ One pinch salt
- ✓ ½ tsp cumin

- ✓ Black pepper
- ✓ 1 tbsp olive oil
- ✓ 1 cup of water
- ✓ 1 tbsp vegetable oil

Directions:

- ❖ In a cup, add chickpea flour, water, and olive oil. Season with salt, cumin, and pepper. Mix all ingredients. Set down at room temperature for two h.
- ❖ Preheat the oven to 450 degrees (230 degrees C). Place a cast-iron skillet in the oven until hot, 5 to 7 minutes. Gently remove the pan from the oven, brush the oil, and pour half of the mixture into the pan, tilting to ensure that it is evenly spread.
- ❖ Bake in a preheated oven bake it for 7 min. Switch the oven on and let it brown for 1 min. Turn off the oven and shift it to a plate. Do the same with the remaining mixture.

Nutrition: Calories: 145.6 kcal Fat: 8.4 g Protein: 4.7 g Carbs:13.8 g Fiber: 0.9 g

104) **EASY BLUEBERRY LEMON BREAKFAST QUINOA**

Preparation Time: 5 minutes   **Cooking Time:** 25 minutes   **Servings: 2**

Ingredients:

- ✓ 3 tbsp maple syrup
- ✓ 1 cup quinoa
- ✓ One pinch salt

- ✓ ½ lemon
- ✓ 2 cup milk
- ✓ 1 cup blueberries
- ✓ 2 tsp flax seed

Directions:

- ❖ Wash quinoa in a fine sieve of ice water to extract bitterness when the water is pure and no stickier. Pour the milk into a pan over medium heat for 2 - 3 mins. Mix the quinoa and salt in the milk; boil over moderate heat once all of the liquid was being consumed, around twenty minutes. In the quinoa mixer, slowly fold the blueberries & add the apple and the lime juice. Serve quinoa mixture in 2 bowls; sprinkle 1 tsp linseed to eat.

Nutrition: Calories: 537.8 kcal Fat: 7.3 g Protein: 21.5 g Carbs: 98.7 g Fiber: 8.9 g

105) EASY CHEESY ARTICHOKE AND SPINACH FRITTATA

Preparation Time: 5 minutes   **Cooking Time:** 40 minutes   **Servings:** 8 slices

Ingredients:

- ✓ 3 tbsp pesto
- ✓ 1/2 cup milk
- ✓ 12 eggs
- ✓ 1/2 cup parmesan cheese, shredded

- ✓ 2 tsp olive oil
- ✓ 14.5 oz artichokes, chopped
- ✓ Two garlic cloves
- ✓ 1 cup cheese
- ✓ 6 cup baby spinach
- ✓ 1/2 tsp kosher salt

Directions:

- ❖ Preheat the oven to 375 F.
- ❖ Take a bowl and put milk, eggs, cheese, salt in it, and whisk together. Dry the artichokes using a paper towel.
- ❖ Take a skillet and heat olive oil in it over medium flame. Sauté the garlic in it for half a minute and put 4 cups of baby spinach in it. Cook them until they become soft, and then add the rest of the spinach in it with artichokes and sauté.
- ❖ Add the egg mixture to the skillet and reduce the flame to medium-low. Cook the eggs for 1 minute without stirring.
- ❖ Once the eggs are cooked, stir it to mix well and top with leftover whole artichokes. Put the skillet in the preheated oven.
- ❖ Bake for about 20 minutes or until its edges start to turn brown and puffed from the top. Take out of the oven and put the pesto on it, and sprinkle with cheese. Bake for five more minutes or until the cheese melts, and a frittata is cooked thoroughly.
- ❖ Sprinkle the black pepper and fresh basil on top.

Nutrition: Calories: 234 kcal Fat: 16 g Protein: 16 g Carbs: 6 g Fiber: 2 g

106) SPECIAL STRAWBERRIES IN BALSAMIC YOGURT SAUCE

Preparation Time: 15 minutes   **Cooking Time:** 180 minutes   **Servings:** 3.2 oz

Ingredients:

- ✓ 1 tbsp honey
- ✓ 1 tbsp balsamic vinegar

- ✓ 1 cup sliced strawberries
- ✓ 1/2 cup yogurt

Directions:

- ❖ Mix all the ingredients in a bowl except strawberries. Put strawberries on top of each serving and refrigerate for 2-3 hours, then serve.

Nutrition: Calories: 51 kcal Fat: g Protein:3 g Carbs: 9 g Fiber:1 g

107) GREEK SPINACH FETA BREAKFAST WRAPS

Preparation Time: 5 minutes   **Cooking Time:** 5 minutes   **Servings:** 1

Ingredients:

- ✓ Two eggs
- ✓ 4 Kalamata olives
- ✓ 1/2 cup spinach
- ✓ 1/4 cup feta cheese 1.5 tbsp butter

- ✓ salt to taste
- ✓ One tortilla
- ✓ Black pepper to taste

Directions:

- ❖ Gather the ingredients. Heat the pan to medium heat. Add 0.5of a tbsp of butter to the pan. Scramble the eggs in a small bowl.Add in the rest of the butter chunks and salt and pepper. Add the egg mixture to the pan.Let the eggs cook for a moment, add in the spinach and mix till the spinach and egg are cooked. Put eggs over the tortilla.Top the eggs with the feta cheese crumbles and chopped Kalamata olives.

Nutrition: Calories:399 kcal Fat: 22.9 g Protein: 19.6 g Carbs: 29.2 g Fiber: 2.3 g

108) ORIGINAL KALE AND GOAT CHEESE FRITTATA CUP

Preparation Time: 15 minutes   **Cooking Time:** 15 minutes   **Servings:** 8

Ingredients:

- ✓ 2 cup kale
- ✓ 3 tbsp olive oil
- ✓ 1/2 tsp dried thyme
- ✓ One clove garlic

- ✓ 1/4 tsp red pepper
- ✓ 1/4 tsp salt
- ✓ 1/4 cup Goat Cheese
- ✓ Eight eggs
- ✓ Black pepper

Directions:

- ❖ Preheat the oven to 350 F.
- ❖ Sauté the garlic in 1 tbsp of oil over medium-high heat, in a non-stick skillet, for 30 sec. Add the red pepper flakes and kale to it. Cook for a few minutes until the kale is soft.
- ❖ Whisk the eggs with pepper and salt in a medium bowl. Add the cooked kale and thyme to it.
- ❖ Take a muffin tin and brush 8 cups with the remaining oil. Put the mixture in it, topping with goat cheese.
- ❖ Put in the preheated oven and bake for about 30 min.
- ❖ Serve hot.

Nutrition: Calories: 110 kcal Fat: 8 g Protein: 8 g Carbs: 3 g Fiber: 1 g

109) TASTY AND FLUFFY LEMON RICOTTA PANCAKES

Preparation Time: 5 minutes   **Cooking Time:** 20 minutes   **Servings:** 6

Ingredients:

- ✓ 1.25 cup ricotta cheese
- ✓ Three eggs
- ✓ One lemon
- ✓ 3/4 cup buttermilk

- ✓ 2 tbsp sugar
- ✓ 1 tbsp baking powder
- 1.25 cup flour
- ✓ 1/4 tsp sea salt
- ✓ Olive oil

Directions:

- ❖ In a mixing bowl, whisk eggs and sugar.
- ❖ Add the buttermilk, salt, and ricotta cheese in it and whisk.
- ❖ In another bowl, mix flour and baking powder, then put it into the cheese mixture.
- ❖ Heat a large non-stick skillet. Spoon batter into the pan. Repeat with the remaining batter.

Nutrition: Calories: 245 kcal Fat: 9 g Protein: 12 g Carbs: 28 g Fiber:1 g

110) SPECIAL SMASHED EGG TOASTS WITH HERBY LEMON YOGURT

Preparation Time: 4 minutes   **Cooking Time:** 15 minutes   **Servings:** 4

Ingredients:

- ✓ Eight eggs
- ✓ One lemon
- ✓ One clove garlic
- ✓ Two fresh basil leaves
- ✓ Four slices of bread
- ✓ 2 tbsp chives

- ✓ 2 tbsp dill
- ✓ 2 cup yogurt
- ✓ 3/4 tsp salt
- ✓ 2 tbsp olive oil
- ✓ 1/2 tsp black pepper
- ✓ 4 tbsp butter

Directions:

- ❖ Boil eight large eggs for exactly 6 minutes and 30 seconds. Let sit in the ice bath for 2 min, then peel the eggs and set aside.
- ❖ In a medium bowl, mince one garlic clove, finely grate the zest one medium lemon, then juice the lemon. Finely chopped 2 tbsp fresh basil leaves, 2 tbsp fresh dill, and 2 tbsp fresh chives. Add 2 cup yogurt, 2 tbsp olive oil, 0.75 tsp kosher salt, and 0.5 tsp black pepper.
- ❖ Cut four crusty bread. Melt 2 tbsp unsalted butter in a large skillet. Add 2 of the slices and cook until crispy, for 2 min per side. Shift to a large platter. Repeat with the remaining.
- ❖ Place the yogurt and eggs on the bread. Drizzle salt and pepper and herbs with oil

Nutrition: Calories: 437 kcal Fat: 35.5 g Protein: 23.5 g Carbs: 7.4 g Fiber: 0.6 g

111) ITALIAN AVOCADO AND EGG BREAKFAST PIZZA

Preparation Time: 5 minutes   **Cooking Time:** 40 minutes   **Servings: 4**

Ingredients:

- 1 Hass avocado
- 1 1/2 tsp lime juice
- 1 tbsp cilantro
- 1/8 tsp salt
- Four eggs
- 1/2 lb pizza dough
- 1 tbsp vegetable oil

Directions:

- Cut the avocado in halves using a spoon, but it's flesh in a bowl. Add the lime juice, cilantro, and salt. Mash well with a fork to form a smooth paste.
- Divide the dough into four equal pieces. Roll each piece into a thin 6-inch circle.
- Place one of the dough circles in the center of the skillet. Cook for 1- 2 min, until it is browned. Turn and cook another side until browned, pressing down with a spatula. Shift it to a plate and repeat.
- Apply 0.5 of the avocado mixture onto each cooked slice of dough.
- Fry eggs to desired doneness and place each one on top of a pizza. Serve immediately.

Nutrition: Calories: 337 kcal Fat: 17.6 g Protein: 12.3 g Carbs: 33.4 g Fiber: 4.9 g

112) TURKISH-STYLE MENEMEN RECIPE

Preparation Time: 5 minutes   **Cooking Time:** 20 minutes   **Servings: 3**

Ingredients:

- 3 tbsp olive oil
- 4 cup tomatoes
- 1/4 tsp black pepper
- Three green peppers
- Four cloves garlic
- 1/2 tsp salt
- Three green onions
- Six eggs

Directions:

- Heat olive oil in a pan, preferably cast iron. Add the chopped onion and green peppers and sauté until tender.
- Add the tomatoes, garlic, and green onions and boil for 10-15 minutes, stirring regularly until cooked down. Sprinkle salt over it.
- Let it boil uncovered until the eggs are gently boiled for 8-10 minutes. Enable the egg whites to cook well with a spoon. If you like hard yolks, cook longer.
- Dress ground black pepper over it.
- Garnish with chopped green onion and mint leaves. Serve in the pan.

Nutrition: Calories:219 kcal Fat:13 g Protein:9 g Carbs: 19.3 g Fiber: 1 g

113) EASY AVOCADO MILKSHAKE

Preparation Time: 10 minutes   **Cooking Time:** 10 minutes   **Servings: 3**

Ingredients:

- 1 cup milk
- One banana
- One avocado
- 3 tbsp honey

Directions:

- Blend milk, avocado, banana, and honey in a blender until smooth

Nutrition: Calories: 246.7 kcal Fat: 11.6 g Protein: 4.5 g Carbs: 33.8 g Fiber: 5.6 g

114) ORIGINAL PUMPKIN OATMEAL WITH SPICES

Preparation Time: 3minutes   **Cooking Time:** 3 minutes   **Servings:** 1

Ingredients:

- ✓ 1/2 cup water
- ✓ ½ cup dried oats
- ✓ 2 tbsp pumpkin puree
- ✓ ½ cup unsweetened almond milk
- ✓ 1/2 tsp pure vanilla extract
- ✓ 1 tbsp maple syrup
- ✓ 1/4 tsp pumpkin pie spice

Directions:

- ❖ Mix all the ingredients in a bow.
- ❖ Microwave them for three minutes.

Nutrition: Calories: 243kcal Fat:4 g Protein: 6g Carbs: 44g Fiber:5 g

115) LOVELY CREAMY OATMEAL WITH FIGS

Preparation Time: **Cooking Time:**   **Servings:** 3

Ingredients:

- ✓ 1 tbsp light butter
- ✓ 1 tbsp honey
- ✓ Five whole figs
- ✓ 1 cup rolled oats
- ✓ 1 cup low fat/skim
- ✓ 1 tsp vanilla extract
- ✓ extra honey to drizzle

Directions:

- ❖ Sauté honey in melted butter and stir in figs. Set aside.
- ❖ Again, melt butter and sauté oats with a few figs and roast for five minutes.
- ❖ Mix in milk and vanilla and boil.
- ❖ Remove the pan from heat when the desired consistency is achieved.
- ❖ Mix roasted figs and oats and serve.

Nutrition: Calories:296 kcal Fat:7 g Protein: 6.3g Carbs:29.3 g Fiber: 3.3g

116) ORIGINAL BREAKFAST SPANAKOPITA

Preparation Time: 10 minutes   **Cooking Time:**   **Servings:** 2

Ingredients:

- ✓ 1 tbsp butter
- ✓ 4 oz Spinach
- ✓ 1 oz feta cheese
- ✓ Two green onions
- ✓ Four eggs
- ✓ 1/4 tsp black pepper
- ✓ 1/2 tsp dill weed
- ✓ 1 oz cheese
- ✓ 1 tbsp chives

Directions:

- ❖ In a medium skillet, melt the butter. Add the dill, onions, and spinach, occasionally stirring.
- ❖ In a container, combine the feta, eggs, dill, cream cheese, and pepper. Transfer the mixture in a skillet over the spinach. Toss and cook for a few minutes.
- ❖ Serve and enjoy it.

Nutrition: Calories:288 kcal Fat: 22g Protein:18 g Carbs:5.3 g Fiber: 1.8g

Soups and Salads Recipes

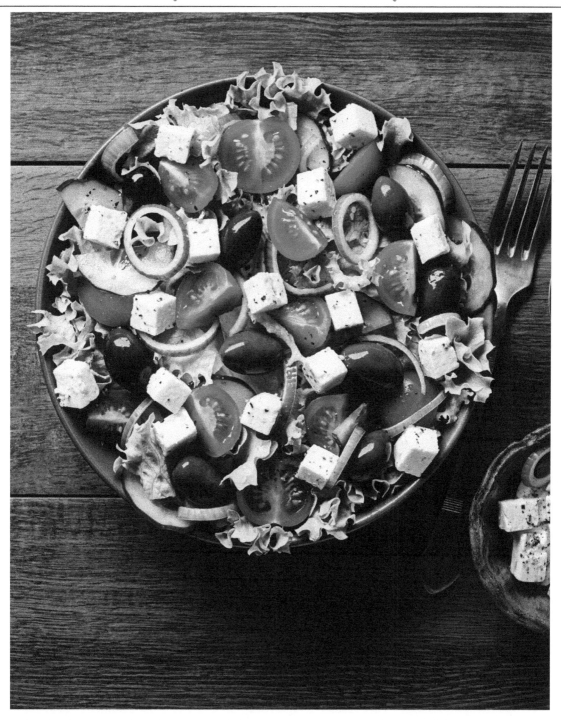

117) CLASSIC MINESTRONE SOUP

Cooking Time: 25 Minutes   **Servings:** 6

Ingredients:

- ✓ 2 tbsp olive oil
- ✓ 3 cloves garlic, minced
- ✓ 1 onion, diced
- ✓ 2 carrots, peeled and diced
- ✓ 2 stalks celery, diced
- ✓ 1 1/2 tsp dried basil
- ✓ 1 tsp dried oregano
- ✓ 1/2 tsp fennel seed
- ✓ 6 cups low sodium chicken broth
- ✓ 1 (28-ounce can diced tomatoes
- ✓ 1 (16-ounce can kidney beans, drained and rinsed
- ✓ 1 zucchini, chopped
- ✓ 1 (3-inch Parmesan rind
- ✓ 1 bay leaf
- ✓ 1 bunch kale leaves, chopped
- ✓ 2 tsp red wine vinegar
- ✓ Kosher salt and black pepper, to taste
- ✓ 1/3 cup freshly grated Parmesan
- 2 tbsp chopped fresh parsley leaves

Directions:

- ❖ Preheat olive oil in the insert of the Instant Pot on Sauté mode.
- ❖ Add carrots, celery, and onion, sauté for 3 minutes.
- ❖ Stir in fennel seeds, oregano, and basil. Stir cook for 1 minute.
- ❖ Add stock, beans, tomatoes, parmesan, bay leaf, and zucchini.
- ❖ Secure and seal the Instant Pot lid then select Manual mode to cook for minutes at high pressure.
- ❖ Once done, release the pressure completely then remove the lid.
- ❖ Add kale and let it sit for 2 minutes in the hot soup.
- ❖ Stir in red wine, vinegar, pepper, and salt.
- ❖ Garnish with parsley and parmesan.
- ❖ Enjoy.

Nutrition: Calories: 805;Carbohydrate: 2.5g;Protein: 124.1g;Fat: 34g;Sugar: 1.4g;Sodium: 634mg

118) SPECIAL KOMBU SEAWEED SALAD

Cooking Time: 40 Minutes   **Servings:** 6

Ingredients:

- ✓ 4 garlic cloves, crushed
- ✓ 1 pound fresh kombu seaweed, boiled and cut into strips
- ✓ 2 tbsp apple cider vinegar
- ✓ Salt, to taste
- ✓ 2 tbsp coconut aminos

Directions:

- ❖ Mix together the kombu, garlic, apple cider vinegar, and coconut aminos in a large bowl.
- ❖ Season with salt and combine well.
- ❖ Dish out in a glass bowl and serve immediately.

Nutrition: Calories: 257;Carbs: 16.9g;Fats: 19.;Proteins: 6.5g;Sodium: 294mg;Sugar: 2.7g

119) TURKEY MEATBALL WITH DITALINI SOUP

Cooking Time: 40 Minutes   **Servings: 4**

Ingredients:

- ✓ meatballs:
- ✓ 1 pound 93% lean ground turkey
- ✓ 1/3 cup seasoned breadcrumbs
- ✓ 3 tbsp grated Pecorino Romano cheese
- ✓ 1 large egg, beaten
- ✓ 1 clove crushed garlic
- ✓ 1 tbsp fresh minced parsley
- ✓ 1/2 tsp kosher salt
- ✓ Soup:
- ✓ cooking spray
- ✓ 1 tsp olive oil
- ✓ 1/2 cup chopped onion
- ✓ 1/2 cup chopped celery
- ✓ 1/2 cup chopped carrot
- ✓ 3 cloves minced garlic
- ✓ 1 can (28 ounces diced San Marzano tomatoes
- ✓ 4 cups reduced sodium chicken broth
- ✓ 4 torn basil leaves
- ✓ 2 bay leaves
- ✓ 1 cup ditalini pasta
- ✓ 1 cup zucchini, diced small
- ✓ Parmesan rind, optional
- ✓ Grated parmesan cheese, optional for serving

Directions:

- ❖ Thoroughly combine turkey with egg, garlic, parsley, salt, pecorino and breadcrumbs in a bowl.
- ❖ Make 30 equal sized meatballs out of this mixture.
- ❖ Preheat olive oil in the insert of the Instant Pot on Sauté mode.
- ❖ Sear the meatballs in the heated oil in batches, until brown.
- ❖ Set the meatballs aside in a plate.
- ❖ Add more oil to the insert of the Instant Pot.
- ❖ Stir in carrots, garlic, celery, and onion. Sauté for 4 minutes.
- ❖ Add basil, bay leaves, tomatoes, and Parmesan rind.
- ❖ Return the seared meatballs to the pot along with the broth.
- ❖ Secure and sear the Instant Pot lid and select Manual mode for 15 minutes at high pressure.
- ❖ Once done, release the pressure completely then remove the lid.
- ❖ Add zucchini and pasta, cook it for 4 minutes on Sauté mode.
- ❖ Garnish with cheese and basil.
- ❖ Serve.

Nutrition: Calories: 261;Carbohydrate: 11.2g;Protein: 36.6g;Fat: 7g;Sugar: 3g;Sodium: 198g

120) LOVELY MINT AVOCADO CHILLED SOUP

Cooking Time: 5 Minutes   **Servings: 2**

Ingredients:

- ✓ 1 cup coconut milk, chilled
- ✓ 1 medium ripe avocado
- ✓ 1 tbsp lime juice
- ✓ Salt, to taste
- ✓ 20 fresh mint leaves

Directions:

- ❖ Put all the ingredients into an immersion blender and blend until a thick mixture is formed.
- ❖ Allow to cool in the fridge for about 10 minutes and serve chilled.

Nutrition: Calories: 286;Carbs: 12.6g;Fats: 26.9g;Proteins: 4.2g;Sodium: 70mg;Sugar: 4.6g

121) CLASSIC SPLIT PEA SOUP

Cooking Time: 30 Minutes   **Servings: 6**

Ingredients:

- ✓ 3 tbsp butter
- ✓ 1 onion diced
- ✓ 2 ribs celery diced
- ✓ 2 carrots diced
- ✓ 6 oz. diced ham
- ✓ 1 lb. dry split peas sorted and rinsed
- ✓ 6 cups chicken stock
- ✓ 2 bay leaves
- ✓ kosher salt and black pepper

Directions:

- ❖ Set your Instant Pot on Sauté mode and melt butter in it.
- ❖ Stir in celery, onion, carrots, salt, and pepper.
- ❖ Sauté them for 5 minutes then stir in split peas, ham bone, chicken stock, and bay leaves.
- ❖ Seal and lock the Instant Pot lid then select Manual mode for 15 minutes at high pressure.
- ❖ Once done, release the pressure completely then remove the lid.
- ❖ Remove the ham bone and separate meat from the bone.
- ❖ Shred or dice the meat and return it to the soup.
- ❖ Adjust seasoning as needed then serve warm.
- ❖ Enjoy.

Nutrition: Calories: 190;Carbohydrate: 30.5g;Protein: 8g;Fat: 3.5g;Sugar: 4.2g;Sodium: 461mg

122) SPECIAL BUTTERNUT SQUASH SOUP

Cooking Time: 40 Minutes   **Servings: 4**

Ingredients:

- ✓ 1 tbsp olive oil
- ✓ 1 medium yellow onion chopped
- ✓ 1 large carrot chopped
- ✓ 1 celery rib chopped
- ✓ 3 cloves of garlic minced
- ✓ 2 lbs. butternut squash, peeled chopped
- ✓ 2 cups vegetable broth
- ✓ 1 green apple peeled, cored, and chopped
- ✓ 1/4 tsp ground cinnamon
- ✓ 1 sprig fresh thyme
- ✓ 1 sprig fresh rosemary
- ✓ 1 tsp kosher salt
- ✓ 1/2 tsp black pepper
- ✓ Pinch of nutmeg optional

Directions:

- ❖ Preheat olive oil in the insert of the Instant Pot on Sauté mode.
- ❖ Add celery, carrots, and garlic, sauté for 5 minutes.
- ❖ Stir in squash, broth, cinnamon, apple nutmeg, rosemary, thyme, salt, and pepper.
- ❖ Mix well gently then seal and secure the lid.
- ❖ Select Manual mode to cook for 10 minutes at high pressure.
- ❖ Once done, release the pressure completely then remove the lid.
- ❖ Puree the soup using an immersion blender.
- ❖ Serve warm.

Nutrition: Calories: 282;Carbohydrate: 50g;Protein: 13g;Fat: 4.7g;Sugar: 12.8g;Sodium: 213mg

123) LOVELY CREAMY CILANTRO LIME COLESLAW

Cooking Time: 10 Minutes   **Servings: 2**

Ingredients:

- ✓ ¾ avocado
- ✓ 1 lime, juiced
- ✓ 1/8 cup water
- ✓ Cilantro, to garnish
- ✓ 6 oz coleslaw, bagged
- ✓ 1/8 cup cilantro leaves
- ✓ 1 garlic clove
- ✓ ¼ tsp salt

Directions:

- ❖ Put garlic and cilantro in a food processor and process until chopped.
- ❖ Add lime juice, avocado and water and pulse until creamy.
- ❖ Put coleslaw in a large bowl and stir in the avocado mixture.
- ❖ Refrigerate for a few hours before serving.

Nutrition: Calories: 240;Carbs: 17.4g;Fats: 19.6g;Proteins: 2.8g;Sodium: 0mg;Sugar: 0.5g

Sauces and Dressings Recipes

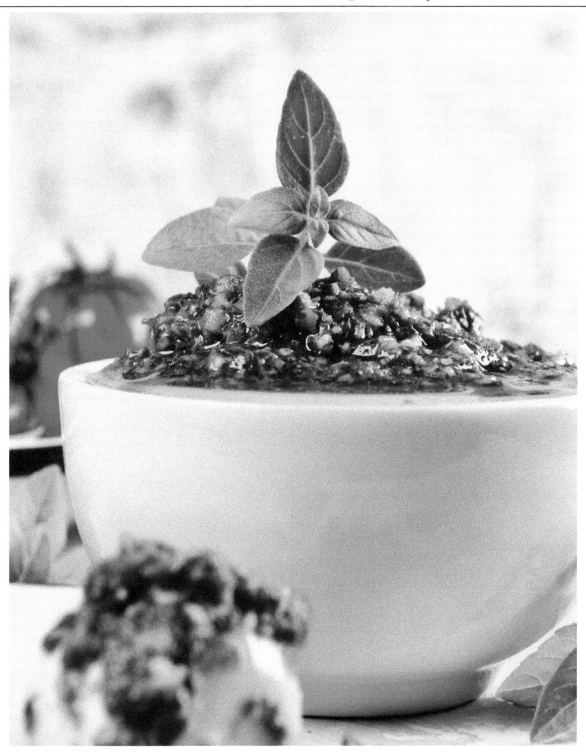

124) EGGPLANT DIP ROAST (BABA GHANOUSH)

Cooking Time: 45 Minutes   **Servings: 2 Cups**

Ingredients:

- ✓ 2 eggplants (close to 1 pound each)
- ✓ 1 tsp chopped garlic
- ✓ 3 tbsp unsalted tahini
- ✓ ¼ cup freshly squeezed lemon juice
- ✓ 1 tbsp olive oil
- ✓ ½ tsp kosher salt

Directions:

- ❖ Preheat the oven to 450°F and line a sheet pan with a silicone baking mat or parchment paper.
- ❖ Prick the eggplants in many places with a fork, place on the sheet pan, and roast in the oven until extremely soft, about 45 minutes. The eggplants should look like they are deflating.
- ❖ When the eggplants are cool, cut them open and scoop the flesh into a large bowl. You may need to use your hands to pull the flesh away from the skin. Discard the skin. Mash the flesh very well with a fork.
- ❖ Add the garlic, tahini, lemon juice, oil, and salt. Taste and adjust the seasoning with additional lemon juice, salt, or tahini if needed.
- ❖ Scoop the dip into a container and refrigerate.
- ❖ STORAGE: Store the covered container in the refrigerator for up to 5 days.

Nutrition: (¼ cup): Total calories: 8 Total fat: 5g; Saturated fat: 1g; Sodium: 156mg; Carbohydrates: 10g; Fiber: 4g; Protein: 2g

125) DELICIOUS HONEY-LEMON VINAIGRETTE

Cooking Time: 5 Minutes   **Servings: ½ Cup**

Ingredients:

- ✓ ¼ cup freshly squeezed lemon juice
- ✓ 1 tsp honey
- ✓ 2 tsp Dijon mustard
- ✓ ⅛ tsp kosher salt
- ✓ ¼ cup olive oil

Directions:

- ❖ Place the lemon juice, honey, mustard, and salt in a small bowl and whisk to combine.
- ❖ Whisk in the oil, pouring it into the bowl in a thin steam.
- ❖ Pour the vinaigrette into a container and refrigerate.
- ❖ STORAGE: Store the covered container in the refrigerator for up to 2 weeks. Allow the vinaigrette to come to room temperature and shake before serving.

Nutrition: (2 tbsp): Total calories: 131; Total fat: 14g; Saturated fat: 2g; Sodium: 133mg; Carbohydrates: 3g; Fiber: <1g; Protein: <1g

126) SPANISH-STYLE ROMESCO SAUCE

Cooking Time: 10 Minutes   **Servings: 1⅔ Cups**

Ingredients:

- ✓ ½ cup raw, unsalted almonds
- ✓ 4 medium garlic cloves (do not peel)
- ✓ 1 (12-ounce) jar of roasted red peppers, drained
- ✓ ½ cup canned diced fire-roasted tomatoes, drained
- ✓ 1 tsp smoked paprika
- ✓ ½ tsp kosher salt
- ✓ Pinch cayenne pepper
- ✓ 2 tsp red wine vinegar
- ✓ 2 tbsp olive oil

Directions:

- ❖ Preheat the oven to 350°F.
- ❖ Place the almonds and garlic cloves on a sheet pan and toast in the oven for 10 minutes. Remove from the oven and peel the garlic when cool enough to handle.
- ❖ Place the almonds in the bowl of a food processor. Process the almonds until they resemble coarse sand, to 45 seconds. Add the garlic, peppers, tomatoes, paprika, salt, and cayenne. Blend until smooth.
- ❖ Once the mixture is smooth, add the vinegar and oil and blend until well combined. Taste and add more vinegar or salt if needed.
- ❖ Scoop the romesco sauce into a container and refrigerate.
- ❖ STORAGE: Store the covered container in the refrigerator for up to 7 days.

Nutrition: (⅓ cup): Total calories: 158; Total fat: 13g; Saturated fat: 1g; Sodium: 292mg; Carbohydrates: 10g; Fiber: 3g; Protein: 4g

127) CARDAMOM MASCARPONE AND STRAWBERRIES

Cooking Time: 10 Minutes   **Servings: 4**

Ingredients:

- ✓ 1 (8-ounce) container mascarpone cheese
- ✓ 2 tsp honey
- ✓ ¼ tsp ground cardamom
- ✓ 2 tbsp milk
- ✓ 1 pound strawberries (should be 24 strawberries in the pack)

Directions:

- ❖ Combine the mascarpone, honey, cardamom, and milk in a medium mixing bowl.
- ❖ Mix the ingredients with a spoon until super creamy, about 30 seconds.
- ❖ Place 6 strawberries and 2 tbsp of the mascarpone mixture in each of 4 containers.
- ❖ STORAGE: Store covered containers in the refrigerator for up to 5 days.

Nutrition: Total calories: 289; Total fat: 2; Saturated fat: 10g; Sodium: 26mg; Carbohydrates: 11g; Fiber: 3g; Protein: 1g

128) SWEET SPICY GREEN PUMPKIN SEEDS

Cooking Time: 15 Minutes   **Servings: 2 Cups**

Ingredients:

- ✓ 2 cups raw green pumpkin seeds (pepitas)
- ✓ 1 egg white, beaten until frothy
- ✓ 3 tbsp honey
- ✓ 1 tbsp chili powder
- ✓ ¼ tsp cayenne pepper
- ✓ 1 tsp ground cinnamon
- ✓ ¼ tsp kosher salt

Directions:

- ❖ Preheat the oven to 350°F. Line a sheet pan with a silicone baking mat or parchment paper.
- ❖ In a medium bowl, mix all the ingredients until the seeds are well coated. Place on the lined sheet pan in a single, even layer.
- ❖ Bake for 15 minutes. Cool the seeds on the sheet pan, then peel clusters from the baking mat and break apart into small pieces.
- ❖ Place ¼ cup of seeds in each of 8 small containers or resealable sandwich bags.
- ❖ STORAGE: Store covered containers or resealable bags at room temperature for up to days.

Nutrition: (¼ cup): Total calories: 209; Total fat: 15g; Saturated fat: 3g; Sodium: 85mg; Carbohydrates: 11g; Fiber: 2g; Protein: 10g

129) DELICIOUS RASPBERRY RED WINE SAUCE

Cooking Time: 20 Minutes   **Servings:** 1 Cup

Ingredients:

- ✓ 2 tsp olive oil
- ✓ 2 tbsp finely chopped shallot
- ✓ 1½ cups frozen raspberries
- ✓ 1 cup dry, fruity red wine
- ✓ 1 tsp thyme leaves, roughly chopped
- ✓ 1 tsp honey
- ✓ ¼ tsp kosher salt
- ✓ ½ tsp unsweetened cocoa powder

Directions:

- ❖ In a -inch skillet, heat the oil over medium heat. Add the shallot and cook until soft, about 2 minutes.
- ❖ Add the raspberries, wine, thyme, and honey and cook on medium heat until reduced, about 15 minutes. Stir in the salt and cocoa powder.
- ❖ Transfer the sauce to a blender and blend until smooth. Depending on how much you can scrape out of your blender, this recipe makes ¾ to 1 cup of sauce.
- ❖ Scoop the sauce into a container and refrigerate.
- ❖ STORAGE: Store the covered container in the refrigerator for up to 7 days.

Nutrition: (¼ cup): Total calories: 107; Total fat: 3g; Saturated fat: <1g; Sodium: 148mg; Carbohydrates: 1g; Fiber: 4g; Protein: 1g

130) ANTIPASTO SHRIMP SKEWERS

Cooking Time: 10 Minutes   **Servings:** 4

Ingredients:

- ✓ 16 pitted kalamata or green olives
- ✓ 16 fresh mozzarella balls (ciliegine)
- ✓ 16 cherry tomatoes
- ✓ 16 medium (41 to 50 per pound) precooked peeled, deveined shrimp
- ✓ 8 (8-inch) wooden or metal skewers

Directions:

- ❖ Alternate 2 olives, 2 mozzarella balls, 2 cherry tomatoes, and 2 shrimp on 8 skewers.
- ❖ Place skewers in each of 4 containers.
- ❖ STORAGE: Store covered containers in the refrigerator for up to 4 days.

Nutrition: Total calories: 108; Total fat: 6g; Saturated fat: 1g; Sodium: 328mg; Carbohydrates: ; Fiber: 1g; Protein: 9g

131) SMOKED PAPRIKA WITH OLIVE OIL–MARINATED CARROTS

Cooking Time: 5 Minutes   **Servings:** 4

Ingredients:

- ✓ 1 (1-pound) bag baby carrots (not the petite size)
- ✓ 2 tbsp olive oil
- ✓ 2 tbsp red wine vinegar
- ✓ ¼ tsp garlic powder
- ✓ ¼ tsp ground cumin
- ✓ ¼ tsp smoked paprika
- ✓ ⅛ tsp red pepper flakes
- ✓ ¼ cup chopped parsley
- ✓ ¼ tsp kosher salt

Directions:

- ❖ Pour enough water into a saucepan to come ¼ inch up the sides. Turn the heat to high, bring the water to a boil, add the carrots, and cover with a lid. Steam the carrots for 5 minutes, until crisp tender.
- ❖ After the carrots have cooled, mix with the oil, vinegar, garlic powder, cumin, paprika, red pepper, parsley, and salt.
- ❖ Place ¾ cup of carrots in each of 4 containers.
- ❖ STORAGE: Store covered containers in the refrigerator for up to 5 days.

Nutrition: Total calories: 109; Total fat: 7g; Saturated fat: 1g; Sodium: 234mg; Carbohydrates: 11g; Fiber: 3g; Protein: 2g

132) GREEK TZATZIKI SAUCE

Cooking Time: 15 Minutes   **Servings:** 2½ Cups

Ingredients:

- ✓ 1 English cucumber
- ✓ 2 cups low-fat (2%) plain Greek yogurt
- ✓ 1 tbsp olive oil
- ✓ 2 tsp freshly squeezed lemon juice
- ✓ ½ tsp chopped garlic
- ✓ ½ tsp kosher salt
- ✓ ⅛ tsp freshly ground black pepper
- ✓ 2 tbsp chopped fresh dill
- ✓ 2 tbsp chopped fresh mint

Directions:

- ❖ Place a sieve over a medium bowl. Grate the cucumber, with the skin, over the sieve. Press the grated cucumber into the sieve with the flat surface of a spatula to press as much liquid out as possible.
- ❖ In a separate medium bowl, place the yogurt, oil, lemon juice, garlic, salt, pepper, dill, and mint and stir to combine.
- ❖ Press on the cucumber one last time, then add it to the yogurt mixture. Stir to combine. Taste and add more salt and lemon juice if necessary.
- ❖ Scoop the sauce into a container and refrigerate.
- ❖ STORAGE: Store the covered container in the refrigerator for up to days.

Nutrition: (¼ cup): Total calories: 51; Total fat: 2g; Saturated fat: 1g; Sodium: 137mg; Carbohydrates: 3g; Fiber: <1g; Protein: 5g

133) SPECIAL FRUIT SALAD WITH MINT AND ORANGE BLOSSOM WATER

Cooking Time: 10 Minutes   **Servings:** 5

Ingredients:

- ✓ 3 cups cantaloupe, cut into 1-inch cubes
- ✓ 2 cups hulled and halved strawberries
- ✓ ½ tsp orange blossom water
- ✓ 2 tbsp chopped fresh mint

Directions:

- ❖ In a large bowl, toss all the ingredients together.
- ❖ Place 1 cup of fruit salad in each of 5 containers.
- ❖ STORAGE: Store covered containers in the refrigerator for up to 5 days.

Nutrition: Total calories: 52; Total fat: 1g; Saturated fat: <1g; Sodium: 10mg; Carbohydrates: 12g; Fiber: 2g; Protein: 1g

134) ROASTED BROCCOLI WITH RED ONIONS AND POMEGRANATE SEEDS

Cooking Time: 20 Minutes   **Servings:** 5

Ingredients:

- ✓ 1 (12-ounce) package broccoli florets (about 6 cups)
- ✓ 1 small red onion, thinly sliced
- ✓ 2 tbsp olive oil
- ✓ ¼ tsp kosher salt
- ✓ 1 (5.3-ounce) container pomegranate seeds (1 cup)

Directions:

- ❖ Preheat the oven to 425°F and line 2 sheet pans with silicone baking mats or parchment paper.
- ❖ Place the broccoli and onion on the sheet pans and toss with the oil and salt. Place the pans in the oven and roast for minutes.
- ❖ After removing the pans from the oven, cool the veggies, then toss with the pomegranate seeds.
- ❖ Place 1 cup of veggies in each of 5 containers.
- ❖ STORAGE: Store covered containers in the refrigerator for up to days.

Nutrition: Total calories: 118; Total fat: ; Saturated fat: 1g; Sodium: 142mg; Carbohydrates: 12g; Fiber: 4g; Protein: 2g

135) DELICIOUS CHERMOULA SAUCE

Cooking Time: 10 Minutes   **Servings: 1 Cup**

Ingredients:

- ✓ 1 cup packed parsley leaves
- ✓ 1 cup cilantro leaves
- ✓ ½ cup mint leaves
- ✓ 1 tsp chopped garlic
- ✓ ½ tsp ground cumin
- ✓ ½ tsp ground coriander
- ✓ ½ tsp smoked paprika
- ✓ ⅛ tsp cayenne pepper
- ✓ ⅛ tsp kosher salt
- ✓ 3 tbsp freshly squeezed lemon juice
- ✓ 3 tbsp water
- ✓ ½ cup extra-virgin olive oil

Directions:

- ❖ Place all the ingredients in a blender or food processor and blend until smooth.
- ❖ Pour the chermoula into a container and refrigerate.
- ❖ STORAGE: Store the covered container in the refrigerator for up to 5 days.

Nutrition: (¼ cup): Total calories: 257; Total fat: 27g; Saturated fat: ; Sodium: 96mg; Carbohydrates: 4g; Fiber: 2g; Protein: 1g

136) DEVILLED EGGS PESTO WITH SUN-DRIED TOMATOES

Cooking Time: 15 Minutes   **Servings: 5**

Ingredients:

- ✓ 5 large eggs
- ✓ 3 tbsp prepared pesto
- ✓ ¼ tsp white vinegar
- ✓ 2 tbsp low-fat (2%) plain Greek yogurt
- ✓ 5 tsp sliced sun-dried tomatoes

Directions:

- ❖ Place the eggs in a saucepan and cover with water. Bring the water to a boil. As soon as the water starts to boil, place a lid on the pan and turn the heat off. Set a timer for minutes.
- ❖ When the timer goes off, drain the hot water and run cold water over the eggs to cool.
- ❖ Peel the eggs, slice in half vertically, and scoop out the yolks. Place the yolks in a medium mixing bowl and add the pesto, vinegar, and yogurt. Mix well, until creamy.
- ❖ Scoop about 1 tbsp of the pesto-yolk mixture into each egg half. Top each with ½ tsp of sun-dried tomatoes.
- ❖ Place 2 stuffed egg halves in each of separate containers.
- ❖ STORAGE: Store covered containers in the refrigerator for up to 5 days.

Nutrition: Total calories: 124; Total fat: 9g; Saturated fat: 2g; Sodium: 204mg; Carbohydrates: 2g; Fiber: <1g; Protein: 8g

137) WHITE BEAN WITH MUSHROOM DIP

Cooking Time: 8 Minutes   **Servings:** 3 Cups

Ingredients:

- ✓ 2 tsp olive oil, plus 2 tbsp
- ✓ 8 ounces button or cremini mushrooms, sliced
- ✓ 1 tsp chopped garlic
- ✓ 1 tbsp fresh thyme leaves
- ✓ 2 (15.5-ounce) cans cannellini beans, drained and rinsed
- ✓ 2 tbsp plus 1 tsp freshly squeezed lemon juice
- ✓ ½ tsp kosher salt

Directions:

- ❖ Heat 2 tsp of oil in a -inch skillet over medium-high heat. Once the oil is shimmering, add the mushrooms and sauté for 6 minutes. Add the garlic and thyme and continue cooking for 2 minutes.
- ❖ While the mushrooms are cooking, place the beans and lemon juice, the remaining tbsp of oil, and the salt in the bowl of a food processor. Add the mushrooms as soon as they are done cooking and blend everything until smooth. Scrape down the sides of the bowl if necessary and continue to process until smooth.
- ❖ Taste and adjust the seasoning with lemon juice or salt if needed.
- ❖ Scoop the dip into a container and refrigerate.
- ❖ STORAGE: Store the covered container in the refrigerator for up to days. Dip can be frozen for up to 3 months.

Nutrition: Total calories: 192; Total fat: ; Saturated fat: 1g; Sodium: 197mg; Carbohydrates: 25g; Fiber: 7g; Protein: 9g

138) NORTH AFRICAN-STYLE SPICED SAUTÉED CABBAGE

Cooking Time: 10 Minutes   **Servings:** 4

Ingredients:

- ✓ 2 tsp olive oil
- ✓ 1 small head green cabbage (about 1½ to 2 pounds), cored and thinly sliced
- ✓ 1 tsp ground coriander
- ✓ 1 tsp garlic powder
- ✓ ½ tsp caraway seeds
- ✓ ½ tsp ground cumin
- ✓ ¼ tsp kosher salt
- ✓ Pinch red chili flakes (optional—if you don't like heat, omit it)
- ✓ 1 tsp freshly squeezed lemon juice

Directions:

- ❖ Heat the oil in a -inch skillet over medium-high heat. Once the oil is hot, add the cabbage and cook down for 3 minutes. Add the coriander, garlic powder, caraway seeds, cumin, salt, and chili flakes (if using) and stir to combine. Continue cooking the cabbage for about 7 more minutes.
- ❖ Stir in the lemon juice and cool.
- ❖ Place 1 heaping cup of cabbage in each of 4 containers.
- ❖ STORAGE: Store covered containers in the refrigerator for up to 5 days.

Nutrition: Total calories: 69; Total fat: 3g; Saturated fat: <1g; Sodium: 178mg; Carbohydrates: 11g; Fiber: 4g; Protein: 3g

139) FLAX, BLUEBERRY, AND SUNFLOWER BUTTER BITES

Cooking Time: 10 Minutes   **Servings:** 6

Ingredients:

- ✓ ¼ cup ground flaxseed
- ✓ ½ cup unsweetened sunflower butter, preferably unsalted
- ✓ ⅓ cup dried blueberries
- ✓ 2 tbsp all-fruit blueberry preserves
- ✓ Zest of 1 lemon
- ✓ 2 tbsp unsalted sunflower seeds
- ✓ ⅓ cup rolled oats

Directions:

- ❖ Mix all the ingredients in a medium mixing bowl until well combined.
- ❖ Form 1balls, slightly smaller than a golf ball, from the mixture and place on a plate in the freezer for about 20 minutes to firm up.
- ❖ Place 2 bites in each of 6 containers and refrigerate.
- ❖ STORAGE: Store covered containers in the refrigerator for up to 5 days. Bites may also be stored in the freezer for up to 3 months.

Nutrition: Total calories: 229; Total fat: 14g; Saturated fat: 1g; Sodium: 1mg; Carbohydrates: 26g; Fiber: 3g; Protein: 7g

140) SPECIAL DIJON RED WINE VINAIGRETTE

Cooking Time: 5 Minutes   **Servings:** ½ **Cup**

Ingredients:

- ✓ 2 tsp Dijon mustard
- ✓ 3 tbsp red wine vinegar
- ✓ 1 tbsp water
- ✓ ¼ tsp dried oregano
- ✓ ¼ tsp chopped garlic
- ✓ ⅛ tsp kosher salt
- ✓ ¼ cup olive oil

Directions:

- ❖ Place the mustard, vinegar, water, oregano, garlic, and salt in a small bowl and whisk to combine.
- ❖ Whisk in the oil, pouring it into the mustard-vinegar mixture in a thin steam.
- ❖ Pour the vinaigrette into a container and refrigerate.
- ❖ STORAGE: Store the covered container in the refrigerator for up to 2 weeks. Allow the vinaigrette to come to room temperature and shake before serving.

Nutrition: (2 tbsp): Total calories: 123; Total fat: 14g; Saturated fat: 2g; Sodium: 133mg; Carbohydrates: 0g; Fiber: 0g; Protein: 0g

141) CLASSIC HUMMUS

Cooking Time: 5 Minutes   **Servings:** 1½ **Cups**

Ingredients:

- ✓ 1 (15-ounce) can low-sodium chickpeas, drained and rinsed
- ✓ ¼ cup unsalted tahini
- ✓ ½ tsp chopped garlic
- ✓ ¼ cup freshly squeezed lemon juice
- ✓ ¼ tsp kosher salt
- ✓ 3 tbsp olive oil
- ✓ 3 tbsp cold water

Directions:

- ❖ Place all the ingredients in a food processor or blender and blend until smooth.
- ❖ Taste and adjust the seasonings if needed.
- ❖ Scoop the hummus into a container and refrigerate.
- ❖ STORAGE: Store the covered container in the refrigerator for up to 5 days.

Nutrition: (¼ cup): Total calories: 192; Total fat: 13g; Saturated fat: 2g; Sodium: 109mg; Carbohydrates: 16g; Fiber: ; Protein: 5g

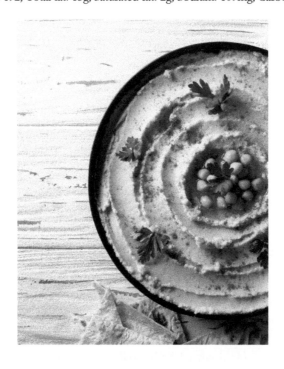

Desserts & Snacks Recipes

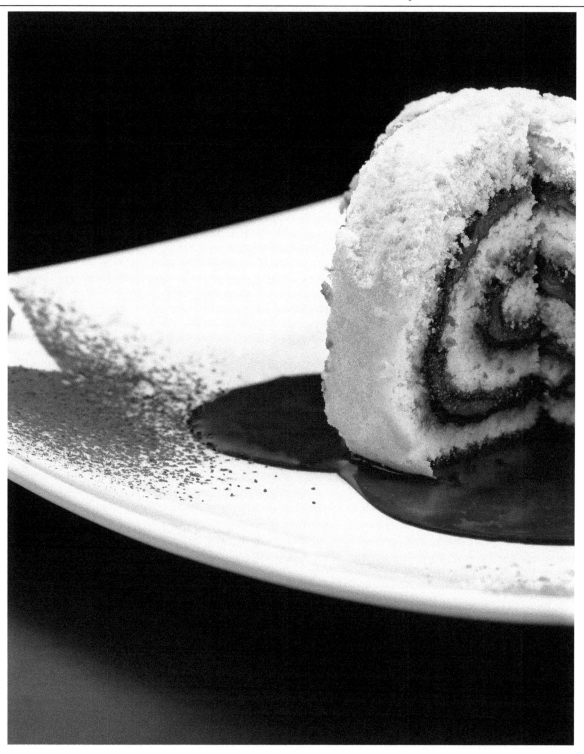

142) **MELON AND GINGER**

Cooking Time: 10 To 15 Minutes **Servings: 4**

Ingredients:

- ✓ ½ cantaloupe, cut into 1-inch chunks
- ✓ 2 cups of watermelon, cut into 1-inch chunks
- ✓ 2 cups honeydew melon, cut into 1-inch chunks
- ✓ 2 tbsp of raw honey
- ✓ Ginger, 2 inches in size, peeled, grated, and preserve the juice

Directions:

- ❖ In a large bowl, combine your cantaloupe, honeydew melon, and watermelon. Gently mix the ingredients.
- ❖ Combine the ginger juice and stir.
- ❖ Drizzle on the honey, serve, and enjoy! You can also chill the mixture for up to an hour before serving.

Nutrition: calories: 91, fats: 0 grams, carbohydrates: 23 grams, protein: 1 gram.

143) **DELICIOUS ALMOND SHORTBREAD COOKIES**

Cooking Time: 25 Minutes **Servings: 16**

Ingredients:

- ✓ ½ cup coconut oil
- ✓ 1 tsp vanilla extract
- ✓ 2 egg yolks
- ✓ 1 tbsp brandy
- ✓ 1 cup powdered sugar
- ✓ 1 cup finely ground almonds
- ✓ 3 ½ cups cake flour
- ✓ ½ cup almond butter
- ✓ 1 tbsp water or rose flower water

Directions:

- ❖ In a large bowl, combine the coconut oil, powdered sugar, and butter. If the butter is not soft, you want to wait until it softens up. Use an electric mixer to beat the ingredients together at high speed.
- ❖ In a small bowl, add the egg yolks, brandy, water, and vanilla extract. Whisk well.
- ❖ Fold the egg yolk mixture into the large bowl.
- ❖ Add the flour and almonds. Fold and mix with a wooden spoon.
- ❖ Place the mixture into the fridge for at least 1 hour and 30 minutes.
- ❖ Preheat your oven to 325 degrees Fahrenheit.
- ❖ Take the mixture, which now looks like dough, and divide it into 1-inch balls.
- ❖ With a piece of parchment paper on a baking sheet, arrange the cookies and flatten them with a fork or your fingers.
- ❖ Place the cookies in the oven for 13 minutes, but watch them so they don't burn.
- ❖ Transfer the cookies onto a rack to cool for a couple of minutes before enjoying!

Nutrition: calories: 250, fats: 14 grams, carbohydrates: 30 grams, protein: 3 grams

144) CLASSIC CHOCOLATE FRUIT KEBABS

Cooking Time: 30 Minutes   **Servings:** 6

Ingredients:

- ✓ 24 blueberries
- ✓ 12 strawberries with the green leafy top part removed
- ✓ 12 green or red grapes, seedless
- ✓ 12 pitted cherries
- ✓ 8 ounces chocolate

Directions:

- ❖ Line a baking sheet with a piece of parchment paper and place 6, -inch long wooden skewers on top of the paper.
- ❖ Start by threading a piece of fruit onto the skewers. You can create and follow any pattern that you like with the ingredients. An example pattern is 1 strawberry, 1 cherry, blueberries, 2 grapes. Repeat the pattern until all of the fruit is on the skewers.
- ❖ In a saucepan on medium heat, melt the chocolate. Stir continuously until the chocolate has melted completely.
- ❖ Carefully scoop the chocolate into a plastic sandwich bag and twist the bag closed starting right above the chocolate.
- ❖ Snip the corner of the bag with scissors.
- ❖ Drizzle the chocolate onto the kebabs by squeezing it out of the bag.
- ❖ Put the baking pan into the freezer for 20 minutes.
- ❖ Serve and enjoy!

Nutrition: calories: 254, fats: 15 grams, carbohydrates: 28 grams, protein: 4 grams.

145) PEACHES AND BLUE CHEESE CREAM

Cooking Time: 20 Hours 10 Minutes   **Servings:** 4

Ingredients:

- ✓ 4 peaches
- ✓ 1 cinnamon stick
- ✓ 4 ounces sliced blue cheese
- ✓ ⅓ cup orange juice, freshly squeezed is best
- ✓ 3 whole cloves
- ✓ 1 tsp of orange zest, taken from the orange peel
- ✓ ¼ tsp cardamom pods
- ✓ ⅔ cup red wine
- ✓ 2 tbsp honey, raw or your preferred variety
- ✓ 1 vanilla bean
- ✓ 1 tsp allspice berries
- ✓ 4 tbsp dried cherries

Directions:

- ❖ Set a saucepan on top of your stove range and add the cinnamon stick, cloves, orange juice, cardamom, vanilla, allspice, red wine, and orange zest. Whisk the ingredients well. Add your peaches to the mixture and poach them for hours or until they become soft.
- ❖ Take a spoon to remove the peaches and boil the rest of the liquid to make the syrup. You want the liquid to reduce itself by at least half.
- ❖ While the liquid is boiling, combine the dried cherries, blue cheese, and honey into a bowl. Once your peaches are cooled, slice them into halves.
- ❖ Top each peach with the blue cheese mixture and then drizzle the liquid onto the top. Serve and enjoy!

Nutrition: calories: 211, fats: 24 grams, carbohydrates: 15 grams, protein: 6 grams

146)   MEDITERRANEAN-STYLE BLACKBERRY ICE CREAM

Cooking Time: 15 Minutes   **Servings: 6**

Ingredients:

- 3 egg yolks
- 1 container of Greek yogurt
- 1 pound mashed blackberries
- ½ tsp vanilla essence
- 1 tsp arrowroot powder
- ¼ tsp ground cloves
- 5 ounces sugar or sweetener substitute
- 1 pound heavy cream

Directions:

- In a small bowl, add the arrowroot powder and egg yolks. Whisk or beat them with an electronic mixture until they are well combined.
- Set a saucepan on top of your stove and turn your heat to medium.
- Add the heavy cream and bring it to a boil.
- Turn off the heat and add the egg mixture into the cream through folding.
- Turn the heat back on to medium and pour in the sugar. Cook the mixture for 10 minutes or until it starts to thicken.
- Remove the mixture from heat and place it in the fridge so it can completely cool. This should take about one hour.
- Once the mixture is cooled, add in the Greek yogurt, ground cloves, blackberries, and vanilla by folding in the ingredients.
- Transfer the ice cream into a container and place it in the freezer for at least two hours.
- Serve and enjoy!

Nutrition: calories: 402, fats: 20 grams, carbohydrates: 52 grams, protein: 8 grams

147)   CLASSIC STUFFED FIGS

Cooking Time: 20 Minutes   **Servings: 6**

Ingredients:

- 10 halved fresh figs
- 20 chopped almonds
- 4 ounces goat cheese, divided
- 2 tbsp of raw honey

Directions:

- Turn your oven to broiler mode and set it to a high temperature.
- Place your figs, cut side up, on a baking sheet. If you like to place a piece of parchment paper on top you can do this, but it is not necessary.
- Sprinkle each fig with half of the goat cheese.
- Add a tbsp of chopped almonds to each fig.
- Broil the figs for 3 to 4 minutes.
- Take them out of the oven and let them cool for 5 to 7 minutes.
- Sprinkle with the remaining goat cheese and honey.

Nutrition: calories: 209, fats: 9 grams, carbohydrates: 26 grams, protein: grams.

148) CHIA PUDDING AND STRAWBERRIES

Cooking Time: 4 Hours 5 Minutes   **Servings:** 4

Ingredients:

- ✓ 2 cups unsweetened almond milk
- ✓ 1 tbsp vanilla extract
- ✓ 2 tbsp raw honey
- ✓ ¼ cup chia seeds
- ✓ 2 cups fresh and sliced strawberries

Directions:

- ❖ In a medium bowl, combine the honey, chia seeds, vanilla, and unsweetened almond milk. Mix well.
- ❖ Set the mixture in the refrigerator for at least 4 hours.
- ❖ When you serve the pudding, top it with strawberries. You can even create a design in a glass serving bowl or dessert dish by adding a little pudding on the bottom, a few strawberries, top the strawberries with some more pudding, and then top the dish with a few strawberries.

Nutrition: calories: 108, fats: grams, carbohydrates: 17 grams, protein: 3 grams

149) SPECIAL CHUNKY MONKEY TRAIL MIX

Cooking Time: 1 Hour 30 Minutes   **Servings:** 6

Ingredients:

- ✓ 1 cup cashews, halved
- ✓ 2 cups raw walnuts, chopped or halved
- ✓ ⅓ cup coconut sugar
- ✓ ½ cup of chocolate chips
- ✓ 1 tsp vanilla extract
- ✓ 1 cup coconut flakes, unsweetened and make sure you have big flakes and not shredded
- ✓ 6 ounces dried banana slices
- ✓ 1 ½ tsp coconut oil at room temperature

Directions:

- ❖ Turn your crockpot to high and add the cashews, walnuts, vanilla, coconut oil, and sugar. Combine until the ingredients are well mixed and then cook for 45 minutes.
- ❖ Reduce the temperature on your crockpot to low.
- ❖ Continue to cook the mixture for another 20 minutes.
- ❖ Place a piece of parchment paper on your counter.
- ❖ Once the mix is done cooking, remove it from the crockpot and set on top of the parchment paper.
- ❖ Let the mixture sit and cool for 20 minutes.
- ❖ Pour the contents into a bowl and add the dried bananas and chocolate chips. Gently mix the ingredients together. You can store the mixture in Ziplock bags for a quick and easy snack.

Nutrition: calories: 250, fats: 6 grams, carbohydrates: 1grams, protein: 4 grams

150) DELICIOUS FIG-PECAN ENERGY BITES

Cooking Time: 20 Minutes   **Servings:** 6

Ingredients:

- ✓ ½ cup chopped pecans
- ✓ 2 tbsp honey
- ✓ ¾ cup dried figs, about 6 to 8, diced
- ✓ 2 tbsp wheat flaxseed
- ✓ ¼ cup quick oats
- ✓ 2 tbsp regular or powdered peanut butter

Directions:

- ❖ Combine the figs, quick oats, pecans, peanut butter, and flaxseed into a bowl. Stir the ingredients well.
- ❖ Drizzle honey onto the ingredients and mix everything with a wooden spoon. Do your best to press all the ingredients into the honey as you are stirring. If you start to struggle because the mixture is too sticky, set it in the freezer for 3 to 5 minutes.
- ❖ Divide the mixture into four sections.
- ❖ Take a wet rag and get your hands damp. You don't want them too wet or they won't work well with the mixture.
- ❖ Divide each of the four sections into 3 separate sections.
- ❖ Take one of the three sections and roll them up. Repeat with each section so you have a dozen energy bites once you are done.
- ❖ If you want to firm them up, you can place them into the freezer for a few minutes. Otherwise, you can enjoy them as soon as they are little energy balls.
- ❖ To store them, you'll want to keep them in a sealed container and set them in the fridge. They can be stored for about a week.

Nutrition: calories: 157, fats: 6 grams, carbohydrates: 26 grams, protein: 3 grams

151) MEDITERRANEAN STYLE BAKED APPLES

Cooking Time: 25 Minutes   **Servings:** 4

Ingredients:

- ✓ ½ lemon, squeezed for juice
- ✓ 1 ½ pounds of peeled and sliced apples
- ✓ ¼ tsp cinnamon

Directions:

- ❖ Set the temperature of your oven to 350 degrees Fahrenheit so it can preheat.
- ❖ Take a piece of parchment paper and lay on top of a baking pan.
- ❖ Combine your lemon juice, cinnamon, and apples into a medium bowl and mix well.
- ❖ Pour the apples onto the baking pan and arrange them so they are not doubled up.
- ❖ Place the pan in the oven and set your timer to 2minutes. The apples should be tender but not mushy.
- ❖ Remove from the oven, plate and enjoy!

Nutrition: calories: 90, fats: 0.3 grams, carbohydrates: 24 grams, protein: 0.5 grams

Meat Recipes

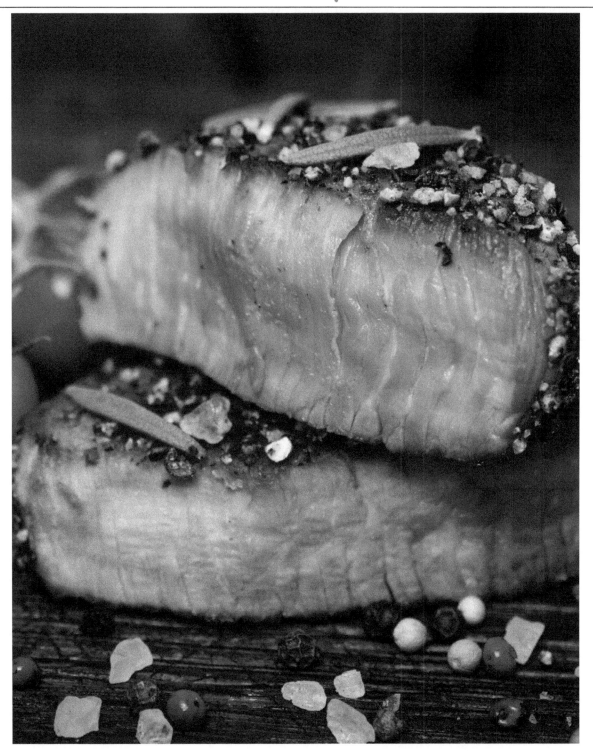

152) TURKEY CHORIZO AND BOK CHOY

Cooking Time: 50 Minutes   **Servings:** 4

Ingredients:

- ✓ 4 mild turkey Chorizo, sliced
- ✓ 1/2 cup full-fat milk
- ✓ 6 ounces Gruyère cheese, preferably freshly grated
- ✓ 1 yellow onion, chopped
- ✓ Coarse salt and ground black pepper, to taste
- ✓ 1 pound Bok choy, tough stem ends trimmed
- ✓ 1 cup cream of mushroom soup
- ✓ 1 tbsp lard, room temperature

Directions:

- ❖ Melt the lard in a nonstick skillet over a moderate flame; cook the Chorizo sausage for about 5 minutes, stirring occasionally to ensure even cooking; reserve.
- ❖ Add in the onion, salt, pepper, Bok choy, and cream of mushroom soup. Continue to cook for 4 minutes longer or until the vegetables have softened.
- ❖ Spoon the mixture into a lightly oiled casserole dish. Top with the reserved Chorizo.
- ❖ In a mixing bowl, thoroughly combine the milk and cheese. Pour the cheese mixture over the sausage.
- ❖ Cover with foil and bake at 36degrees F for about 35 minutes.
- ❖ Storing
- ❖ Cut your casserole into four portions. Place each portion in an airtight container; keep in your refrigerator for 3 to 4 days.
- ❖ For freezing, wrap your portions tightly with heavy-duty aluminum foil or freezer wrap. Freeze up to 1 to 2 months. Defrost in the refrigerator. Enjoy!

Nutrition: 18Calories; 12g Fat; 2.6g Carbs; 9.4g Protein; 1g Fiber

153) CLASSIC SPICY CHICKEN BREASTS

Cooking Time: 30 Minutes   **Servings:** 6

Ingredients:

- ✓ 1 ½ pounds chicken breasts
- ✓ 1 bell pepper, deveined and chopped
- ✓ 1 leek, chopped
- ✓ 1 tomato, pureed
- ✓ 2 tbsp coriander
- ✓ 2 garlic cloves, minced
- ✓ 1 tsp cayenne pepper
- ✓ 1 tsp dry thyme
- ✓ 1/4 cup coconut aminos
- ✓ Sea salt and ground black pepper, to taste

Directions:

- ❖ Rub each chicken breasts with the garlic, cayenne pepper, thyme, salt and black pepper. Cook the chicken in a saucepan over medium-high heat.
- ❖ Sear for about 5 minutes until golden brown on all sides.
- ❖ Fold in the tomato puree and coconut aminos and bring it to a boil. Add in the pepper, leek, and coriander.
- ❖ Reduce the heat to simmer. Continue to cook, partially covered, for about 20 minutes.
- ❖ Storing
- ❖ Place the chicken breasts in airtight containers or Ziploc bags; keep in your refrigerator for 3 to 4 days.
- ❖ For freezing, place the chicken breasts in airtight containers or heavy-duty freezer bags. It will maintain the best quality for about 4 months. Defrost in the refrigerator. Bon appétit!

Nutrition: 239 Calories; 6g Fat; 5.5g Carbs; 34.3g Protein; 1g Fiber

154) DELICIOUS SAUCY BOSTON BUTT

Cooking Time: 1 Hour 20 Minutes   **Servings:** 8

Ingredients:

- ✓ 1 tbsp lard, room temperature
- ✓ 2 pounds Boston butt, cubed
- ✓ Salt and freshly ground pepper
- ✓ 1/2 tsp mustard powder
- ✓ A bunch of spring onions, chopped
- ✓ 2 garlic cloves, minced
- ✓ 1/2 tbsp ground cardamom
- ✓ 2 tomatoes, pureed
- ✓ 1 bell pepper, deveined and chopped
- ✓ 1 jalapeno pepper, deveined and finely chopped
- ✓ 1/2 cup unsweetened coconut milk
- ✓ 2 cups chicken bone broth

Directions:

- ❖ In a wok, melt the lard over moderate heat. Season the pork belly with salt, pepper and mustard powder.
- ❖ Sear the pork for 8 to 10 minutes, stirring periodically to ensure even cooking; set aside, keeping it warm.
- ❖ In the same wok, sauté the spring onions, garlic, and cardamom. Spoon the sautéed vegetables along with the reserved pork into the slow cooker.
- ❖ Add in the remaining ingredients, cover with the lid and cook for 1 hour 10 minutes over low heat.
- ❖ Storing
- ❖ Divide the pork and vegetables between airtight containers or Ziploc bags; keep in your refrigerator for up to 3 to 5 days.
- ❖ For freezing, place the pork and vegetables in airtight containers or heavy-duty freezer bags. Freeze up to 4 months. Defrost in the refrigerator. Bon appétit!

Nutrition: 369 Calories; 20.2g Fat; 2.9g Carbs; 41.3g Protein; 0.7g Fiber

155) OLD-FASHIONED HUNGARIAN GOULASH

Cooking Time: 9 Hours 10 Minutes   **Servings:** 4

Ingredients:

- ✓ 1 ½ pounds pork butt, chopped
- ✓ 1 tsp sweet Hungarian paprika
- ✓ 2 Hungarian hot peppers, deveined and minced
- ✓ 1 cup leeks, chopped
- ✓ 1 ½ tbsp lard
- ✓ 1 tsp caraway seeds, ground
- ✓ 4 cups vegetable broth
- ✓ 2 garlic cloves, crushed
- ✓ 1 tsp cayenne pepper
- ✓ 2 cups tomato sauce with herbs
- ✓ 1 ½ pounds pork butt, chopped
- ✓ 1 tsp sweet Hungarian paprika
- ✓ 2 Hungarian hot peppers, deveined and minced
- ✓ 1 cup leeks, chopped
- ✓ 1 ½ tbsp lard
- ✓ 1 tsp caraway seeds, ground
- ✓ 4 cups vegetable broth
- ✓ 2 garlic cloves, crushed
- ✓ 1 tsp cayenne pepper
- ✓ 2 cups tomato sauce with herbs

Directions:

- ❖ Melt the lard in a heavy-bottomed pot over medium-high heat. Sear the pork for 5 to 6 minutes until just browned on all sides; set aside.
- ❖ Add in the leeks and garlic; continue to cook until they have softened.
- ❖ Place the reserved pork along with the sautéed mixture in your crock pot. Add in the other ingredients and stir to combine.
- ❖ Cover with the lid and slow cook for 9 hours on the lowest setting.
- ❖ Storing
- ❖ Spoon your goulash into four airtight containers or Ziploc bags; keep in your refrigerator for up to 3 to 4 days.
- ❖ For freezing, place the goulash in airtight containers. Freeze up to 4 to 6 months. Defrost in the refrigerator. Enjoy!

Nutrition: 456 Calories; 27g Fat; 6.7g Carbs; 32g Protein; 3.4g Fiber

156)   FLATBREAD AND CHICKEN LIVER PÂTÉ

Cooking Time: 2 Hours 15 Minutes   **Servings:** 4

Ingredients:

- ✓ 1 yellow onion, finely chopped
- ✓ 10 ounces chicken livers
- ✓ 1/2 tsp Mediterranean seasoning blend
- ✓ 4 tbsp olive oil
- ✓ 1 garlic clove, minced

- ✓ For Flatbread:
- ✓ 1 cup lukewarm water
- ✓ 1/2 stick butter
- ✓ 1/2 cup flax meal
- ✓ 1 ½ tbsp psyllium husks
- ✓ 1 ¼ cups almond flour

Directions:

- ❖ Pulse the chicken livers along with the seasoning blend, olive oil, onion and garlic in your food processor; reserve.
- ❖ Mix the dry ingredients for the flatbread. Mix in all the wet ingredients. Whisk to combine well.
- ❖ Let it stand at room temperature for 2 hours. Divide the dough into 8 balls and roll them out on a flat surface.
- ❖ In a lightly greased pan, cook your flatbread for 1 minute on each side or until golden.
- ❖ Storing
- ❖ Wrap the chicken liver pate in foil before packing it into airtight containers; keep in your refrigerator for up to 7 days.
- ❖ For freezing, place the chicken liver pate in airtight containers or heavy-duty freezer bags. Freeze up to 2 months. Defrost overnight in the refrigerator.
- ❖ As for the keto flatbread, wrap them in foil before packing them into airtight containers; keep in your refrigerator for up to 4 days.
- ❖ Bon appétit!

Nutrition: 395 Calories; 30.2g Fat; 3.6g Carbs; 17.9g Protein; 0.5g Fiber

157)   SATURDAY CHICKEN WITH CAULIFLOWER SALAD

Cooking Time: 20 Minutes   **Servings:** 2

Ingredients:

- ✓ 1 tsp hot paprika
- ✓ 2 tbsp fresh basil, snipped
- ✓ 1/2 cup mayonnaise
- ✓ 1 tsp mustard
- ✓ 2 tsp butter
- ✓ 2 chicken wings

- ✓ 1/2 cup cheddar cheese, shredded
- ✓ Sea salt and ground black pepper, to taste
- ✓ 2 tbsp dry sherry
- ✓ 1 shallot, finely minced
- ✓ 1/2 head of cauliflower

Directions:

- ❖ Boil the cauliflower in a pot of salted water until it has softened; cut into small florets and place in a salad bowl.
- ❖ Melt the butter in a saucepan over medium-high heat. Cook the chicken for about 8 minutes or until the skin is crisp and browned. Season with hot paprika salt, and black pepper.
- ❖ Whisk the mayonnaise, mustard, dry sherry, and shallot and dress your salad. Top with cheddar cheese and fresh basil.
- ❖ Storing
- ❖ Place the chicken wings in airtight containers or Ziploc bags; keep in your refrigerator for up 3 to 4 days.
- ❖ Keep the cauliflower salad in your refrigerator for up 3 days.
- ❖ For freezing, place the chicken wings in airtight containers or heavy-duty freezer bags. Freeze up to 3 months. Once thawed in the refrigerator, reheat in a saucepan until thoroughly warmed.

Nutrition: 444 Calories; 36g Fat; 5.7g Carbs; 20.6g Protein; 4.3g Fiber

158) SPECIAL KANSAS-STYLE MEATLOAF

Cooking Time: 1 Hour 10 Minutes   **Servings:** 8

Ingredients:

- ✓ 2 pounds ground pork
- ✓ 2 eggs, beaten
- ✓ 1/2 cup onions, chopped
- ✓ 1/2 cup marinara sauce, bottled
- ✓ 8 ounces Colby cheese, shredded
- ✓ 1 tsp granulated garlic
- ✓ Sea salt and freshly ground black pepper, to taste
- ✓ 1 tsp lime zest
- ✓ 1 tsp mustard seeds
- ✓ 1/2 cup tomato puree
- ✓ 1 tbsp Erythritol

Directions:

- ❖ Mix the ground pork with the eggs, onions, marinara salsa, cheese, granulated garlic, salt, pepper, lime zest, and mustard seeds; mix to combine.
- ❖ Press the mixture into a lightly-greased loaf pan. Mix the tomato paste with the Erythritol and spread the mixture over the top of your meatloaf.
- ❖ Bake in the preheated oven at 5 degrees F for about 1 hour 10 minutes, rotating the pan halfway through the cook time. Storing Wrap your meatloaf tightly with heavy-duty aluminum foil or plastic wrap. Then, keep in your refrigerator for up to 3 to 4 days.
- ❖ For freezing, wrap your meatloaf tightly to prevent freezer burn. Freeze up to 3 to 4 months. Defrost in the refrigerator. Bon appétit!

Nutrition: 318 Calories; 14. Fat; 6.2g Carbs; 39.3g Protein; 0.3g Fiber

159) ORIGINAL TURKEY KEBABS

Cooking Time: 30 Minutes   **Servings:** 6

Ingredients:

- ✓ 1 ½ pounds turkey breast, cubed
- ✓ 3 Spanish peppers, sliced
- ✓ 2 zucchinis, cut into thick slices
- ✓ 1 onion, cut into wedges
- ✓ 2 tbsp olive oil, room temperature
- ✓ 1 tbsp dry ranch seasoning

Directions:

- ❖ Thread the turkey pieces and vegetables onto bamboo skewers. Sprinkle the skewers with dry ranch seasoning and olive oil.
- ❖ Grill your kebabs for about 10 minutes, turning them periodically to ensure even cooking.
- ❖ Storing
- ❖ Wrap your kebabs in foil before packing them into airtight containers; keep in your refrigerator for up to 3 to days.
- ❖ For freezing, place your kebabs in airtight containers or heavy-duty freezer bags. Freeze up to 2-3 months. Defrost in the refrigerator. Bon appétit!

Nutrition: 2 Calories; 13.8g Fat; 6.7g Carbs; 25.8g Protein; 1.2g Fiber

160) ORIGINAL MEXICAN-STYLE TURKEY BACON BITES

Cooking Time: 5 Minutes   **Servings:** 4

Ingredients:

- ✓ 4 ounces turkey bacon, chopped
- ✓ 4 ounces Neufchatel cheese
- ✓ 1 tbsp butter, cold
- ✓ 1 jalapeno pepper, deveined and minced
- ✓ 1 tsp Mexican oregano
- ✓ 2 tbsp scallions, finely chopped

Directions:

- ❖ Thoroughly combine all ingredients in a mixing bowl.
- ❖ Roll the mixture into 8 balls.
- ❖ Storing
- ❖ Divide the turkey bacon bites between two airtight containers or Ziploc bags; keep in your refrigerator for up 3 to days.

Nutrition: 19Calories; 16.7g Fat; 2.2g Carbs; 8.8g Protein; 0.3g Fiber

161) ORIGINAL MUFFINS WITH GROUND PORK

Cooking Time: 25 Minutes **Servings: 6**

Ingredients:

- ✓ 1 stick butter
- ✓ 3 large eggs, lightly beaten
- ✓ 2 tbsp full-fat milk
- ✓ 1/2 tsp ground cardamom
- ✓ 3 ½ cups almond flour
- ✓ 2 tbsp flaxseed meal
- ✓ 1 tsp baking powder
- ✓ 2 cups ground pork
- ✓ Salt and pepper, to your liking
- ✓ 1/2 tsp dried basil

Directions:

- ❖ In the preheated frying pan, cook the ground pork until the juices run clear, approximately 5 minutes.
- ❖ Add in the remaining ingredients and stir until well combined.
- ❖ Spoon the mixture into lightly greased muffin cups. Bake in the preheated oven at 5 degrees F for about 17 minutes.
- ❖ Allow your muffins to cool down before unmolding and storing.
- ❖ Storing
- ❖ Place your muffins in the airtight containers or Ziploc bags; keep in the refrigerator for a week.
- ❖ For freezing, divide your muffins among Ziploc bags and freeze up to 3 months. Defrost in your microwave for a couple of minutes. Bon appétit!

Nutrition: 330 Calories; 30.3g Fat; 2.3g Carbs; 19g Protein; 1.2g Fiber

162) TYPICAL MEDITERRANEAN-STYLE CHEESY PORK LOIN

Cooking Time: 25 Minutes **Servings: 4**

Ingredients:

- ✓ 1 pound pork loin, cut into 1-inch-thick pieces
- ✓ 1 tsp Mediterranean seasoning mix
- ✓ Salt and pepper, to taste
- ✓ 1 onion, sliced
- ✓ 1 tsp fresh garlic, smashed
- ✓ 2 tbsp black olives, pitted and sliced
- ✓ 2 tbsp balsamic vinegar
- ✓ 1/2 cup Romano cheese, grated
- ✓ 2 tbsp butter, room temperature
- ✓ 1 tbsp curry paste
- ✓ 1 cup roasted vegetable broth
- ✓ 1 tbsp oyster sauce

Directions:

- ❖ In a frying pan, melt the butter over a moderately high heat. Once hot, cook the pork until browned on all sides; season with salt and black pepper and set aside.
- ❖ In the pan drippings, cook the onion and garlic for 4 to 5 minutes or until they've softened.
- ❖ Add in the Mediterranean seasoning mix, curry paste, and vegetable broth. Continue to cook until the sauce has thickened and reduced slightly or about 10 minutes. Add in the remaining ingredients along with the reserved pork.
- ❖ Top with cheese and cook for 10 minutes longer or until cooked through.
- ❖ Storing
- ❖ Divide the pork loin between four airtight containers; keep in your refrigerator for 3 to 5 days.
- ❖ For freezing, place the pork loin in airtight containers or heavy-duty freezer bags. Freeze up to 4 to 6 months. Defrost in the refrigerator. Enjoy!

Nutrition: 476 Calories; 35.3g Fat; 6.2g Carbs; 31.1g Protein; 1.4g Fiber

Sides & Appetizers Recipes

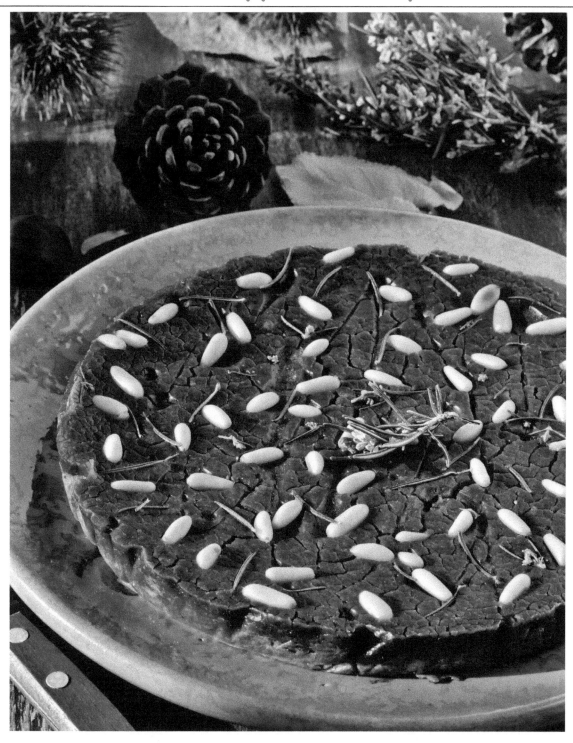

163) ARTICHOKE OLIVE PASTA

Cooking Time: 25 Minutes   **Servings: 4**

Ingredients:

- ✓ salt
- ✓ pepper
- ✓ 2 tbsp olive oil, divided
- ✓ 2 garlic cloves, thinly sliced
- ✓ 1 can artichoke hearts, drained, rinsed, and quartered lengthwise
- ✓ 1-pint grape tomatoes, halved lengthwise, divided
- ✓ ½ cup fresh basil leaves, torn apart
- ✓ 12 ounces whole-wheat spaghetti
- ✓ ½ medium onion, thinly sliced
- ✓ ½ cup dry white wine
- ✓ 1/3 cup pitted Kalamata olives, quartered lengthwise
- ✓ ¼ cup grated Parmesan cheese, plus extra for serving

Directions:

- ❖ Fill a large pot with salted water.
- ❖ Pour the water to a boil and cook your pasta according to package instructions until al dente.
- ❖ Drain the pasta and reserve 1 cup of the cooking water.
- ❖ Return the pasta to the pot and set aside.
- ❖ Heat 1 tbsp of olive oil in a large skillet over medium-high heat.
- ❖ Add onion and garlic, season with pepper and salt, and cook well for about 3-4 minutes until nicely browned.
- ❖ Add wine and cook for 2 minutes until evaporated.
- ❖ Stir in artichokes and keep cooking 2-3 minutes until brown.
- ❖ Add olives and half of your tomatoes.
- ❖ Cook well for 1-2 minutes until the tomatoes start to break down.
- ❖ Add pasta to the skillet.
- ❖ Stir in the rest of the tomatoes, cheese, basil, and remaining oil.
- ❖ Thin the mixture with the reserved pasta water if needed.
- ❖ Place in containers and sprinkle with extra cheese.
- ❖ Enjoy!

Nutrition: 340, Total Fat: 11.9 g, Saturated Fat: 3.3 g, Cholesterol: 10 mg, Sodium: 278 mg, Total Carbohydrate: 35.8 g, Dietary Fiber: 7.8 g, Total Sugars: 4.8 g, Protein: 11.6 g, Vitamin D: 0 mcg, Calcium: 193 mg, Iron: 3 mg, Potassium: 524 mg

164) MEDITERRANEAN OLIVE TUNA PASTA

Cooking Time: 20 Minutes   **Servings:** 4

Ingredients:

- ✓ 8 ounces of tuna steak, cut into 3 pieces
- ✓ ¼ cup green olives, chopped
- ✓ 3 cloves garlic, minced
- ✓ 2 cups grape tomatoes, halved
- ✓ ½ cup white wine
- ✓ 2 tbsp lemon juice
- ✓ 6 ounces pasta - whole wheat gobetti, rotini, or penne
- ✓ 1 10-ounce package frozen artichoke hearts, thawed and squeezed dry
- ✓ 4 tbsp extra-virgin olive oil, divided
- ✓ 2 tsp fresh grated lemon zest
- ✓ 2 tsp fresh rosemary, chopped, divided
- ✓ ½ tsp salt, divided
- ✓ ¼ tsp fresh ground pepper
- ✓ ¼ cup fresh basil, chopped

Directions:

- ❖ Preheat grill to medium-high heat.
- ❖ Take a large pot of water and put it on to boil.
- ❖ Place the tuna pieces in a bowl and add 1 tbsp of oil, 1 tsp of rosemary, lemon zest, a ¼ tsp of salt, and pepper.
- ❖ Grill the tuna for about 3 minutes per side.
- ❖ Transfer tuna to a plate and allow it to cool.
- ❖ Place the pasta in boiling water and cook according to package instructions.
- ❖ Drain the pasta.
- ❖ Flake the tuna into bite-sized pieces.
- ❖ In a large skillet, heat remaining oil over medium heat.
- ❖ Add artichoke hearts, garlic, olives, and remaining rosemary.
- ❖ Cook for about 3-4 minutes until slightly browned.
- ❖ Add tomatoes, wine, and bring the mixture to a boil.
- ❖ Cook for about 3 minutes until the tomatoes are broken down.
- ❖ Stir in pasta, lemon juice, tuna, and remaining salt.
- ❖ Cook for 1-2 minutes until nicely heated.
- ❖ Spread over the containers.
- ❖ Before eating, garnish with some basil and enjoy!

Nutrition: 455, Total Fat: 21.2 g, Saturated Fat: 3.5 g, Cholesterol: 59 mg, Sodium: 685 mg, Total Carbohydrate: 38.4 g, Dietary Fiber: 6.1 g, Total Sugars: 3.5 g, Protein: 25.5 g, Vitamin D: 0 mcg, Calcium: 100 mg, Iron: 5 mg, Potassium: 800 mg

165) SPECIAL BRAISED ARTICHOKES

Cooking Time: 30 Minutes   **Servings:** 6

Ingredients:

- ✓ 6 tbsp olive oil
- ✓ 2 pounds baby artichokes, trimmed
- ✓ ½ cup lemon juice
- ✓ 4 garlic cloves, thinly sliced
- ✓ ½ tsp salt
- ✓ 1½ pounds tomatoes, seeded and diced
- ✓ ½ cup almonds, toasted and sliced

Directions:

- ❖ Heat oil in a skillet over medium heat.
- ❖ Add artichokes, garlic, and lemon juice, and allow the garlic to sizzle.
- ❖ Season with salt.
- ❖ Reduce heat to medium-low, cover, and simmer for about 15 minutes.
- ❖ Uncover, add tomatoes, and simmer for another 10 minutes until the tomato liquid has mostly evaporated.
- ❖ Season with more salt and pepper.
- ❖ Sprinkle with toasted almonds.
- ❖ Enjoy!

Nutrition: Calories: 265, Total Fat: 1g, Saturated Fat: 2.6 g, Cholesterol: 0 mg, Sodium: 265 mg, Total Carbohydrate: 23 g, Dietary Fiber: 8.1 g, Total Sugars: 12.4 g, Protein: 7 g, Vitamin D: 0 mcg, Calcium: 81 mg, Iron: 2 mg, Potassium: 1077 mg

166) DELICIOUS FRIED GREEN BEANS

Cooking Time: 15 Minutes   **Servings:** 2

Ingredients:

- ✓ ½ pound green beans, trimmed
- ✓ 1 egg
- ✓ 2 tbsp olive oil
- ✓ 1¼ tbsp almond flour
- ✓ 2 tbsp parmesan cheese
- ✓ ½ tsp garlic powder
- ✓ sea salt or plain salt
- ✓ freshly ground black pepper

Directions:

- ❖ Start by beating the egg and olive oil in a bowl.
- ❖ Then, mix the remaining Ingredients: in a separate bowl and set aside.
- ❖ Now, dip the green beans in the egg mixture and then coat with the dry mix.
- ❖ Finally, grease a baking pan, then transfer the beans to the pan and bake at 5 degrees F for about 12-15 minutes or until crisp.
- ❖ Serve warm.

Nutrition: Calories: 334, Total Fat: 23 g, Saturated Fat: 8.3 g, Cholesterol: 109 mg, Sodium: 397 mg, Total Carbohydrate: 10.9 g, Dietary Fiber: 4.3 g, Total Sugars: 1.9 g, Protein: 18.1 g, Vitamin D: 8 mcg, Calcium: 398 mg, Iron: 2 mg, Potassium: 274 mg

167) VEGGIE MEDITERRANEAN-STYLE PASTA

Cooking Time: 2 Hours   **Servings:** 4

Ingredients:

- ✓ 1 tbsp olive oil
- ✓ 1 small onion, finely chopped
- ✓ 2 small garlic cloves, finely chopped
- ✓ 2 14-ounce cans diced tomatoes
- ✓ 1 tbsp sun-dried tomato paste
- ✓ 1 bay leaf
- ✓ 1 tsp dried thyme
- ✓ 1 tsp dried basil
- ✓ 1 tsp oregano
- ✓ 1 tsp dried parsley
- ✓ bread of your choice
- ✓ ½ tsp salt
- ✓ ½ tsp brown sugar
- ✓ freshly ground black pepper
- ✓ 1 piece aubergine
- ✓ 2 pieces courgettes
- ✓ 2 pieces red peppers, de-seeded
- ✓ 2 garlic cloves, peeled
- ✓ 2-3 tbsp olive oil
- ✓ 12 small vine-ripened tomatoes
- ✓ 16 ounces of pasta of your preferred shape, such as Gigli, conchiglie, etc.
- ✓ 3½ ounces parmesan cheese

Directions:

- ❖ Heat oil in a pan over medium heat.
- ❖ Add onions and fry them until tender.
- ❖ Add garlic and stir-fry for 1 minute.
- ❖ Add the remaining Ingredients: listed under the sauce and bring to a boil.
- ❖ Reduce the heat, cover, and simmer for 60 minutes.
- ❖ Season with black pepper and salt as needed. Set aside.
- ❖ Preheat oven to 350 degrees F.
- ❖ Chop up courgettes, aubergine and red peppers into 1-inch pieces.
- ❖ Place them on a roasting pan along with whole garlic cloves.
- ❖ Drizzle with olive oil and season with salt and black pepper.
- ❖ Mix the veggies well and roast in the oven for 45 minutes until they are tender.
- ❖ Add tomatoes just before 20 minutes to end time.
- ❖ Cook your pasta according to package instructions.
- ❖ Drain well and stir into the sauce.
- ❖ Divide the pasta sauce between 4 containers and top with vegetables.
- ❖ Grate some parmesan cheese on top and serve with bread.
- ❖ Enjoy!

Nutrition: Calories: 211, Total Fat: 14.9 g, Saturated Fat: 2.1 g, Cholesterol: 0 mg, Sodium: 317 mg, Total Carbohydrate: 20.1 g, Dietary Fiber: 5.7 g, Total Sugars: 11.7 g, Protein: 4.2 g, Vitamin D: 0 mcg, Calcium: 66 mg, Iron: 2 mg, Potassium: 955 mg

168) CLASSIC BASIL PASTA

Cooking Time: 40 Minutes   **Servings:** 4

Ingredients:

- ✓ 2 red peppers, de-seeded and cut into chunks
- ✓ 2 red onions cut into wedges
- ✓ 2 mild red chilies, de-seeded and diced
- ✓ 3 garlic cloves, coarsely chopped
- ✓ 1 tsp golden caster sugar
- ✓ 2 tbsp olive oil, plus extra for serving
- ✓ 2 pounds small ripe tomatoes, quartered
- ✓ 12 ounces pasta
- ✓ a handful of basil leaves, torn
- ✓ 2 tbsp grated parmesan
- ✓ salt
- ✓ pepper

Directions:

- ❖ Preheat oven to 390 degrees F.
- ❖ On a large roasting pan, spread peppers, red onion, garlic, and chilies.
- ❖ Sprinkle sugar on top.
- ❖ Drizzle olive oil and season with salt and pepper.
- ❖ Roast the veggies for 1minutes.
- ❖ Add tomatoes and roast for another 15 minutes.
- ❖ In a large pot, cook your pasta in salted boiling water according to instructions.
- ❖ Once ready, drain pasta.
- ❖ Remove the veggies from the oven and carefully add pasta.
- ❖ Toss everything well and let it cool.
- ❖ Spread over the containers.
- ❖ Before eating, place torn basil leaves on top, and sprinkle with parmesan.
- ❖ Enjoy!

Nutrition: Calories: 384, Total Fat: 10.8 g, Saturated Fat: 2.3 g, Cholesterol: 67 mg, Sodium: 133 mg, Total Carbohydrate: 59.4 g, Dietary Fiber: 2.3 g, Total Sugars: 5.7 g, Protein: 1 g, Vitamin D: 0 mcg, Calcium: 105 mg, Iron: 4 mg, Potassium: 422 mg

169) ORIGINAL RED ONION KALE PASTA

Cooking Time: 25 Minutes   **Servings:** 4

Ingredients:

- ✓ 2½ cups vegetable broth
- ✓ ¾ cup dry lentils
- ✓ ½ tsp of salt
- ✓ 1 bay leaf
- ✓ ¼ cup olive oil
- ✓ 1 large red onion, chopped
- ✓ 1 tsp fresh thyme, chopped
- ✓ ½ tsp fresh oregano, chopped
- ✓ 1 tsp salt, divided
- ✓ ½ tsp black pepper
- ✓ 8 ounces vegan sausage, sliced into ¼-inch slices
- ✓ 1 bunch kale, stems removed and coarsely chopped
- ✓ 1 pack rotini

Directions:

- ❖ Add vegetable broth, ½ tsp of salt, bay leaf, and lentils to a saucepan over high heat and bring to a boil.
- ❖ Reduce the heat to medium-low and allow to cook for about minutes until tender.
- ❖ Discard the bay leaf. Take another skillet and heat olive oil over medium-high heat.
- ❖ Stir in thyme, onions, oregano, ½ a tsp of salt, and pepper; cook for 1 minute.
- ❖ Add sausage and reduce heat to medium-low.
- ❖ Cook for 10 minutes until the onions are tender.
- ❖ Bring water to a boil in a large pot, and then add rotini pasta and kale.
- ❖ Cook for about 8 minutes until al dente.
- ❖ Remove a bit of the cooking water and put it to the side.
- ❖ Drain the pasta and kale and return to the pot.
- ❖ Stir in both the lentils mixture and the onions mixture.
- ❖ Add the reserved cooking liquid to add just a bit of moistness.
- ❖ Spread over containers.

Nutrition: Calories: 508, Total Fat: 17 g, Saturated Fat: 3 g, Cholesterol: 0 mg, Sodium: 2431 mg, Total Carbohydrate: 59.3 g, Dietary Fiber: 6 g, Total Sugars: 4.8 g, Protein: 30.9 g, Vitamin D: 0 mcg, Calcium: 256 mg, Iron: 8 mg, Potassium: 1686 mg

170) ITALIAN SCALLOPS PEA FETTUCCINE

Cooking Time: 15 Minutes   **Servings:** 5

Ingredients:

- ✓ 8 ounces whole-wheat fettuccine (pasta, macaroni)
- ✓ 1 pound large sea scallops
- ✓ ¼ tsp salt, divided
- ✓ 1 tbsp extra virgin olive oil
- ✓ 1 8-ounce bottle of clam juice
- ✓ 1 cup low-fat milk
- ✓ ¼ tsp ground white pepper
- ✓ 3 cups frozen peas, thawed
- ✓ ¾ cup finely shredded Romano cheese, divided
- ✓ 1/3 cup fresh chives, chopped
- ✓ ½ tsp freshly grated lemon zest
- ✓ 1 tsp lemon juice

Directions:

- ❖ Boil water in a large pot and cook fettuccine according to package instructions.
- ❖ Drain well and put it to the side.
- ❖ Heat oil in a large, non-stick skillet over medium-high heat.
- ❖ Pat the scallops dry and sprinkle them with 1/8 tsp of salt.
- ❖ Add the scallops to the skillet and cook for about 2-3 minutes per side until golden brown. Remove scallops from pan.
- ❖ Add clam juice to the pan you removed the scallops from.
- ❖ In another bowl, whisk in milk, white pepper, flour, and remaining 1/8 tsp of salt.
- ❖ Once the mixture is smooth, whisk into the pan with the clam juice.
- ❖ Bring the entire mix to a simmer and keep stirring for about 1-2 minutes until the sauce is thick.
- ❖ Return the scallops to the pan and add peas. Bring it to a simmer.
- ❖ Stir in fettuccine, chives, ½ a cup of Romano cheese, lemon zest, and lemon juice.
- ❖ Mix well until thoroughly combined.
- ❖ Cool and spread over containers.
- ❖ Before eating, serve with remaining cheese sprinkled on top.
- ❖ Enjoy!

Nutrition: Calories: 388, Total Fat: 9.2 g, Saturated Fat: 3.7 g, Cholesterol: 33 mg, Sodium: 645 mg, Total Carbohydrate: 50.1 g, Dietary Fiber: 10.4 g, Total Sugars: 8.7 g, Protein: 24.9 g, Vitamin D: 25 mcg, Calcium: 293 mg, Iron: 4 mg, Potassium: 247 mg

171) TUSCAN BAKED MUSHROOMS

Cooking Time: 20 Minutes   **Servings:** 2

Ingredients:

- ✓ ½ pound mushrooms (sliced)
- ✓ 2 tbsp olive oil (onion and garlic flavored)
- ✓ 1 can tomatoes
- ✓ 1 cup Parmesan cheese
- ✓ ½ tsp oregano
- ✓ 1 tbsp basil
- ✓ sea salt or plain salt
- ✓ freshly ground black pepper

Directions:

- ❖ Heat the olive oil in the pan and add the mushrooms, salt, and pepper. Cook for about 2 minutes.
- ❖ Then, transfer the mushrooms into a baking dish.
- ❖ Now, in a separate bowl mix the tomatoes, basil, oregano, salt, and pepper, and layer it on the mushrooms. Top it with Parmesan cheese.
- ❖ Finally, bake the dish at 0 degrees F for about 18-22 minutes or until done.
- ❖ Serve warm.

Nutrition: Calories: 358, Total Fat: 27 g, Saturated Fat: 10.2 g, Cholesterol: 40 mg, Sodium: 535 mg, Total Carbohydrate: 13 g, Dietary Fiber: 3.5 g, Total Sugars: 6.7 g, Protein: 23.2 g, Vitamin D: 408 mcg, Calcium: 526 mg, Iron: 4 mg, Potassium: 797 mg

PART II-INTRODUCTION

The Mediterranean diet is the most popular and healthy regimen in the world. It is an eating pattern based on the traditional diets of the southern European regions surrounding the Mediterranean Sea. The health benefits will reduce the risk of heart disease, diabetes, some types of cancer, and weight problems. This diet is easy to follow since it is based on whole foods and contains no processed or refined foods. It also promotes a large amount of fiber. The diet focuses on eating lots of fruits, vegetables, whole grains, legumes, nuts, olive oil, and fish. These are all foods that are usually very healthy and delicious, and not too many people have trouble finding them. This book will focus on the main components plus some extra tips to help you if you are trying to eat for a healthier lifestyle or even live a healthier life in general. Many people say they know about the Mediterranean Diet but don't know what it is. If you're new to the Mediterranean Diet or want guidance on how to start eating better, you've come to the right place. Whether you're starting from scratch or already trying to eat healthier, there are several benefits to following this method.

Read these tips and tricks to get started with the Mediterranean Diet today. Many people who have tried the Mediterranean Diet Cookbook have told us that it has made their lives much more manageable. So, to help you get started, here's an overview of some of the features and benefits of the Mediterranean Diet. It doesn't take much to save a few calories and a few inches, which is the goal of the Mediterranean Diet. This comprehensive collection of recipes will show you how to prepare a delicious Mediterranean Diet treat. Remember that there is no particular rule for what you can and cannot eat on a Mediterranean Diet. It's all about moderation. Try our recipes and find out if they are right for you! Today many people, especially teenagers, fill their plates with pizza, white bread, refined sugar, and processed food with lots of preservatives.

But analysis and research on processed foods such as frozen food, white bread, and carbonated beverages have led to surprising facts. Habitual consumption of these foods can tax the body. Excessive consumption can lead to elevated insulin production. This can cause diabetes, obesity, and coronary artery malfunction.

The reality of animal fats is not much different. The saturated fats in these foods can harm our bodies. They cause the accumulation of extra fat in our body and disturb our body mass index. Saturated fat in animal products like milk and butter increases lousy cholesterol or LDL. In short, it can damage the health of the coronary arteries.

In this technologically advanced society, when we can perform our tasks with little effort, physical activities are negligible. Poor health conveniently comes into play. It becomes essential to switch to a healthier diet that meets our body's nutritional needs while keeping us full.

The Mediterranean diet can do this. It is an eating pattern that overflows with whole grains, a plant-based diet in which olive oil is a source of fat. This diet has no room for processed foods loaded with sugar or artificial sweeteners. The low amount of fat keeps your heart healthy and provides both essential nutrients and agility. Try it, and you won't look back. You'll leap into a healthy future.

I wish you all the best in healthy eating.

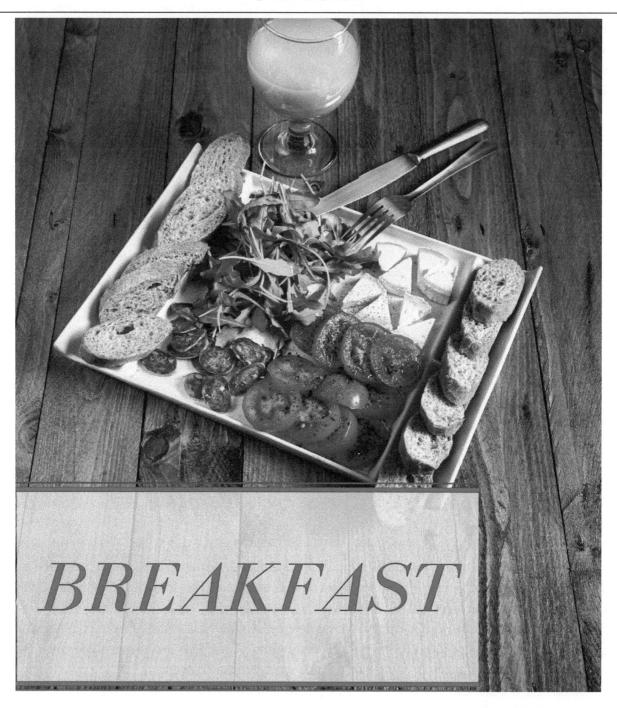

BREAKFAST

172) BREAKFAST WITH MEDITERRANEAN-STYLE BURRITO

Cooking Time: 5 Minutes   **Servings:** 6

Ingredients:

- ✓ 9 eggs whole
- ✓ 6 tortillas whole 10 inch, regular or sun-dried tomato
- ✓ 3 tbsp sun-dried tomatoes, chopped
- ✓ 1/2 cup feta cheese I use light/low-fat feta
- ✓ 2 cups baby spinach washed and dried
- ✓ 3 tbsp black olives, sliced
- ✓ 3/4 cup refried beans, canned
- ✓ Garnish:
- ✓ Salsa

Directions:

- ❖ Spray a medium frying pan with non- stick spray, add the eggs and scramble and toss for about 5 minutes, or until eggs are no longer liquid
- ❖ Add in the spinach, black olives, sun-dried tomatoes and continue to stir and toss until no longer wet
- ❖ Add in the feta cheese and cover, cook until cheese is melted
- ❖ Add 2 tbsp of refried beans to each tortilla
- ❖ Top with egg mixture, dividing evenly between all burritos, and wrap
- ❖ Frying in a pan until lightly browned
- ❖ Allow to cool completely before slicing
- ❖ Wrap the slices in plastic wrap and then aluminum foil and place in the freezer for up to 2 months or fridge for 2 days
- ❖ To Serve: Remove the aluminum foil and plastic wrap, and microwave for 2 minutes, then allow to rest for 30 seconds, enjoy! Enjoy hot with salsa and fruit

Nutrition: Calories:252;Total Carbohydrates: 21g;Total Fat: 11g;Protein: 14g |

173) SHAKSHUKA AND FETA

Cooking Time: 40 Minutes   **Servings:** 4-6

Ingredients:

- ✓ 6 large eggs
- ✓ 3 tbsp extra-virgin olive oil
- ✓ 1 large onion, halved and thinly sliced
- ✓ 1 large red bell pepper, seeded and thinly sliced
- ✓ 3 garlic cloves, thinly sliced
- ✓ 1 tsp ground cumin
- ✓ 1 tsp sweet paprika
- ✓ ⅛ tsp cayenne, or to taste
- ✓ 1 (28-ounce) can whole plum tomatoes with juices, coarsely chopped
- ✓ ¾ tsp salt, more as needed
- ✓ ¼ tsp black pepper, more as needed
- ✓ 5 oz feta cheese, crumbled, about 1 1/4 cups
- ✓ To Serve:
- ✓ Chopped cilantro
- ✓ Hot sauce

Directions:

- ❖ Preheat oven to 375 degrees F
- ❖ In a large skillet over medium-low heat, add the oil
- ❖ Once heated, add the onion and bell pepper, cook gently until very soft, about 20 minutes
- ❖ Add in the garlic and cook until tender, 1 to 2 minutes, then stir in cumin, paprika and cayenne, and cook 1 minute
- ❖ Pour in tomatoes, season with 3/4 tsp salt and 1/4 tsp pepper, simmer until tomatoes have thickened, about 10 minutes
- ❖ Then stir in crumbled feta
- ❖ Gently crack eggs into skillet over tomatoes, season with salt and pepper
- ❖ Transfer skillet to oven
- ❖ Bake until eggs have just set, 7 to 10 minutes
- ❖ Allow to cool and distribute among the containers, store in the fridge for 2-3 days
- ❖ To Serve: Reheat in the oven at 360 degrees F for 5 minutes or until heated through

Nutrition: Calories:337;Carbs: 17g;Total Fat: 25g;Protein

174)   SPINACH, FETA WITH EGG BREAKFAST QUESADILLAS

Cooking Time: 15 Minutes   **Servings: 5**

Ingredients:

- ✓ 8 eggs (optional)
- ✓ 2 tsp olive oil
- ✓ 1 red bell pepper
- ✓ 1/2 red onion
- ✓ 1/4 cup milk
- ✓ 4 handfuls of spinach leaves
- ✓ 1 1/2 cup mozzarella cheese
- ✓ 5 sun-dried tomato tortillas
- ✓ 1/2 cup feta
- ✓ 1/4 tsp salt
- ✓ 1/4 tsp pepper
- ✓ Spray oil

Directions:

- ❖ In a large non-stick pan over medium heat, add the olive oil
- ❖ Once heated, add the bell pepper and onion, cook for 4-5 minutes until soft
- ❖ In the meantime, whisk together the eggs, milk, salt and pepper in a bowl
- ❖ Add in the egg/milk mixture into the pan with peppers and onions, stirring frequently, until eggs are almost cooked through
- ❖ Add in the spinach and feta, fold into the eggs, stirring until spinach is wilted and eggs are cooked through
- ❖ Remove the eggs from heat and plate
- ❖ Spray a separate large non-stick pan with spray oil, and place over medium heat
- ❖ Add the tortilla, on one half of the tortilla, spread about ½ cup of the egg mixture
- ❖ Top the eggs with around ⅓ cup of shredded mozzarella cheese
- ❖ Fold the second half of the tortilla over, then cook for 2 minutes, or until golden brown
- ❖ Flip and cook for another minute until golden brown
- ❖ Allow the quesadilla to cool completely, divide among the container, store for 2 days or wrap in plastic wrap and foil, and freeze for up to 2 months
- ❖ To Serve: Reheat in oven at 375 for 3-5 minutes or until heated through

Nutrition: (1/2 quesadilla): Calories:213;Total Fat: 11g;Total Carbs: 15g;Protein: 15g

175) BREAKFAST COBBLER

Cooking Time: 12 Minutes   **Servings:** 4

Ingredients:

- ✓ 2 lbs apples, cut into chunks
- ✓ 1 1/2 cups water
- ✓ 1/4 tsp nutmeg
- ✓ 1 1/2 tsp cinnamon
- ✓ 1/2 cup dry buckwheat
- ✓ 1/2 cup dates, chopped
- ✓ Pinch of ground ginger

Directions:

- ❖ Spray instant pot from inside with cooking spray.
- ❖ Add all ingredients into the instant pot and stir well.
- ❖ Seal pot with a lid and select manual and set timer for 12 minutes.
- ❖ Once done, release pressure using quick release. Remove lid.
- ❖ Stir and serve.

Nutrition: Calories: 195;Fat: 0.9 g;Carbohydrates: 48.3 g;Sugar: (35.8)g;Protein: 3.3 g;Cholesterol: 0 mg

177) EGG-TOPPED QUINOA BOWL AND KALE

Cooking Time: 5 Minutes   **Servings:** 2

Ingredients:

- ✓ 1-ounce pancetta, chopped
- ✓ 1 bunch kale, sliced
- ✓ ½ cup cherry tomatoes, halved
- ✓ 1 tsp red wine vinegar
- ✓ 1 cup cooked quinoa
- ✓ 1 tsp olive oil
- ✓ 2 eggs
- ✓ 1/3 cup avocado, sliced
- ✓ sea salt or plain salt
- ✓ fresh black pepper

Directions:

- ❖ Start by heating pancetta in a skillet until golden brown. Add in kale and further cook for 2 minutes.
- ❖ Then, stir in tomatoes, vinegar, and salt and remove from heat.
- ❖ Now, divide this mixture into 2 bowls, add avocado to both, and then set aside.
- ❖ Finally, cook both the eggs and top each bowl with an egg.
- ❖ Serve hot with toppings of your choice.

Nutrition: Calories: 547, Total Fat: 22., Saturated Fat: 5.3, Cholesterol: 179 mg, Sodium: 412 mg, Total Carbohydrate: 62.5 g, Dietary Fiber: 8.6 g, Total Sugars: 1.7 g, Protein: 24.7 g, Vitamin D: 15 mcg, Calcium: 117 mg, Iron: 6 mg, Potassium: 1009 mg

178) COCONUT BANANA MIX

Cooking Time: 4 Minutes   **Servings:** 4

Ingredients:

- ✓ 1 cup coconut milk
- ✓ 1 banana
- ✓ 1 cup dried coconut
- ✓ 2 tbsp ground flax seed
- ✓ 3 tbsp chopped raisins
- ✓ ⅛ tsp nutmeg
- ✓ ⅛ tsp cinnamon
- ✓ Salt to taste

Directions:

- ❖ Set a large skillet on the stove and set it to low heat.
- ❖ Chop up the banana.
- ❖ Pour the coconut milk, nutmeg, and cinnamon into the skillet.
- ❖ Pour in the ground flaxseed while stirring continuously.
- ❖ Add the dried coconut and banana. Mix the ingredients until combined well.
- ❖ Allow the mixture to simmer for 2 to 3 minutes while stirring occasionally.
- ❖ Set four airtight containers on the counter.
- ❖ Remove the pan from heat and sprinkle enough salt for your taste buds.
- ❖ Divide the mixture into the containers and place them into the fridge overnight. They can remain in the fridge for up to 3 days.
- ❖ Before you set this tasty mixture in the microwave to heat up, you need to let it thaw on the counter for a bit.

Nutrition: calories: 279, fats: 22 grams, carbohydrates: 25 grams, protein: 6.4 grams

179) OLIVE OIL RASPBERRY-LEMON MUFFINS

Cooking Time: 20 Minutes   **Servings:** 12

Ingredients:

- ✓ Cooking spray to grease baking liners
- ✓ 1 cup all-purpose flour
- ✓ 1 cup whole-wheat flour
- ✓ ½ cup tightly packed light brown sugar
- ✓ ½ tsp baking soda
- ✓ ½ tsp aluminum-free baking powder
- ✓ ⅛ tsp kosher salt
- ✓ 1¼ cups buttermilk
- ✓ 1 large egg
- ✓ ¼ cup extra-virgin olive oil
- ✓ 1 tbsp freshly squeezed lemon juice
- ✓ Zest of 2 lemons
- ✓ 1¼ cups frozen raspberries (do not thaw)

Directions:

- ❖ Preheat the oven to 400°F and line a muffin tin with baking liners. Spray the liners lightly with cooking spray.
- ❖ In a large mixing bowl, whisk together the all-purpose flour, whole-wheat flour, brown sugar, baking soda, baking powder, and salt.
- ❖ In a medium bowl, whisk together the buttermilk, egg, oil, lemon juice, and lemon zest.
- ❖ Pour the wet ingredients into the dry ingredients and stir just until blended. Do not overmix.
- ❖ Fold in the frozen raspberries.
- ❖ Scoop about ¼ cup of batter into each muffin liner and bake for 20 minutes, or until the tops look browned and a paring knife comes out clean when inserted. Remove the muffins from the tin to cool.
- ❖ STORAGE: Store covered containers at room temperature for up to 4 days. To freeze muffins for up to 3 months, wrap them in foil and place in an airtight resealable bag.

Nutrition: Total calories: 166; Total fat: 5g; Saturated fat: 1g; Sodium: 134mg; Carbohydrates: 30g; Fiber: 3g; Protein: 4g

180) BREAKFAST MEDITERRANEAN-STYLE SALAD

Cooking Time: 10 Minutes   **Servings:** 2

Ingredients:

- ✓ 4 eggs (optional)
- ✓ 10 cups arugula
- ✓ 1/2 seedless cucumber, chopped
- ✓ 1 cup cooked quinoa, cooled
- ✓ 1 large avocado
- ✓ 1 cup natural almonds, chopped
- ✓ 1/2 cup mixed herbs like mint and dill, chopped
- ✓ 2 cups halved cherry tomatoes and/or heirloom tomatoes cut into wedges
- ✓ Extra virgin olive oil
- ✓ 1 lemon
- ✓ Sea salt, to taste
- ✓ Freshly ground black pepper, to taste

Directions:

- ❖ Cook the eggs by soft-boiling them - Bring a pot of water to a boil, then reduce heat to a simmer. Gently lower all the eggs into water and allow them to simmer for 6 minutes. Remove the eggs from water and run cold water on top to stop the cooking, process set aside and peel when ready to use
- ❖ In a large bowl, combine the arugula, tomatoes, cucumber, and quinoa
- ❖ Divide the salad among 2 containers, store in the fridge for 2 days
- ❖ To Serve: Garnish with the sliced avocado and halved egg, sprinkle herbs and almonds over top. Drizzle with olive oil, season with salt and pepper, toss to combine. Season with more salt and pepper to taste, a squeeze of lemon juice, and a drizzle of olive oil

Nutrition: Calories:2;Carbs: 18g;Total Fat: 16g;Protein: 10g

181) GREEK YOGURT BLUEBERRY PANCAKES

Cooking Time: 15 Minutes **Servings:** 6

Ingredients:

- ✓ 1 1/4 cup all-purpose flour
- ✓ 2 tsp baking powder
- ✓ 1 tsp baking soda
- ✓ 1/4 tsp salt
- ✓ 1/4 cup sugar
- ✓ 3 eggs
- ✓ 3 tbsp vegan butter unsalted, melted
- ✓ 1/2 cup milk
- ✓ 1 1/2 cups Greek yogurt plain, non-fat
- ✓ 1/2 cup blueberries optional
- ✓ Toppings:
- ✓ Greek yogurt
- ✓ Mixed berries – blueberries, raspberries and blackberries

Directions:

- ❖ In a large bowl, whisk together the flour, salt, baking powder and baking soda
- ❖ In a separate bowl, whisk together butter, sugar, eggs, Greek yogurt, and milk until the mixture is smooth
- ❖ Then add in the Greek yogurt mixture from step to the dry mixture in step 1, mix to combine, allow the patter to sit for 20 minutes to get a smooth texture – if using blueberries fold them into the pancake batter
- ❖ Heat the pancake griddle, spray with non-stick butter spray or just brush with butter
- ❖ Pour the batter, in 1/4 cupful's, onto the griddle
- ❖ Cook until the bubbles on top burst and create small holes, lift up the corners of the pancake to see if they're golden browned on the bottom
- ❖ With a wide spatula, flip the pancake and cook on the other side until lightly browned
- ❖ Distribute the pancakes in among the storage containers, store in the fridge for 3 day or in the freezer for 2 months
- ❖ To Serve: Reheat microwave for 1 minute (until 80% heated through) or on the stove top, drizzle warm syrup on top, scoop of Greek yogurt, and mixed berries (including blueberries, raspberries, blackberries)

Nutrition: Calories:258;Total Carbohydrates: 33g;Total Fat: 8g;Protein: 11g

182) BREAKFAST VEGETABLE BOWL

Cooking Time: 5 Minutes **Servings:** 2

Ingredients:

- ✓ Breakfast Bowl:
- ✓ 1 ½ cups cooked quinoa
- ✓ 1 lb asparagus[1], cut into bite-sized pieces, ends trimmed and discarded
- ✓ 1 tbsp avocado oil or olive oil
- ✓ 3 cups shredded kale leaves
- ✓ 1 batch lemony dressing
- ✓ 3 cups shredded, uncooked Brussels sprouts
- ✓ 1 avocado, peeled, pitted and thinly-sliced
- ✓ 4 eggs, cooked to your preference (optional)
- ✓ Garnishes:
- ✓ Toasted sesame seeds
- ✓ Crushed red pepper
- ✓ Sunflower seeds
- ✓ Sliced almonds
- ✓ Hummus
- ✓ Lemon Dressing:
- ✓ 2 tsp Dijon mustard
- ✓ 1 garlic clove, minced
- ✓ 2 tbsp avocado oil or olive oil
- ✓ 2 tbsp freshly-squeezed lemon juice
- ✓ Salt, to taste
- ✓ Freshly-cracked black pepper, to taste

Directions:

- ❖ In a large sauté pan over medium-high heat, add the oil
- ❖ Once heated, add the asparagus and sauté for 4-5 minutes, stirring occasionally, until tender. Remove from heat and set side
- ❖ Add the Brussels sprouts, quinoa, and cooked asparagus, and toss until combined
- ❖ Distribute among the container, store in fridge for 2-3 days
- ❖ To serve: In a large, mixing bowl combine the kale and lemony dressing. Use your fingers to massage the dressing into the kale for 2-3 minutes, or until the leaves are dark and softened, set aside. In a small mixing bowl, combine the avocado, lemon juice, dijon mustard, garlic clove, salt, and pepper. Assemble the bowls by smearing a spoonful of hummus along the side of each bowl, then portion the kale salad evenly between the four bowls. Top with the avocado slices, egg, and your desired garnishes
- ❖ Recipe Note: Feel free to sub the asparagus with your favorite vegetable(s), sautéing or roasting them until cooked

Nutrition: Calories:632;Carbs: 52g;Total Fat: 39g;Protein: 24g

183) SPICED PEACH AND ORANGE COMPOTE WITH WHOLE-WHEAT PANCAKES

Cooking Time: 15 Minutes   **Servings:** 6

Ingredients:

- 1½ cups whole-wheat flour
- 1 tsp baking powder
- ½ tsp baking soda
- ½ tsp ground cinnamon
- ⅛ tsp kosher salt
- 1 large egg
- 1 cup low-fat (2%) plain Greek yogurt
- 1 tbsp honey
- 1 cup low-fat (2%) milk
- 2 tsp olive oil, divided
- 1 (10-ounce) package frozen sliced peaches
- ½ cup orange juice
- ¼ tsp pumpkin pie spice

Directions:

- TO MAKE THE PANCAKES
- Combine the flour, baking powder, baking soda, cinnamon, and salt in a large mixing bowl and whisk to make sure everything is distributed evenly. In a separate bowl, whisk together the egg, yogurt, honey, and milk. Pour the liquid ingredients into the dry ingredients and stir until just combined. Do not overmix.
- Heat ½ tsp of oil in a 12-inch skillet or griddle over medium heat. Once the pan is hot, spoon ¼ cup of pancake batter into the pan. You should be able to fit pancakes in a 12-inch skillet. Cook each side for about 1 minute and 30 seconds, watching carefully and checking the underside for a golden but not burnt color before flipping. Repeat until all the batter has been used.
- Place 2 pancakes in each of 6 containers.
- TO MAKE THE COMPOTE
- Thaw the peaches in the microwave just to the point that they can be cut, about 30 seconds on high. Cut the peaches into 1-inch pieces.
- Bring the peaches, orange juice, and pumpkin pie spice to a boil in a saucepan. As soon as bubbles appear, lower the heat to medium-low and cook for 12 minutes, until the juice has thickened and the peaches are very soft. Allow to cool, then mash with a potato masher.
- Place 2 tbsp of compote in each of 6 sauce containers.
- STORAGE: Store covered pancake containers in the refrigerator for up to 5 days or in the freezer for up to 2 months. Peach compote will last up to 2 weeks in the refrigerator and up to 2 months in the freezer.

Nutrition: Total calories: 209; Total fat: 5g; Saturated fat: 2g; Sodium: 289mg; Carbohydrates: 34g; Fiber: 4g; Protein: 11g

184) BANANA PEANUT BUTTER GREEK YOGURT

Cooking Time: 5 Minutes   **Servings:** 4

Ingredients:

- 3 cups vanilla Greek yogurt
- 2 medium bananas sliced
- 1/4 cup creamy natural peanut butter
- 1/4 cup flaxseed meal
- 1 tsp nutmeg

Directions:

- Divide yogurt between four jars with lids
- Top with banana slices
- In a bowl, melt the peanut butter in a microwave safe bowl for -40 seconds and drizzle one tbsp on each bowl on top of the bananas
- Store in the fridge for up to 3 days
- When ready to serve, sprinkle with flaxseed meal and ground nutmeg
- Enjoy!

Nutrition: Calories:3;Carbs: 47g;Total Fat: 10g;Protein: 22g

185) **SPICED PEACH AND ORANGE COMPOTE WITH WHOLE-WHEAT PANCAKES**

Cooking Time: 15 Minutes **Servings: 6**

Ingredients:

- ✓ 1½ cups whole-wheat flour
- ✓ 1 tsp baking powder
- ✓ ½ tsp baking soda
- ✓ ½ tsp ground cinnamon
- ✓ ⅛ tsp kosher salt
- ✓ 1 large egg
- ✓ 1 cup low-fat (2%) plain Greek yogurt
- ✓ 1 tbsp honey
- ✓ 1 cup low-fat (2%) milk
- ✓ 2 tsp olive oil, divided
- ✓ 1 (10-ounce) package frozen sliced peaches
- ✓ ½ cup orange juice
- ✓ ¼ tsp pumpkin pie spice

Directions:

- ❖ TO MAKE THE PANCAKES
- ❖ Combine the flour, baking powder, baking soda, cinnamon, and salt in a large mixing bowl and whisk to make sure everything is distributed evenly. In a separate bowl, whisk together the egg, yogurt, honey, and milk. Pour the liquid ingredients into the dry ingredients and stir until just combined. Do not overmix.
- ❖ Heat ½ tsp of oil in a 12-inch skillet or griddle over medium heat. Once the pan is hot, spoon ¼ cup of pancake batter into the pan. You should be able to fit pancakes in a 12-inch skillet. Cook each side for about 1 minute and 30 seconds, watching carefully and checking the underside for a golden but not burnt color before flipping. Repeat until all the batter has been used.
- ❖ Place 2 pancakes in each of 6 containers.
- ❖ TO MAKE THE COMPOTE
- ❖ Thaw the peaches in the microwave just to the point that they can be cut, about 30 seconds on high. Cut the peaches into 1-inch pieces.
- ❖ Bring the peaches, orange juice, and pumpkin pie spice to a boil in a saucepan. As soon as bubbles appear, lower the heat to medium-low and cook for 12 minutes, until the juice has thickened and the peaches are very soft. Allow to cool, then mash with a potato masher.
- ❖ Place 2 tbsp of compote in each of 6 sauce containers.
- ❖ STORAGE: Store covered pancake containers in the refrigerator for up to 5 days or in the freezer for up to 2 months. Peach compote will last up to 2 weeks in the refrigerator and up to 2 months in the freezer.

Nutrition: Total calories: 209; Total fat: 5g; Saturated fat: 2g; Sodium: 289mg; Carbohydrates: 34g; Fiber: 4g; Protein: 11g

186) **BANANA PEANUT BUTTER GREEK YOGURT**

Cooking Time: 5 Minutes **Servings: 4**

Ingredients:

- ✓ 3 cups vanilla Greek yogurt
- ✓ 2 medium bananas sliced
- ✓ 1/4 cup creamy natural peanut butter
- ✓ 1/4 cup flaxseed meal
- ✓ 1 tsp nutmeg

Directions:

- ❖ Divide yogurt between four jars with lids
- ❖ Top with banana slices
- ❖ In a bowl, melt the peanut butter in a microwave safe bowl for -40 seconds and drizzle one tbsp on each bowl on top of the bananas
- ❖ Store in the fridge for up to 3 days
- ❖ When ready to serve, sprinkle with flaxseed meal and ground nutmeg
- ❖ Enjoy!

Nutrition: Calories:3;Carbs: 47g;Total Fat: 10g;Protein: 22g

187) SPICED PEACH AND ORANGE COMPOTE WITH WHOLE-WHEAT PANCAKES

Cooking Time: 15 Minutes   **Servings:** 6

Ingredients:

- 1½ cups whole-wheat flour
- 1 tsp baking powder
- ½ tsp baking soda
- ½ tsp ground cinnamon
- ⅛ tsp kosher salt
- 1 large egg
- 1 cup low-fat (2%) plain Greek yogurt
- 1 tbsp honey
- 1 cup low-fat (2%) milk
- 2 tsp olive oil, divided
- 1 (10-ounce) package frozen sliced peaches
- ½ cup orange juice
- ¼ tsp pumpkin pie spice

Directions:

- TO MAKE THE PANCAKES
- Combine the flour, baking powder, baking soda, cinnamon, and salt in a large mixing bowl and whisk to make sure everything is distributed evenly. In a separate bowl, whisk together the egg, yogurt, honey, and milk. Pour the liquid ingredients into the dry ingredients and stir until just combined. Do not overmix.
- Heat ½ tsp of oil in a 12-inch skillet or griddle over medium heat. Once the pan is hot, spoon ¼ cup of pancake batter into the pan. You should be able to fit pancakes in a 12-inch skillet. Cook each side for about 1 minute and 30 seconds, watching carefully and checking the underside for a golden but not burnt color before flipping. Repeat until all the batter has been used.
- Place 2 pancakes in each of 6 containers.
- TO MAKE THE COMPOTE
- Thaw the peaches in the microwave just to the point that they can be cut, about 30 seconds on high. Cut the peaches into 1-inch pieces.
- Bring the peaches, orange juice, and pumpkin pie spice to a boil in a saucepan. As soon as bubbles appear, lower the heat to medium-low and cook for 12 minutes, until the juice has thickened and the peaches are very soft. Allow to cool, then mash with a potato masher.
- Place 2 tbsp of compote in each of 6 sauce containers.
- STORAGE: Store covered pancake containers in the refrigerator for up to 5 days or in the freezer for up to 2 months. Peach compote will last up to 2 weeks in the refrigerator and up to 2 months in the freezer.

Nutrition: Total calories: 209; Total fat: 5g; Saturated fat: 2g; Sodium: 289mg; Carbohydrates: 34g; Fiber: 4g; Protein: 11g

188) BANANA PEANUT BUTTER GREEK YOGURT

Cooking Time: 5 Minutes   **Servings:** 4

Ingredients:

- 3 cups vanilla Greek yogurt
- 2 medium bananas sliced
- 1/4 cup creamy natural peanut butter
- 1/4 cup flaxseed meal
- 1 tsp nutmeg

Directions:

- Divide yogurt between four jars with lids
- Top with banana slices
- In a bowl, melt the peanut butter in a microwave safe bowl for -40 seconds and drizzle one tbsp on each bowl on top of the bananas
- Store in the fridge for up to 3 days
- When ready to serve, sprinkle with flaxseed meal and ground nutmeg
- Enjoy!

Nutrition: Calories:3;Carbs: 47g;Total Fat: 10g;Protein: 22g

189) BREAKFAST BARS WITH APPLE QUINOA

Cooking Time: 40 Minutes   **Servings: 12**

Ingredients:

- ✓ 2 eggs
- ✓ 1 apple peeled and chopped into ½ inch chunks
- ✓ 1 cup unsweetened apple sauce
- ✓ 1 ½ cups cooked & cooled quinoa
- ✓ 1 ½ cups rolled oats
- ✓ 1/4 cup peanut butter
- ✓ 1 tsp vanilla
- ✓ 1/2 tsp cinnamon
- ✓ 1/4 cup coconut oil
- ✓ ½ tsp baking powder

Directions:

- ❖ Heat oven to 350 degrees F
- ❖ Spray an 8x8 inch baking dish with oil, set aside
- ❖ In a large bowl, stir together the apple sauce, cinnamon, coconut oil, peanut butter, vanilla and eggs
- ❖ Add in the cooked quinoa, rolled oats and baking powder, mix until completely incorporated
- ❖ Fold in the apple chunks
- ❖ Spread the mixture into the prepared baking dish, spreading it to each corner
- ❖ Bake for 40 minutes, or until a toothpick comes out clean
- ❖ Allow to cool before slicing
- ❖ Wrap the bars individually in plastic wrap. Store in an airtight container or baggie in the freezer for up to a month.
- ❖ To serve: Warm up in the oven at 350 F for 5 minutes or microwave for up to 30 seconds

Nutrition: (1 bar): Calories:230;Total Fat: 10g;Total Carbs: 31g;Protein: 7g

190) KALE, PEPPER, AND CHICKPEA SHAKSHUKA

Cooking Time: 35 Minutes   **Servings: 5**

Ingredients:

- ✓ 1 tbsp olive oil
- ✓ 1 small red onion, thinly sliced
- ✓ 1 red bell pepper, thinly sliced
- ✓ 1 green bell pepper, thinly sliced
- ✓ 1 bunch kale, stemmed and roughly chopped
- ✓ ½ cup packed cilantro leaves, chopped
- ✓ ½ tsp kosher salt
- ✓ 1 tsp smoked paprika
- ✓ 1 (14.5-ounce) can diced tomatoes
- ✓ 1 (14-ounce) can low-sodium chickpeas, drained and rinsed
- ✓ ⅔ cup water
- ✓ 5 eggs
- ✓ 2½ whole-wheat pitas (optional)

Directions:

- ❖ Preheat the oven to 375°F.
- ❖ Heat the oil in an oven-safe 1inch skillet over medium-high heat. Once the oil is shimmering, add the onions and red and green bell peppers. Sauté for 5 minutes, then cover, leaving the lid slightly ajar. Cook for 5 more minutes, then add the kale and cover, leaving the lid slightly ajar. Cook for 10 more minutes, stirring occasionally.
- ❖ Add the cilantro, salt, paprika, tomatoes, chickpeas, and water, and stir to combine.
- ❖ Make 5 wells in the mixture. Break an egg into a small bowl and pour it into a well. Repeat with the remaining eggs.
- ❖ Place the pan in the oven and bake until the egg whites are opaque and the eggs still jiggle a little when the pan is shaken, about 12 to 1minutes, but start checking at 8 minutes.
- ❖ When the shakshuka is cool, scoop about 1¼ cups of veggies into each of 5 containers, along with 1 egg each. If using, place ½ pita in each of 5 resealable bags.
- ❖ STORAGE: Store covered containers in the refrigerator for up to 5 days.

Nutrition: Total calories: 244; Total fat: 9g; Saturated fat: 2g; Sodium: 529mg; Carbohydrates: 29g; Fiber: ; Protein: 14g

191)   BACON BRIE OMELETTE WITH RADISH SALAD

Cooking Time: 10 Minutes   **Servings: 6**

Ingredients:

- ✓ 200 g smoked lardons
- ✓ 3 tsp olive oil, divided
- ✓ 7 ounces smoked bacon
- ✓ 6 lightly beaten eggs
- ✓ small bunch chives, snipped up
- ✓ 3½ ounces sliced brie
- ✓ 1 tsp red wine vinegar
- ✓ 1 tsp Dijon mustard
- ✓ 1 cucumber, deseeded, halved, and sliced up diagonally
- ✓ 7 ounces radish, quartered

Directions:

- ❖ Heat up the grill.
- ❖ Add 1 tsp of oil to a small pan and heat on the grill.
- ❖ Add lardons and fry them until nice and crisp.
- ❖ Drain the lardon on kitchen paper.
- ❖ Heat the remaining 2 tsp of oil in a non-sticking pan on the grill.
- ❖ Add lardons, eggs, chives, and ground pepper, and cook over low heat until semi-set.
- ❖ Carefully lay the Brie on top, and grill until it has set and is golden in color.
- ❖ Remove from pan and cut into wedges.
- ❖ Make the salad by mixing olive oil, mustard, vinegar, and seasoning in a bowl.
- ❖ Add cucumber and radish and mix well.
- ❖ Serve the salad alongside the Omelette wedges in containers.
- ❖ Enjoy!

Nutrition: Calories: 620, Total Fat: 49.3g, Saturated Fat: 22.1, Cholesterol: 295 mg, Sodium: 1632 mg, Total Carbohydrate: 4.3g, Dietary Fiber: 0.9 g, Total Sugars: 2.5 g, Protein: 39.2 g, Vitamin D: 41 mcg, Calcium: 185 mg, Iron: 2 mg, Potassium: 527 mg

192)   OATMEAL WITH CRANBERRIES

Cooking Time: 6 Minutes   **Servings: 2**

Ingredients:

- ✓ 1/2 cup steel-cut oats
- ✓ 1 cup unsweetened almond milk
- ✓ 1 1/2 tbsp maple syrup
- ✓ 1/4 tsp cinnamon
- ✓ 1/4 tsp vanilla
- ✓ 1/4 cup dried cranberries
- ✓ 1 cup of water
- ✓ 1 tsp lemon zest, grated
- ✓ 1/4 cup orange juice

Directions:

- ❖ Add all ingredients into the heat-safe dish and stir well.
- ❖ Pour 1 cup of water into the instant pot then place the trivet in the pot.
- ❖ Place dish on top of the trivet.
- ❖ Seal pot with lid and cook on high for 6 minutes.
- ❖ Once done, allow to release pressure naturally for 10 minutes then release remaining using quick release. Remove lid.
- ❖ Serve and enjoy.

Nutrition: Calories: 161;Fat: 3.2 g;Carbohydrates: 29.9 g;Sugar: 12.4 g;Protein: 3.4 g;Cholesterol: 0 mg

193)   FIG TOAST WITH RICOTTA

Cooking Time: 15 Minutes   **Servings: 1**

Ingredients:

- ✓ 2 slices whole-wheat toast
- ✓ 1 tsp honey
- ✓ ¼ cup ricotta (partly skimmed)
- ✓ 1 dash cinnamon
- ✓ 2 figs (sliced)
- ✓ 1 tsp sesame seeds

Directions:

- ❖ Start by mixing ricotta with honey and dash of cinnamon.
- ❖ Then, spread this mixture on the toast.
- ❖ Now, top with fig and sesame seeds.
- ❖ Serve.

Nutrition: Calories: 372, Total Fat: 8.8g, Saturated Fat: 3.8, Cholesterol: 19 mg, Sodium: 373 mg, Total Carbohydrate: .7 g, Dietary Fiber: 8.8 g, Total Sugars: 27.1 g, Protein: 17 g, Vitamin D: 0 mcg, Calcium: 328 mg, Iron: 3 mg, Potassium: 518 mg

194) MOROCCAN FISH

Cooking Time: 1 Hour 25 Minutes   **Servings: 12**

Ingredients:

- ✓ Garbanzo beans (15 oz. Can)
- ✓ Red bell peppers (2)
- ✓ Large carrot (1)
- ✓ Vegetable oil (1 tbsp.)
- ✓ Onion (1)
- ✓ Garlic (1 clove)
- ✓ Tomatoes (3 chopped/14.5 oz can)
- ✓ Olives (4 chopped)
- ✓ Chopped fresh parsley (.25 cup)
- ✓ Ground cumin (.25 cup)
- ✓ Paprika (3 tbsp.)
- ✓ Chicken bouillon granules (2 tbsp.)
- ✓ Cayenne pepper (1 tsp.)
- ✓ Salt (to your liking)
- ✓ Tilapia fillets (5 lb.)

Directions:

- ❖ Drain and rinse the beans. Thinly slice the carrot and onion. Mince the garlic and chop the olives. Discard the seeds from the peppers and slice them into strips.
- ❖ Warm the oil in a frying pan using the medium temperature setting. Toss in the onion and garlic. Simmer them for approximately five minutes.
- ❖ Fold in the bell peppers, beans, tomatoes, carrots, and olives.
- ❖ Continue sautéing them for about five additional minutes.
- ❖ Sprinkle the veggies with the cumin, parsley, salt, chicken bouillon, paprika, and cayenne.
- ❖ Stir thoroughly and place the fish on top of the veggies.
- ❖ Pour in water to cover the veggies.
- ❖ Lower the heat setting and cover the pan to slowly cook until the fish is flaky (about 40 min..

Nutrition: Calories: 268;Protein: 42 grams;Fat: 5 grams

195) SARDINES WITH NIÇOISE-INSPIRED SALAD

Cooking Time: 15 Minutes   **Servings: 4**

Ingredients:

- ✓ 4 eggs
- ✓ 12 ounces baby red potatoes (about 12 potatoes)
- ✓ 6 ounces green beans, halved
- ✓ 4 cups baby spinach leaves or mixed greens
- ✓ 1 bunch radishes, quartered (about 1⅓ cups)
- ✓ 1 cup cherry tomatoes
- ✓ 20 kalamata or niçoise olives (about ⅓ cup)
- ✓ 3 (3.75-ounce) cans skinless, boneless sardines packed in olive oil, drained
- ✓ 8 tbsp Dijon Red Wine Vinaigrette

Directions:

- ❖ Place the eggs in a saucepan and cover with water. Bring the water to a boil. As soon as the water starts to boil, place a lid on the pan and turn the heat off. Set a timer for minutes.
- ❖ When the timer goes off, drain the hot water and run cold water over the eggs to cool. Peel the eggs when cool and cut in half.
- ❖ Prick each potato a few times with a fork. Place them on a microwave-safe plate and microwave on high for 4 to 5 minutes, until the potatoes are tender. Let cool and cut in half.
- ❖ Place green beans on a microwave-safe plate and microwave on high for 1½ to 2 minutes, until the beans are crisp-tender. Cool.
- ❖ Place 1 egg, ½ cup of green beans, 6 potato halves, 1 cup of spinach, ⅓ cup of radishes, ¼ cup of tomatoes, olives, and 3 sardines in each of 4 containers. Pour 2 tbsp of vinaigrette into each of 4 sauce containers.
- ❖ STORAGE: Store covered containers in the refrigerator for up to 4 days.

Nutrition: Total calories: 450; Total fat: 32g; Saturated fat: 5g; Sodium: 6mg; Carbohydrates: 22g; Fiber: 5g; Protein: 21g

196) POMODORO LETTUCE SALAD

Cooking Time: 15 Minutes   **Servings:** 6

Ingredients:

- ✓ 1 heart of Romaine lettuce, chopped
- ✓ 3 Roma tomatoes, diced
- ✓ 1 English cucumber, diced
- ✓ 1 small red onion, finely chopped
- ✓ ½ cup curly parsley, finely chopped

- ✓ 2 tbsp virgin olive oil
- ✓ lemon juice, ½ large lemon
- ✓ 1 tsp garlic powder
- ✓ salt
- ✓ pepper

Directions:

- ❖ Add all Ingredients: to a large bowl.
- ❖ Toss well and transfer them to containers.
- ❖ Enjoy!

Nutrition: Calories: 68, Total Fat: 9 g, Saturated Fat: 0.8 g, Cholesterol: 0 mg, Sodium: 7 mg, Total Carbohydrate: 6 g, Dietary Fiber: 1.5 g, Total Sugars: 3.3 g, Protein: 1.3 g, Vitamin D: 0 mcg, Calcium: 18 mg, Iron: 1 mg, Potassium: 309 mg

197) MEDITERRANEAN-STYLE CHICKEN PASTA BAKE

Cooking Time: 30 Minutes   **Servings:** 4

Ingredients:

- ✓ Marinade:
- ✓ 1½ lbs. boneless, skinless chicken thighs, cut into bite-sized pieces*
- ✓ 2 garlic cloves, thinly sliced
- ✓ 2-3 tbsp. marinade from artichoke hearts
- ✓ 4 sprigs of fresh oregano, leaves stripped
- ✓ Olive oil
- ✓ Red wine vinegar
- ✓ Pasta:
- ✓ 1 lb whole wheat fusilli pasta
- ✓ 1 red onion, thinly sliced
- ✓ 1 pint grape or cherry tomatoes, whole

- ✓ ½ cup marinated artichoke hearts, roughly chopped
- ✓ ½ cup white beans, rinsed + drained (I use northern white beans)
- ✓ ½ cup Kalamata olives, roughly chopped
- ✓ ⅓ cup parsley and basil leaves, roughly chopped
- ✓ 2-3 handfuls of part-skim shredded mozzarella cheese
- ✓ Salt, to taste
- ✓ Pepper, to taste
- ✓ Garnish:
- ✓ Parsley
- ✓ Basil leaves

Directions:

- ❖ Create the chicken marinade by drain the artichoke hearts reserving the juice
- ❖ In a large bowl, add the artichoke juice, garlic, chicken, and oregano leaves, drizzle with olive oil, a splash of red wine vinegar, and mix well to coat
- ❖ Marinate for at least 1 hour, maximum hours
- ❖ Cook the pasta in boiling salted water, drain and set aside
- ❖ Preheat your oven to 42degrees F
- ❖ In a casserole dish, add the sliced onions and tomatoes, toss with olive oil, salt and pepper. Then cook, stirring occasionally, until the onions are soft and the tomatoes start to burst, about 15-20 minutes
- ❖ In the meantime, in a large skillet over medium heat, add 1 tsp of olive oil
- ❖ Remove the chicken from the marinade, pat dry, and season with salt and pepper
- ❖ Working in batches, brown the chicken on both sides, leaving slightly undercooked
- ❖ Remove the casserole dish from the oven, add in the cooked pasta, browned chicken, artichoke hearts, beans, olives, and chopped herbs, stir to combine
- ❖ Top with grated cheese
- ❖ Bake for an additional 5-7 minutes, until the cheese is brown and bubbling
- ❖ Remove from the oven and allow the dish to cool completely
- ❖ Distribute among the containers, store for 2-3 days
- ❖ To Serve: Reheat in the microwave for 1-2 minutes or until heated through.
- ❖ Garnish with fresh herbs and serve

Nutrition: Calories:487;Carbs: 95g;Total Fat: 5g;Protein: 22g

198) LEEKS, GREENS, AND POTATOES IN GREEK-STYLE BRAISED PORK

Cooking Time: 1 Hour 40 Minutes   **Servings: 4**

Ingredients:

- ✓ 1 tbsp olive oil, plus 2 tsp
- ✓ 1¼ pounds boneless pork loin chops, fat cap removed and cut into 1-inch pieces
- ✓ 2 leeks, white and light green parts quartered vertically and thinly sliced
- ✓ 1 bulb fennel, quartered and thinly sliced
- ✓ 1 cup chopped onion
- ✓ 1 tsp chopped garlic
- ✓ 2 cups reduced-sodium chicken broth
- ✓ 1 tsp fennel seed
- ✓ 1 tsp dried oregano
- ✓ ½ tsp kosher salt
- ✓ 1 pound baby red potatoes, halved
- ✓ 1 bunch chard, including stems, chopped
- ✓ 2 tbsp freshly squeezed lemon juice

Directions:

- ❖ Heat tbsp of oil in a soup pot or Dutch oven over medium-high heat. When the oil is shimmering, add the pork cubes and brown for about 6 minutes, turning the cubes over after 3 minutes. Remove the pork to a plate.
- ❖ Add the remaining tsp of oil to the same pot and add the leeks, fennel, onion, and garlic. Cook for 3 minutes.
- ❖ Pour the broth into the pan, scraping up any browned bits on the bottom. Add the fennel seed, oregano, and salt, and add the pork, plus any juices that may have accumulated on the plate. Make sure the pork is submerged in the liquid. Place the potatoes on top, then place the chard on top of the potatoes.
- ❖ Cover, turn down the heat to low, and simmer for 1½ hours, until the pork is tender. When the pork is done cooking, add the lemon juice. Taste and add more salt if needed. Cool.
- ❖ Scoop 2 cups of the mixture into each of 4 containers.
- ❖ STORAGE: Store covered containers in the refrigerator for up to 5 days.

Nutrition: Total calories: 3; Total fat: 13g; Saturated fat: 3g; Sodium: 1,607mg; Carbohydrates: 33g; Fiber: 8g; Protein: 34g

199) AVOCADO ARUGULA SALAD

Cooking Time: 15 Minutes   **Servings: 4**

Ingredients:

- ✓ 4 cups packed baby arugula
- ✓ 4 green onions, tops trimmed, chopped
- ✓ 1½ cups shelled fava beans
- ✓ 3 Persian cucumbers, chopped
- ✓ 2 cups grape tomatoes, halved
- ✓ 1 jalapeno pepper, sliced
- ✓ 1 avocado, cored, peeled, and roughly chopped
- ✓ lemon juice, 1½ lemons
- ✓ ½ cup extra virgin olive oil
- ✓ salt
- ✓ pepper
- ✓ 1 garlic clove, finely chopped
- ✓ 2 tbsp fresh cilantro, finely chopped
- ✓ 2 tbsp fresh mint, finely chopped

Directions:

- ❖ Place the lemon-honey vinaigrette Ingredients: in a small bowl and whisk them well.
- ❖ In a large mixing bowl, add baby arugula, fava beans, green onions, tomatoes, cucumbers, and jalapeno.
- ❖ Divide the whole salad among four containers.
- ❖ Before serving, dress the salad with the vinaigrette and toss.
- ❖ Add the avocado to the salad.
- ❖ Enjoy!

Nutrition: Calories: 229, Total Fat: 11.1 g, Saturated Fat: 2.5 g, Cholesterol: 0 mg, Sodium: 24 mg, Total Carbohydrate: 32.1 g, Dietary Fiber: 12 g, Total Sugars: 10.1 g, Protein: 3 g, Vitamin D: 0 mcg, Calcium: 163 mg, Iron: 3 mg, Potassium: 1166 mg

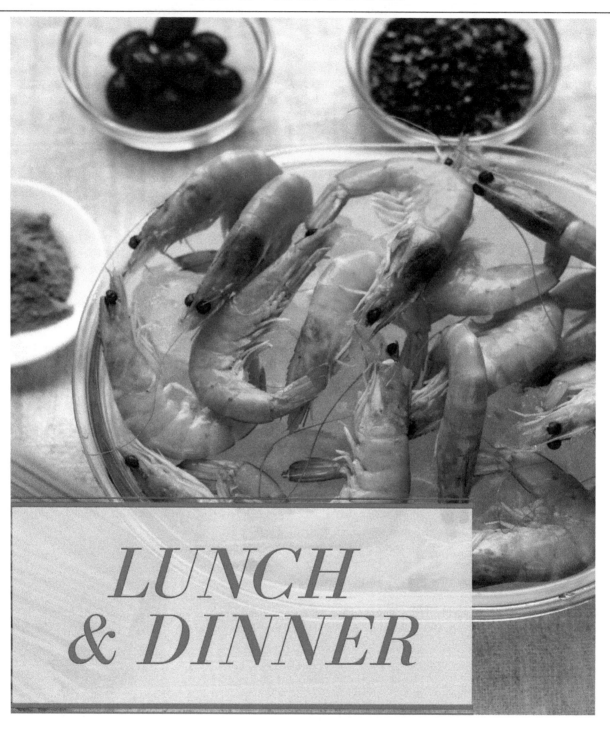

LUNCH
& DINNER

200) MEDITERRANEAN-STYLE SNAPPER

Cooking Time: 12 Minutes   **Servings: 4**

Ingredients:

- ✓ non-stick cooking spray
- ✓ 2 tbsp extra virgin olive oil
- ✓ 1 medium onion, chopped
- ✓ 2 garlic cloves, minced
- ✓ 1 tsp oregano
- ✓ 1 14-ounce can diced tomatoes, undrained
- ✓ ½ cup black olives, sliced
- ✓ 4 4-ounce red snapper fillets
- ✓ salt
- ✓ pepper
- ✓ ¼ cup crumbled feta cheese
- ✓ ¼ cup fresh parsley, minced

Directions:

- ❖ Preheat oven to 425 degrees Fahrenheit.
- ❖ Grease a 13x9 baking dish with non-stick cooking spray.
- ❖ Heat oil in a large skillet over medium heat.
- ❖ Add onion, oregano, garlic, and sauté for 2 minutes.
- ❖ Add can of tomatoes and olives, and bring mixture to a boil; remove from heat.
- ❖ Season both sides of fillets with salt and pepper and place in the baking dish.
- ❖ Spoon the tomato mixture evenly over the fish.
- ❖ Bake for 10 minutes.
- ❖ Remove from oven and sprinkle with parsley and feta.
- ❖ Enjoy!

Nutrition: Calories: 257, Total Fat: g, Saturated Fat: 1.7 g, Cholesterol: 53 mg, Sodium: 217 mg, Total Carbohydrate: 8.2 g, Dietary Fiber: 2.5 g, Total Sugars: 3.8 g, Protein: 31.3 g, Vitamin D: 0 mcg, Calcium: 85 mg, Iron: 1 mg, Potassium: 881 mg

201) ITALIAN SKILLET CHICKEN AND MUSHROOMS WITH TOMATOES

Cooking Time: 20 Minutes   **Servings: 4**

Ingredients:

- ✓ 4 large chicken cutlets, boneless skinless chicken breasts cut into 1/4-inch thin cutlets
- ✓ 1 tbsp dried oregano, divided
- ✓ 1/2 cup all-purpose flour, more for later
- ✓ 8 oz Baby Bella mushrooms, cleaned, trimmed, and sliced
- ✓ 14 oz grape tomatoes, halved
- ✓ 2 tbsp chopped fresh garlic
- ✓ Extra Virgin Olive Oil
- ✓ 1/2 cup white wine
- ✓ 1 tbsp freshly squeezed lemon juice, juice of 1/2 lemon
- ✓ 1 tsp salt, divided
- ✓ 1 tsp black pepper, divided
- ✓ 3/4 cup chicken broth
- ✓ Handful baby spinach, optional

Directions:

- ❖ Pat the chicken cutlets dry, season both sides with 2 tsp salt, 1/2 tsp black pepper, 1/2 tbsp dried oregano,
- ❖ Coat the chicken cutlets with the flour, gently dust-off excess and set aside
- ❖ In a large cast iron skillet with a lid, heat 2 tbsp olive oil
- ❖ Once heated, brown the chicken cutlets on both sides, for about 3 minutes, then transfer the chicken cutlets to plate
- ❖ In the same skillet, add more olive oil if needed,
- ❖ Once heated, add in the mushrooms and sauté on medium-high for about 1 minute
- ❖ Then add the tomatoes, garlic, the remaining 1/2 tbsp oregano, 1/2 tsp salt, and 1/2 tsp pepper, and 2 tsp flour, cook for 3 minutes or so, stirring regularly
- ❖ Add in the white wine, cook briefly to reduce, then add the lemon juice and chicken broth
- ❖ Bring the liquid to a boil, then transfer the chicken back into the skillet, cook over high heat for 3-4 minutes, then reduce the heat to medium-low, cover and cook for another 8 minutes or until the chicken is cooked through
- ❖ Allow the dish to cool completely
- ❖ Distribute among the containers, store for 3 days
- ❖ To Serve: Reheat in the microwave for 1-2 minutes or until heated through. Serve with baby spinach, your favorite small pasta and a crusty Italian bread!

Nutrition: Calories:218;Carbs: 16g;Total Fat: 6g;Protein: 23g

202) VEGETABLE QUINOA BOWL ROAST

Cooking Time: 20 Minutes   **Servings:** 2

Ingredients:

- ✓ Quinoa:
- ✓ ¾ cup quinoa, rinsed
- ✓ 1 ½ cups
- ✓ vegetable broth
- ✓ Chili-Lime Kale
- ✓ 1/2 tsp chili powder
- ✓ pinch salt
- ✓ pinch pepper
- ✓ 2 cups packed kale, de-stemmed and chopped
- ✓ 1 tsp olive, coconut or canola oil
- ✓ Juice of 1/4 lime
- ✓ Garlic Roasted Broccoli:
- ✓ 2 cups broccoli,
- ✓ 2 tsp olive or canola oil
- ✓ 2 cloves garlic, minced
- ✓ Pinch of salt
- ✓ Black pepper
- ✓ Curry Roasted Sweet Potatoes:
- ✓ 1 small sweet potato
- ✓ 1 tsp olive or canola oil
- ✓ 1 tsp curry powder
- ✓ 1 tsp sriracha
- ✓ Pinch salt
- ✓ Spicy Roasted Chickpeas:
- ✓ 1 ½ cups (cooked) chickpeas
- ✓ 1 tsp olive or canola oil
- ✓ 2 tsp sriracha
- ✓ 2 tsp soy sauce
- ✓ Optional:
- ✓ Lime
- ✓ Avocado
- ✓ Hummus
- ✓ Red pepper flakes
- ✓ Guacamole

Directions:

- ❖ Preheat the oven to 400-degree F
- ❖ Line a large baking sheet with parchment paper
- ❖ Prepare the vegetables by chopping the broccoli into medium sized florets, de-stemming and chopping the kale, scrubbing and slicing the sweet potato into ¼" wide rounds
- ❖ Take the broccoli florets and massage with oil, garlic, salt and pepper - making sure to work the ingredients into the tops of each florets - Place the florets in a row down in the center third of a large baking sheet
- ❖ Using the same bowl, the broccoli in, mix together the chickpeas, oil, sriracha and soy sauce, then spread them out in a row next to the broccoli
- ❖ In the same bowl combine the oil, curry powder, salt, and sriracha, add the sliced sweet potato and toss to coat, then lay the rounds on the remaining third of the baking tray
- ❖ Bake for 10 minutes, flip the sweet potatoes and broccoli, and redistribute the chickpeas to cook evenly Bake for another 8-12 minutes
- ❖ For the Quinoa: Prepare the quinoa by rinsing and draining it. Add the rinsed quinoa and vegetable broth to a small saucepan and bring to a boil over high heat. Turn the heat down to medium-low, cover and allow to simmer for about 15 minutes. Once cooked, fluff with a fork and set aside
- ❖ In the meantime, place a large skillet with 1 tsp oil, add in the kale and cook for about 5 minutes, or until nearly tender
- ❖ Add in the salt, chili powder, and lime juice, toss to coat and cook for another 2-3 minutes
- ❖ Allow all the ingredient to cool
- ❖ Distribute among the containers – Add ½ to 1 cup of quinoa into each bowl, top with ½ of the broccoli, ½ kale, ½ the chickpeas and ½ sweet potatoes
- ❖ To Serve: Reheat in the microwave for 1-2 minutes or until heated through. Enjoy

Nutrition: Calories:611;Carbs: 93g;Total Fat: 17g;Protein: 24g

203) MEDITERRANEAN-STYLE SALMON

Cooking Time: 15 Minutes   **Servings: 4**

Ingredients:

- ✓ ½ cup of olive oil
- ✓ ¼ cup balsamic vinegar
- ✓ 4 garlic cloves, pressed
- ✓ 4 pieces salmon fillets
- ✓ 1 tbsp fresh cilantro, chopped
- ✓ 1 tbsp fresh basil, chopped
- ✓ 1½ tsp garlic salt

Directions:

- ❖ Combine olive oil and balsamic vinegar.
- ❖ Add salmon fillets to a shallow baking dish.
- ❖ Rub the garlic onto the fillets.
- ❖ Pour vinegar and oil all over, making sure to turn them once to coat them.
- ❖ Season with cilantro, garlic salt, and basil.
- ❖ Set aside and allow to marinate for about 10 minutes.
- ❖ Preheat the broiler to your oven.
- ❖ Place the baking dish with the salmon about 6 inches from the heat source.
- ❖ Broil for 15 minutes until both sides are evenly browned and can be flaked with a fork.
- ❖ Make sure to keep brushing with sauce from the pan.
- ❖ Enjoy!

Nutrition: Calories: 459, Total Fat: 36.2 g, Saturated Fat: 5.2 g, Cholesterol: 78 mg, Sodium: 80 mg, Total Carbohydrate: 1.2 g, Dietary Fiber: 0.1 g, Total Sugars: 0.1 g, Protein: 34.8 g, Vitamin D: 0 mcg, Calcium: 71 mg, Iron: 1 mg, Potassium: 710 mg

204) HEARTTHROB MEDITERRANEAN-STYLE TILAPIA

Cooking Time: 15 Minutes   **Servings: 4**

Ingredients:

- ✓ 3 tbsp sun-dried tomatoes, packed in oil, drained and chopped
- ✓ 1 tbsp capers, drained
- ✓ 2 tilapia fillets
- ✓ 1 tbsp oil from sun-dried tomatoes
- ✓ 1 tbsp lemon juice
- ✓ 2 tbsp kalamata olives, chopped and pitted

Directions:

- ❖ Pre-heat your oven to 372-degree Fahrenheit
- ❖ Take a small sized bowl and add sun-dried tomatoes, olives, capers and stir well
- ❖ Keep the mixture on the side
- ❖ Take a baking sheet and transfer the tilapia fillets and arrange them side by side
- ❖ Drizzle olive oil all over them
- ❖ Drizzle lemon juice
- ❖ Bake in your oven for 10-15 minutes
- ❖ After 10 minutes, check the fish for a "Flaky" texture
- ❖ Once cooked properly, top the fish with tomato mix and serve!
- ❖ Meal Prep/Storage Options: Store in airtight containers in your fridge for 1-3 days.

Nutrition: Calories: 183;Fat: 8g;Carbohydrates: 18g;Protein:183g

205)   GARLIC WITH CAJUN SHRIMP BOWL AND NOODLES

Cooking Time: 15 Minutes   **Servings: 2**

Ingredients:

- ✓ 1 sliced onion
- ✓ 1 tbsp almond butter, but you can use regular butter as well
- ✓ 1 tsp onion powder
- ✓ ½ tsp salt
- ✓ 1 sliced red pepper
- ✓ 3 cloves of minced garlic
- ✓ 1 tsp paprika
- ✓ 20 jumbo shrimp, deveined and shells removed
- ✓ 3 tbsp of ghee
- ✓ 2 zucchini, 3 if they are smaller in size, cut into noodles
- ✓ Red pepper flakes and cayenne pepper, as desired

Directions:

- ❖ In a small bowl, mix the pepper flakes, paprika, onion powder, salt, and cayenne pepper.
- ❖ Toss the shrimp into the cajun mixture and coat the seafood thoroughly.
- ❖ Add the ghee to a medium or large skillet and place on medium-low heat.
- ❖ Once the ghee is melted, add the garlic and saute for minutes.
- ❖ Carefully add the shrimp into the skillet and cook until they are opaque. Set the pan aside.
- ❖ In a new pan, add the butter and allow it to melt.
- ❖ Combine the zucchini noodles and cook on medium-low heat for 3 to 4 minutes.
- ❖ Turn off the heat and place the zucchini noodles on serving dishes. Add the shrimp to the top and enjoy.

Nutrition: calories: 712, fats: 30 grams, carbohydrates: 20.1 grams, protein: grams.

206)   MARINATED CHICKEN WITH GARLIC

Cooking Time: 15 Minutes   **Servings: 3**

Ingredients:

- ✓ 1 ½ lbs. boneless skinless chicken breasts,
- ✓ 1/4 cup olive oil
- ✓ 1/4 cup lemon juice
- ✓ 3 cloves garlic, minced
- ✓ 1/2 tbsp dried oregano
- ✓ 1/2 tsp salt
- ✓ Freshly cracked pepper
- ✓ To Serve:
- ✓ Rice or cauliflower rice
- ✓ Roasted vegetables, such as carrots, asparagus, or green beans

Directions:

- ❖ In a large Ziplock bag or dish, add in the olive oil, lemon juice, garlic, oregano, salt, and pepper
- ❖ Close the bag and shake the ingredients to combine, or stir the ingredients in the dish until well combined
- ❖ Filet each chicken breast into two thinner pieces and place the pieces in the bag or dish - make sure the chicken is completely covered in marinade and allow to marinate for up to minutes up to 8 hours, turn occasionally to maximize the marinade flavors
- ❖ Once ready, heat a large skillet over medium heat
- ❖ Once heated, transfer the chicken from the marinade to the hot skillet and cook on each side cooked through, about 7 minutes each side, depending on the size - Discard of any excess marinade
- ❖ Transfer the cooked chicken from the skillet to a clean cutting board, allow to rest for five minutes before slicing
- ❖ Distribute the chicken, cooked rice and vegetables among the containers. Store in the fridge for up to 4 days. To Serve: Reheat in the microwave for 1-2 minutes or until heated through and enjoy!

Nutrition: Calories:446;Total Fat: 24g;Total Carbs: 4g;Fiber: 0g;Protein: 52g

207) TABOULI SALAD

Cooking Time: 30 Minutes   **Servings:** 6

Ingredients:

- ✓ ½ cup extra fine bulgar wheat
- ✓ 4 firm Roma tomatoes, finely chopped, juice drained
- ✓ 1 English cucumber, finely chopped
- ✓ 2 bunches fresh parsley, stems removed, finely chopped
- ✓ 12-15 fresh mint leaves, finely chopped
- ✓ 4 green onions, finely chopped (white and green)
- ✓ salt
- ✓ 3-4 tbsp lime juice
- ✓ 3-4 tbsp extra virgin olive oil
- ✓ Romaine lettuce leaves
- ✓ pita bread

Directions:

- ❖ Wash bulgur wheat thoroughly and allow it to soak under water for 5 minutes.
- ❖ Drain bulgur wheat well and set aside.
- ❖ Add all vegetables, green onions, and herbs to a dish.
- ❖ Add bulgur and season the mixture with salt.
- ❖ Add limejuice and olive oil. Mix well.
- ❖ Put to the jars and refrigerate.
- ❖ Transfer to a serving platter and serve with sides of pita and romaine lettuce.

Nutrition: Calories: 136, Total Fat: 7.6 g, Saturated Fat: 1.1 g, Cholesterol: 0 mg, Sodium: 72 mg, Total Carbohydrate: 15.6 g, Dietary Fiber: 3.7 g, Total Sugars: 3.6 g, Protein: 3.4 g, Vitamin D: 0 mcg, Calcium: 71 mg, Iron: 3 mg, Potassium: 439 mg

208) MEDITERRANEAN-STYLE FLOUNDER

Cooking Time: 45 Minutes   **Servings:** 4

Ingredients:

- ✓ Roma or plum tomatoes (5)
- ✓ Extra-virgin olive oil (2 tbsp.)
- ✓ Spanish onion (half of 1)
- ✓ Garlic (2 cloves)
- ✓ Italian seasoning (1 pinch)
- ✓ Kalamata olives (24)
- ✓ White wine (.25 cup)
- ✓ Capers (.25 cup)
- ✓ Lemon juice (1 tsp.)
- ✓ Chopped basil (6 leaves)
- ✓ Freshly grated parmesan cheese (3 tbsp.)
- ✓ Flounder fillets (1 lb.)
- ✓ Freshly torn basil (6 leaves)

Directions:

- ❖ Set the oven to reach 425° Fahrenheit. Remove the pit and chop the olives (set aside.
- ❖ Pour water into a saucepan and bring to boiling. Plunge the tomatoes into the water and remove immediately. Add to a dish of ice water and drain. Remove the skins, chop, and set to the side for now.
- ❖ Heat a skillet with the oil using the medium temperature heat setting. Chop and toss in the onions. Sauté them for around four minutes.
- ❖ Dice and add the garlic, tomatoes, and seasoning. Simmer for five to seven minutes.
- ❖ Stir in the capers, wine, olives, half of the basil, and freshly squeezed lemon juice.
- ❖ Lower the heat setting and blend in the cheese. Simmer it until the sauce is thickened (15 min..
- ❖ Arrange the flounder into a shallow baking tin. Add the sauce and garnish with the remainder of the basil leaves.
- ❖ Set the timer to bake it for 12 minutes until the fish is easily flaked.

Nutrition: Calories: 282;Protein: 24.4 grams;Fat: 15.4 grams

209) LEMON GREEK CHICKEN SOUP

Cooking Time: 20 Minutes   **Servings: 8**

Ingredients:

- ✓ 10 cups chicken broth
- ✓ 3 tbsp olive oil
- ✓ 8 cloves garlic, minced
- ✓ 1 sweet onion
- ✓ 1 large lemon, zested
- ✓ 2 boneless skinless chicken breasts
- ✓ 1 cup Israeli couscous (pearl)
- ✓ 1/2 tsp crushed red pepper
- ✓ 2 oz crumbled feta
- ✓ 1/3 cup chopped chive
- ✓ Salt, to taste
- ✓ Pepper, to taste

Directions:

- ❖ In a large 6-8-quart sauce pot over medium-low heat, add the olive oil
- ❖ Once heated, sauté the onion and minced the garlic for 3-4 minutes to soften
- ❖ Then add in the chicken broth, raw chicken breasts, lemon zest, and crushed red pepper to the pot Raise the heat to high, cover, and bring to a boil
- ❖ Once boiling, reduce the heat to medium, then simmer for 5 minutes Stir in the couscous, 1 tsp salt, and black pepper to taste
- ❖ Simmer another 5 minute, then turn the heat off Using tongs, remove the two chicken breasts from the pot and transfer to a plate
- ❖ Use a fork and the tongs to shred the chicken, then return to the pot
- ❖ Stir in the crumbled feta cheese and chopped chive Season to taste with salt and pepper as needed
- ❖ Allow the soup to cool completely Distribute among the containers, store for 2-3 days
- ❖ To Serve: Reheat in the microwave for 1-2 minutes or until heated through, or reheat on the stove

Nutrition: Calories:2Carbs: 23g;Total Fat: g;Protein: 11g

210) TUNA WITH HERBS SALAD WRAPS

Cooking Time: 15 Minutes   **Servings: 4**

Ingredients:

- ✓ 1 (11-ounce) pouch tuna in water
- ✓ 1 cup parsley leaves, chopped
- ✓ ¼ cup mint leaves, chopped
- ✓ ¼ cup minced shallot
- ✓ 1½ tsp sumac
- ✓ 1 tsp Dijon mustard
- ✓ 1 tbsp olive oil
- ✓ 1 tbsp freshly squeezed lemon juice
- ✓ ¼ cup unsalted sunflower seeds
- ✓ 16 large or medium romaine or bibb lettuce leaves
- ✓ 1 red bell pepper, cut into thin sticks (3 to 4 inches long)
- ✓ 3 Persian cucumbers, cut into thin sticks (3 to 4 inches long)

Directions:

- ❖ In a large bowl, mix together the tuna, parsley, mint, shallot, sumac, mustard, oil, lemon juice, and sunflower seeds.
- ❖ Place ¾ cup of tuna salad in each of 4 containers. Place 4 lettuce leaves, one quarter of the peppers, and one quarter of the cucumbers in each of 4 separate containers so that they don't get soggy from the tuna salad.
- ❖ STORAGE: Store covered containers in the refrigerator for up to 4 days.
- ❖ TIP Tuna in pouches is preferable to cans, because pouches don't need to be drained and the tuna isn't soggy. You can substitute canned salmon, canned sardines, or even shredded rotisserie chicken for the tuna in this salad.

Nutrition: Total calories: 223; Total fat: 9g; Saturated fat: 1g; Sodium: 422mg; Carbohydrates: 12g; Fiber: 4g; Protein: 24g

211) MEDITERRANEAN-STYLE STEAMED SALMON WITH FRESH HERBS AND LEMON

Cooking Time: 15 Minutes   **Servings:** 4

Ingredients:

- ✓ 1 yellow onion, halved and sliced
- ✓ 4 green onions spring onions, trimmed and sliced lengthwise, divided
- ✓ 1 lb skin-on salmon fillet (such as wild Alaskan), cut into 4 portions
- ✓ 1/2 tsp Aleppo pepper
- ✓ 4 to 5 garlic cloves, chopped
- ✓ Extra virgin olive oil
- ✓ A large handful fresh parsley
- ✓ 1 lemon, thinly sliced
- ✓ 1 tsp ground coriander
- ✓ 1 tsp ground cumin
- ✓ 1/2 cup white wine (or you can use water or low-sodium broth, if you prefer)
- ✓ Kosher salt, to taste
- ✓ Black pepper, to taste

Directions:

- ❖ Prepare a large piece of wax paper or parchment paper (about 2 feet long) and place it right in the center of a -inch deep pan or braiser
- ❖ Place the sliced yellow onions and a sprinkle a little bit of green onions the onions on the bottom of the braiser
- ❖ Arrange the salmon, skin-side down, on top, season with kosher salt and black pepper
- ❖ In a small bowl, mix together the coriander, cumin, and Aleppo pepper, coat top of salmon with the spice mixture, and drizzle with a little bit of extra virgin olive oil
- ❖ Then add garlic, parsley and the remaining green onions on top of the salmon (make sure that everything is arrange evenly over the salmon portions.)
- ❖ Arrange the lemon slices on top of the salmon
- ❖ Add another drizzle of extra virgin olive oil, then add the white wine
- ❖ Fold the parchment paper over to cover salmon, secure the edges and cover the braiser with the lid
- ❖ Place the braising pan over medium-high heat, cook for 5 minutes
- ❖ Lower the heat to medium, cook for another 8 minutes, covered still
- ❖ Remove from heat and allow to rest undisturbed for about 5 minutes.
- ❖ Remove the lid and allow the salmon to cool completely
- ❖ Distribute among the containers, store for 2-3 days
- ❖ To Serve: Reheat in the microwave for 1-2 minutes or until heated through.
- ❖ Recipe Notes: The pan or braiser you use needs to have a lid to allow the steamed salmon.

Nutrition: Calories:321;Carbs: g;Total Fat: 18g;Protein: 28g

212) BEEF-BASED SAUSAGE PANCAKES

Cooking Time: 30 Minutes   **Servings:** 2

Ingredients:

- ✓ 4 gluten-free Italian beef sausages, sliced
- ✓ 1 tbsp olive oil
- ✓ 1/3 large red bell peppers, seeded and sliced thinly
- ✓ 1/3 cup spinach
- ✓ ¾ tsp garlic powder
- ✓ 1/3 large green bell peppers, seeded and sliced thinly
- ✓ ¾ cup heavy whipped cream
- ✓ Salt and black pepper, to taste

Directions:

- ❖ Mix together all the ingredients in a bowl except whipped cream and keep aside.
- ❖ Put butter and half of the mixture in a skillet and cook for about 6 minutes on both sides.
- ❖ Repeat with the remaining mixture and dish out.
- ❖ Beat whipped cream in another bowl until smooth.
- ❖ Serve the beef sausage pancakes with whipped cream.
- ❖ For meal prepping, it is compulsory to gently slice the sausages before mixing with other ingredients.

Nutrition: Calories: 415 ;Carbohydrates: ;Protein: 29.5g;Fat: 31.6g ;Sugar: 4.3g;Sodium: 1040mg

213)   LOBSTER SALAD

Cooking Time: 15 Minutes   **Servings: 2**

Ingredients:

- ✓ ¼ yellow onion, chopped
- ✓ ¼ yellow bell pepper, seeded and chopped
- ✓ ¾ pound cooked lobster meat, shredded
- ✓ 1 celery stalk, chopped
- ✓ Black pepper, to taste
- ✓ ¼ cup avocado mayonnaise

Directions:

- ❖ Mix together all the ingredients in a bowl and stir until well combined.
- ❖ Refrigerate for about 3 hours and serve chilled.
- ❖ Put the salad into a container for meal prepping and refrigerate for about 2 days.

Nutrition: Calories: 336 ;Carbohydrates: 2g;Protein: 27.2g;Fat: 25.2g ;Sugar: 1.2g;Sodium: 926mg

214)   MEDITERRANEAN-STYLE PESTO CHICKEN

Cooking Time: 40 Minutes   **Servings: 4**

Ingredients:

- ✓ 1 pound chicken breasts (2 large breasts), butterflied and cut in half to make 4 pieces
- ✓ 1 (6-ounce) jar prepared pesto
- ✓ 1 tsp olive oil
- ✓ 12 ounces baby spinach leaves
- ✓ Chunky Roasted Cherry Tomato and Basil Sauce

Directions:

- ❖ Place the chicken and pesto in a gallon-size resealable bag. Marinate for at least hour.
- ❖ Preheat the oven to 350°F and rub a 13-by-9-inch glass or ceramic baking dish with the oil, or spray with cooking spray.
- ❖ Place the spinach in the pan, then place the chicken on top of the spinach. Pour the pesto from the bag into the dish. Cover the pan with aluminum foil and bake for 20 minutes. Remove the foil and bake for another 15 to 20 minutes. Cool.
- ❖ Place 1 piece of chicken, one quarter of the spinach, and ⅓ cup of chunky tomato sauce in each of separate containers.
- ❖ STORAGE: Store covered containers in the refrigerator for up to days.

Nutrition: Total calories: 531; Total fat: 43g; Saturated fat: 7g; Sodium: 1,243mg; Carbohydrates: 13g; Fiber: 4g; Protein: 29g

215)   CRISPY AND BAKED CHICKEN

Cooking Time: 40 Minutes   **Servings: 2**

Ingredients:

- ✓ 2 chicken breasts, skinless and boneless
- ✓ 2 tbsp butter
- ✓ ¼ tsp turmeric powder
- ✓ Salt and black pepper, to taste
- ✓ ¼ cup sour cream

Directions:

- ❖ Preheat the oven to 360 degrees F and grease a baking dish with butter.
- ❖ Season the chicken with turmeric powder, salt and black pepper in a bowl.
- ❖ Put the chicken on the baking dish and transfer it in the oven.
- ❖ Bake for about 10 minutes and dish out to serve topped with sour cream.
- ❖ Transfer the chicken in a bowl and set aside to cool for meal prepping. Divide it into 2 containers and cover the containers. Refrigerate for up to 2 days and reheat in microwave before serving.

Nutrition: Calories: 304 ;Carbohydrates: 1.4g;Protein: 21g;Fat: 21.6g ;Sugar: 0.1g;Sodium: 137mg

216) MARINATED TUNA STEAK SPECIAL

Cooking Time: 15-20 Minutes   **Servings: 4**

Ingredients:

- ✓ Olive oil (2 tbsp.)
- ✓ Orange juice (.25 cup)
- ✓ Soy sauce (.25 cup)
- ✓ Lemon juice (1 tbsp.)
- ✓ Fresh parsley (2 tbsp.)
- ✓ Garlic clove (1)
- ✓ Ground black pepper (.5 tsp.)
- ✓ Fresh oregano (.5 tsp.)
- ✓ Tuna steaks (4 - 4 oz. Steaks)

Directions:

- ❖ Mince the garlic and chop the oregano and parsley.
- ❖ In a glass container, mix the pepper, oregano, garlic, parsley, lemon juice, soy sauce, olive oil, and orange juice.
- ❖ Warm the grill using the high heat setting. Grease the grate with oil.
- ❖ Add to tuna steaks and cook for five to six minutes. Turn and baste with the marinated sauce.
- ❖ Cook another five minutes or until it's the way you like it. Discard the remaining marinade.

Nutrition: Calories: 200;Protein: 27.4 grams;Fat: 7.9 grams

217) SHRIMP AND GARLIC PASTA

Cooking Time: 15 Minutes   **Servings: 4**

Ingredients:

- ✓ 6 ounces whole wheat spaghetti
- ✓ 12 ounces raw shrimp, peeled and deveined, cut into 1-inch pieces
- ✓ 1 bunch asparagus, trimmed
- ✓ 1 large bell pepper, thinly sliced
- ✓ 1 cup fresh peas
- ✓ 3 garlic cloves, chopped
- ✓ 1 and ¼ tsp kosher salt
- ✓ ½ and ½ cups non-fat plain yogurt
- ✓ 3 tbsp lemon juice
- ✓ 1 tbsp extra-virgin olive oil
- ✓ ½ tsp fresh ground black pepper
- ✓ ¼ cup pine nuts, toasted

Directions:

- ❖ Take a large sized pot and bring water to a boil
- ❖ Add your spaghetti and cook them for about minutes less than the directed package instruction
- ❖ Add shrimp, bell pepper, asparagus and cook for about 2-4 minutes until the shrimp are tender
- ❖ Drain the pasta and the contents well
- ❖ Take a large bowl and mash garlic until a paste form
- ❖ Whisk in yogurt, parsley, oil, pepper and lemon juice into the garlic paste
- ❖ Add pasta mix and toss well
- ❖ Serve by sprinkling some pine nuts!
- ❖ Enjoy!
- ❖ Meal Prep/Storage Options: Store in airtight containers in your fridge for 1-3 days.

Nutrition: Calories: 406;Fat: 22g;Carbohydrates: 28g;Protein: 26g

218) BUTTER PAPRIKA SHRIMPS

Cooking Time: 30 Minutes   **Servings: 2**

Ingredients:

- ✓ ¼ tbsp smoked paprika
- ✓ 1/8 cup sour cream
- ✓ ½ pound tiger shrimps
- ✓ 1/8 cup butter
- ✓ Salt and black pepper, to taste

Directions:

- ❖ Preheat the oven to 390 degrees F and grease a baking dish.
- ❖ Mix together all the ingredients in a large bowl and transfer into the baking dish.
- ❖ Place in the oven and bake for about 15 minutes.
- ❖ Place paprika shrimp in a dish and set aside to cool for meal prepping. Divide it in 2 containers and cover the lid. Refrigerate for 1-2 days and reheat in microwave before serving.

Nutrition: Calories: 330 ;Carbohydrates: 1.;Protein: 32.6g;Fat: 21.5g;Sugar: 0.2g;Sodium: 458mg

219) MOROCCAN FISH

Cooking Time: 1 Hour 25 Minutes   **Servings: 12**

Ingredients:

- ✓ Garbanzo beans (15 oz. Can)
- ✓ Red bell peppers (2)
- ✓ Large carrot (1)
- ✓ Vegetable oil (1 tbsp.)
- ✓ Onion (1)
- ✓ Garlic (1 clove)
- ✓ Tomatoes (3 chopped/14.5 oz can)
- ✓ Olives (4 chopped)
- ✓ Chopped fresh parsley (.25 cup)
- ✓ Ground cumin (.25 cup)
- ✓ Paprika (3 tbsp.)
- ✓ Chicken bouillon granules (2 tbsp.)
- ✓ Cayenne pepper (1 tsp.)
- ✓ Salt (to your liking)
- ✓ Tilapia fillets (5 lb.)

Directions:

- ❖ Drain and rinse the beans. Thinly slice the carrot and onion. Mince the garlic and chop the olives. Discard the seeds from the peppers and slice them into strips.
- ❖ Warm the oil in a frying pan using the medium temperature setting. Toss in the onion and garlic. Simmer them for approximately five minutes.
- ❖ Fold in the bell peppers, beans, tomatoes, carrots, and olives.
- ❖ Continue sautéing them for about five additional minutes.
- ❖ Sprinkle the veggies with the cumin, parsley, salt, chicken bouillon, paprika, and cayenne.
- ❖ Stir thoroughly and place the fish on top of the veggies.
- ❖ Pour in water to cover the veggies.
- ❖ Lower the heat setting and cover the pan to slowly cook until the fish is flaky (about 40 min..

Nutrition: Calories: 268;Protein: 42 grams;Fat: 5 grams

220) SARDINES WITH NIÇOISE-INSPIRED SALAD

Cooking Time: 15 Minutes   **Servings: 4**

Ingredients:

- ✓ 4 eggs
- ✓ 12 ounces baby red potatoes (about 12 potatoes)
- ✓ 6 ounces green beans, halved
- ✓ 4 cups baby spinach leaves or mixed greens
- ✓ 1 bunch radishes, quartered (about 1⅓ cups)
- ✓ 1 cup cherry tomatoes
- ✓ 20 kalamata or niçoise olives (about ⅓ cup)
- ✓ 3 (3.75-ounce) cans skinless, boneless sardines packed in olive oil, drained
- ✓ 8 tbsp Dijon Red Wine Vinaigrette

Directions:

- ❖ Place the eggs in a saucepan and cover with water. Bring the water to a boil. As soon as the water starts to boil, place a lid on the pan and turn the heat off. Set a timer for minutes.
- ❖ When the timer goes off, drain the hot water and run cold water over the eggs to cool. Peel the eggs when cool and cut in half.
- ❖ Prick each potato a few times with a fork. Place them on a microwave-safe plate and microwave on high for 4 to 5 minutes, until the potatoes are tender. Let cool and cut in half.
- ❖ Place green beans on a microwave-safe plate and microwave on high for 1½ to 2 minutes, until the beans are crisp-tender. Cool.
- ❖ Place 1 egg, ½ cup of green beans, 6 potato halves, 1 cup of spinach, ⅓ cup of radishes, ¼ cup of tomatoes, olives, and 3 sardines in each of 4 containers. Pour 2 tbsp of vinaigrette into each of 4 sauce containers.
- ❖ STORAGE: Store covered containers in the refrigerator for up to 4 days.

Nutrition: Total calories: 450; Total fat: 32g; Saturated fat: 5g; Sodium: 6mg; Carbohydrates: 22g; Fiber: 5g; Protein: 21g

221) POMODORO LETTUCE SALAD

Cooking Time: 15 Minutes   **Servings: 6**

Ingredients:

- 1 heart of Romaine lettuce, chopped
- 3 Roma tomatoes, diced
- 1 English cucumber, diced
- 1 small red onion, finely chopped
- ½ cup curly parsley, finely chopped
- 2 tbsp virgin olive oil
- lemon juice, ½ large lemon
- 1 tsp garlic powder
- salt
- pepper

Directions:

- Add all Ingredients: to a large bowl.
- Toss well and transfer them to containers.
- Enjoy!

Nutrition: Calories: 68, Total Fat: 9 g, Saturated Fat: 0.8 g, Cholesterol: 0 mg, Sodium: 7 mg, Total Carbohydrate: 6 g, Dietary Fiber: 1.5 g, Total Sugars: 3.3 g, Protein: 1.3 g, Vitamin D: 0 mcg, Calcium: 18 mg, Iron: 1 mg, Potassium: 309 mg

222) MEDITERRANEAN-STYLE CHICKEN PASTA BAKE

Cooking Time: 30 Minutes   **Servings: 4**

Ingredients:

- Marinade:
- 1½ lbs. boneless, skinless chicken thighs, cut into bite-sized pieces*
- 2 garlic cloves, thinly sliced
- 2-3 tbsp. marinade from artichoke hearts
- 4 sprigs of fresh oregano, leaves stripped
- Olive oil
- Red wine vinegar
- Pasta:
- 1 lb whole wheat fusilli pasta
- 1 red onion, thinly sliced
- 1 pint grape or cherry tomatoes, whole
- ½ cup marinated artichoke hearts, roughly chopped
- ½ cup white beans, rinsed + drained (I use northern white beans)
- ½ cup Kalamata olives, roughly chopped
- ⅓ cup parsley and basil leaves, roughly chopped
- 2-3 handfuls of part-skim shredded mozzarella cheese
- Salt, to taste
- Pepper, to taste
- Garnish:
- Parsley
- Basil leaves

Directions:

- Create the chicken marinade by drain the artichoke hearts reserving the juice
- In a large bowl, add the artichoke juice, garlic, chicken, and oregano leaves, drizzle with olive oil, a splash of red wine vinegar, and mix well to coat
- Marinate for at least 1 hour, maximum hours
- Cook the pasta in boiling salted water, drain and set aside
- Preheat your oven to 42degrees F
- In a casserole dish, add the sliced onions and tomatoes, toss with olive oil, salt and pepper. Then cook, stirring occasionally, until the onions are soft and the tomatoes start to burst, about 15-20 minutes
- In the meantime, in a large skillet over medium heat, add 1 tsp of olive oil
- Remove the chicken from the marinade, pat dry, and season with salt and pepper
- Working in batches, brown the chicken on both sides, leaving slightly undercooked
- Remove the casserole dish from the oven, add in the cooked pasta, browned chicken, artichoke hearts, beans, olives, and chopped herbs, stir to combine
- Top with grated cheese
- Bake for an additional 5-7 minutes, until the cheese is brown and bubbling
- Remove from the oven and allow the dish to cool completely
- Distribute among the containers, store for 2-3 days
- To Serve: Reheat in the microwave for 1-2 minutes or until heated through.
- Garnish with fresh herbs and serve

Nutrition: Calories:487;Carbs: 95g;Total Fat: 5g;Protein: 22g

223)   VEGETABLE FLATBREAD ROAST

Cooking Time: 25 Minutes   **Servings: 12**

Ingredients:

- ✓ 16 oz pizza dough, homemade or frozen
- ✓ 6 oz soft goat cheese, divided
- ✓ ¾ cup grated Parmesan cheese divided
- ✓ 3 tbsp chopped fresh dill, divided
- ✓ 1 small red onion, sliced thinly
- ✓ 1 small zucchini, sliced thinly
- ✓ 2 small tomatoes, thinly sliced
- ✓ 1 small red pepper, thinly sliced into rings
- ✓ Olive oil
- ✓ Salt, to taste
- ✓ Pepper, to taste

Directions:

- ❖ Preheat the oven to 400 degrees F
- ❖ Roll the dough into a large rectangle, and then place it on a piece of parchment paper sprayed with non-stick spray
- ❖ Take a knife and spread half the goat cheese onto one half of the dough, then sprinkle with half the dill and half the Parmesan cheese
- ❖ Carefully fold the other half of the dough on top of the cheese, spread and sprinkle the remaining parmesan and goat cheese
- ❖ Layer the thinly sliced vegetables over the top
- ❖ Brush the olive oil over the top of the veggies and sprinkle with salt, pepper, and the remaining dill
- ❖ Bake for 22-25 minutes, until the edges are medium brown, cut in half, lengthwise
- ❖ Then slice the flatbread in long 2-inch slices and allow to cool
- ❖ Distribute among the containers, store for 2 days
- ❖ To Serve: Reheat in the oven at 375 degrees for 5 minutes or until hot. Enjoy with a fresh salad.

Nutrition: Calories:170;Carbs: 21g;Total Fat: 6g;Protein: 8g

224)   COBB SALAD WITH STEAK

Cooking Time: 15 Minutes   **Servings: 4**

Ingredients:

- ✓ 6 large eggs
- ✓ 2 tbsp unsalted butter
- ✓ 1 lb steak
- ✓ 2 tbsp olive oil
- ✓ 6 cups baby spinach
- ✓ 1 cup cherry tomatoes, halved
- ✓ 1 cup pecan halves
- ✓ 1/2 cup crumbled feta cheese
- ✓ Kosher salt, to taste
- ✓ Freshly ground black pepper, to taste

Directions:

- ❖ In a large skillet over medium high heat, melt butter
- ❖ Using paper towels, pat the steak dry, then drizzle with olive oil and season with salt and pepper, to taste
- ❖ Once heated, add the steak to the skillet and cook, flipping once, until cooked through to desired doneness, - cook for 4 minutes per side for a medium-rare steak
- ❖ Transfer the steak to a plate and allow it to cool before dicing
- ❖ Place the eggs in a large saucepan and cover with cold water by 1 inch
- ❖ Bring to a boil and cook for 1 minute, cover the eggs with a tight-fitting lid and remove from heat, set aside for 8-10 minutes, then drain well and allow to cool before peeling and dicing
- ❖ Assemble the salad in the container by placing the spinach at the bottom of the container, top with arranged rows of steak, eggs, feta, tomatoes, and pecans
- ❖ To Serve: Top with the balsamic vinaigrette, or desired dressing
- ❖ Recipe Note: You can also use New York, rib-eye or filet mignon for this recipe

Nutrition: Calories:640;Total Fat: 51g;Total Carbs: 9.8g;Fiber: 5g;Protein: 38.8g

225) LAMB CHOPS GRILL

Cooking Time: 10 Minutes   **Servings: 4**

Ingredients:

- ✓ 4 8-ounce lamb shoulder chops
- ✓ 2 tbsp Dijon mustard
- ✓ 2 tbsp balsamic vinegar
- ✓ 1 tbsp chopped garlic
- ✓ ¼ tsp ground black pepper
- ✓ ½ cup olive oil
- ✓ 2 tbsp fresh basil, shredded

Directions:

- ❖ Pat the lamb chops dry and arrange them in a shallow glass-baking dish.
- ❖ Take a bowl and whisk in Dijon mustard, garlic, balsamic vinegar, and pepper.
- ❖ Mix well to make the marinade.
- ❖ Whisk oil slowly into the marinade until it is smooth.
- ❖ Stir in basil.
- ❖ Pour the marinade over the lamb chops, making sure to coat both sides.
- ❖ Cover, refrigerate and allow the chops to marinate for anywhere from 1-4 hours.
- ❖ Remove the chops from the refrigerator and leave out for 30 minutes or until room temperature.
- ❖ Preheat grill to medium heat and oil grate.
- ❖ Grill the lamb chops until the center reads 145 degrees F and they are nicely browned, about 5-minutes per side.
- ❖ Enjoy!

Nutrition: Calories: 1587, Total Fat: 97.5 g, Saturated Fat: 27.6 g, Cholesterol: 600 mg, Sodium: 729 mg, Total Carbohydrate: 1.3 g, Dietary Fiber: 0.4 g, Total Sugars: 0.1 g, Protein: 176.5 g, Vitamin D: 0 mcg, Calcium: 172 mg, Iron: 15 mg, Potassium: 30 mg

226) FLATBREAD AND ROASTED VEGETABLES

Cooking Time: 45 Minutes   **Servings: 12**

Ingredients:

- ✓ 5 ounces goat cheese
- ✓ 1 thinly sliced onion
- ✓ 2 thinly sliced tomatoes
- ✓ Olive oil
- ✓ ¼ tsp pepper
- ✓ ⅛ tsp salt
- ✓ 16 ounces homemade or frozen pizza dough
- ✓ ¾ tbsp chopped dill, fresh is better
- ✓ 1 thinly sliced zucchini
- ✓ 1 red pepper, cup into rings

Directions:

- ❖ Set your oven to 400 degrees Fahrenheit.
- ❖ Set the dough on a large piece of parchment paper. Use a rolling pin to roll the dough into a large rectangle.
- ❖ Spread half of the goat cheese on ½ of the pizza dough.
- ❖ Sprinkle half of the dill on the other half of the dough.
- ❖ Fold the dough so the half with the dill is on top of the cheese.
- ❖ Spread the remaining goat cheese on the pizza dough and then sprinkle the rest of the dill over the cheese.
- ❖ Layer the vegetables on top in any arrangement you like.
- ❖ Drizzle olive oil on top of the vegetables.
- ❖ Sprinkle salt and pepper over the olive oil.
- ❖ Set the piece of parchment paper on a pizza pan or baking pan and place it in the oven.
- ❖ Set the timer for 22 minutes. If the edges are not a medium brown, leave the flatbread in the oven for another couple of minutes.
- ❖ Remove the pizza from the oven when it is done and cut the flatbread in half lengthwise.
- ❖ Slice the flatbread into 2-inch long pieces and enjoy!

Nutrition: calories: 170, fats: 5 grams, carbohydrates: 20 grams, protein: 8 grams.

227) SEAFOOD RICE

Cooking Time: 40 Minutes   **Servings:** 4-5

Ingredients:

- ✓ 4 small lobster tails (6-12 oz each)
- ✓ Water
- ✓ 3 tbsp Extra Virgin Olive Oil
- ✓ 1 large yellow onion, chopped
- ✓ 2 cups Spanish rice or short grain rice, soaked in water for 15 minutes and then drained
- ✓ 4 garlic cloves, chopped
- ✓ 2 large pinches of Spanish saffron threads soaked in 1/2 cup water
- ✓ 1 tsp Sweet Spanish paprika
- ✓ 1 tsp cayenne pepper
- ✓ 1/2 tsp aleppo pepper flakes
- ✓ Salt, to taste
- ✓ 2 large Roma tomatoes, finely chopped
- ✓ 6 oz French green beans, trimmed
- ✓ 1 lb prawns or large shrimp or your choice, peeled and deveined
- ✓ 1/4 cup chopped fresh parsley

Directions:

- ❖ In a large pot, add 3 cups of water and bring it to a rolling boil
- ❖ Add in the lobster tails and allow boil briefly, about 1-minutes or until pink, remove from heat
- ❖ Using tongs transfer the lobster tails to a plate and Do not discard the lobster cooking water
- ❖ Allow the lobster is cool, then remove the shell and cut into large chunks.
- ❖ In a large deep pan or skillet over medium-high heat, add 3 tbsp olive oil
- ❖ Add the chopped onions, sauté the onions for 2 minutes and then add the rice, and cook for 3 more minutes, stirring regularly
- ❖ Then add in the lobster cooking water and the chopped garlic and, stir in the saffron and its soaking liquid, cayenne pepper, aleppo pepper, paprika, and salt
- ❖ Gently stir in the chopped tomatoes and green beans, bring to a boil and allow the liquid slightly reduce, then cover (with lid or tightly wrapped foil) and cook over low heat for 20 minutes
- ❖ Once done, uncover and spread the shrimp over the rice, push it into the rice slightly, add in a little water, if needed
- ❖ Cover and cook for another 15 minutes until the shrimp turn pink
- ❖ Then add in the cooked lobster chunks
- ❖ Once the lobster is warmed through, remove from heat allow the dish to cool completely
- ❖ Distribute among the containers, store for 2 days
- ❖ To Serve: Reheat in the microwave for 1-2 minutes or until heated through. Garnish with parsley and enjoy!
- ❖ Recipe Notes: Remember to soak your rice if needed to help with the cooking process

Nutrition: Calories:536;Carbs: 56g;Total Fat: 26g;Protein: 50g

228)   MEDITERRANEAN-STYLE PASTA SALAD

Cooking Time: 25 Minutes   **Servings:** 8

Ingredients:

- Salad:
- 8 oz pasta, I used farfalle, any smallish pasta works great!
- 1 cup rotisserie chicken, chopped
- 1/2 cup sun-dried tomatoes packed in oil, drained and coarsely chopped
- 1/2 cup jarred marinated artichoke hearts, drained and coarsely chopped
- 1/2 of 1 full English cucumber, chopped
- 1/3 cup kalamata olives, coarsely chopped
- 2 cups lightly packed fresh arugula
- 1/4 cup fresh flat leaf Italian parsley, coarsely chopped
- 1 small avocado, pit removed and coarsely chopped
- 1/3 cup feta cheese

- Dressing:
- 4 tbsp red wine vinegar
- 1 ½ tbsp dijon mustard, do not use regular mustard
- 1/2 tsp dried oregano
- 1 tsp dried basil
- 1 clove garlic, minced
- 1-2 tsp honey
- 1/2 cup olive oil
- 3 tbsp freshly squeezed lemon juice
- Fine sea salt, to taste
- Freshly cracked pepper, to taste

Directions:

- Prepare the pasta according to package directions until al dente, drain the pasta and allow it to completely cool to room temperature, then add it to a large bowl
- Add in the chopped rotisserie chicken, chopped cucumber, coarsely chopped kalamata olives, coarsely chopped sun-dried tomatoes, coarsely chopped artichoke hearts, arugula, and parsley, toss
- Distribute the salad among the containers, store for 2-days
- Prepare the dressing - In a mason jar with a lid, combine the red wine vinegar, Dijon mustard, garlic, 1/2 tsp salt (or to taste), dried oregano, dried basil and 1/tsp pepper (or to taste, honey (add to sweetness preference), olive oil, and freshly squeezed lemon juice, place the lid on the mason jar and shake to combine, store in fridge
- To Serve: Add in the avocado and feta cheese to the salad, drizzle with the dressing, adjust any seasonings salt and pepper to taste, serve

Nutrition: Calories:32Carbs: 24g;Total Fat: 21g;Protein: 8g

229)   DELIZIOSA BROCCOLI TORTELLINI SALAD

Cooking Time: 20 To 25 Minutes   **Servings:** 12

Ingredients:

- 1 cup sunflower seeds, or any of your favorite seeds
- 3 heads of broccoli, fresh is best!
- ½ cup sugar
- 20 ounces cheese-filled tortellini

- 1 onion
- 2 tsp cider vinegar
- ½ cup mayonnaise
- 1 cup raisins-optional

Directions:

- Cut your broccoli into florets and chop the onion.
- Follow the directions to make the cheese-filled tortellini. Once they are cooked, drain and rinse them with cold water.
- In a bowl, combine your mayonnaise, sugar, and vinegar. Whisk well to give the ingredients a dressing consistency.
- In a separate large bowl, toss in your seeds, onion, tortellini, raisins, and broccoli.
- Pour the salad dressing into the large bowl and toss the ingredients together. You will want to ensure everything is thoroughly mixed as you'll want a taste of the salad dressing with every bite!

Nutrition: calories: 272, fats: 8.1 grams, carbohydrates: 38.grams, protein: 5 grams.

230) AVOCADO LEMON HERB CHICKEN SALAD

Cooking Time: 15 Minutes **Servings: 4**

Ingredients:

- Marinade/ Dressing:
- 2 tbsp olive oil
- 1/4 cup fresh lemon juice
- 2 tbsp water
- 2 tbsp fresh chopped parsley
- 2 tsp garlic, minced
- 1 tsp each dried thyme and dried rosemary
- 1 tsp salt
- 1/4 tsp cracked pepper, or to taste

- ✓ 1 pound skinless & boneless chicken thigh fillets or chicken breasts Salad:
- ✓ 4 cups Romaine lettuce leaves, washed and dried
- ✓ 1 large avocado, pitted, peeled and sliced
- ✓ 8 oz feta cheese
- ✓ 1 cup grape tomatoes, halved
- ✓ 1/4 of a red onion, sliced, optional
- ✓ 1/4 cup diced bacon, trimmed of rind and fat (optional)
- ✓ Lemon wedges, to serve

Directions:

- In a large jug, whisk together the olive oil, lemon juice, water, chopped parsley, garlic, thyme, rosemary, salt, and pepper
- Pour half of the marinade into a large, shallow dish and refrigerate the remaining marinade to use as the dressing
- Add the chicken to the marinade in the bowl, allow the chicken to marinade for 15- minutes (or up to two hours in the refrigerator if you can)
- In the meantime,
- Once the chicken is ready, place a skillet or grill over medium-high heat add 1 tbsp of oil in, sear the chicken on both sides until browned and cooked through about 7 minutes per side, depending on thickness, and discard of the marinade
- Allow the chicken to rest for 5 minutes, slice and then allow the chicken to cool
- Distribute among the containers, and keep in the refrigerator
- To Serve: Reheat the chicken in the microwave for 30 seconds to 1 minutes. In a bowl, add the romaine lettuce, avocado, feta cheese, grape tomatoes, red onion and bacon, mix to combine. Arrange the chicken over salad. Drizzle the salad with the Untouched dressing. Serve with lemon wedges and enjoy!

Nutrition: Calories:378;Carbs: 6g;Total Fat: 22g;Protein: 31g

231) AVOCADO ARUGULA SALAD

Cooking Time: 15 Minutes **Servings: 4**

Ingredients:

- 4 cups packed baby arugula
- 4 green onions, tops trimmed, chopped
- 1½ cups shelled fava beans
- 3 Persian cucumbers, chopped
- 2 cups grape tomatoes, halved
- 1 jalapeno pepper, sliced
- 1 avocado, cored, peeled, and roughly chopped

- ✓ lemon juice, 1½ lemons
- ✓ ½ cup extra virgin olive oil
- ✓ salt
- ✓ pepper
- ✓ 1 garlic clove, finely chopped
- ✓ 2 tbsp fresh cilantro, finely chopped
- ✓ 2 tbsp fresh mint, finely chopped

Directions:

- Place the lemon-honey vinaigrette Ingredients: in a small bowl and whisk them well.
- In a large mixing bowl, add baby arugula, fava beans, green onions, tomatoes, cucumbers, and jalapeno.
- Divide the whole salad among four containers.
- Before serving, dress the salad with the vinaigrette and toss.
- Add the avocado to the salad.
- Enjoy!

Nutrition: Calories: 229, Total Fat: 11.1 g, Saturated Fat: 2.5 g, Cholesterol: 0 mg, Sodium: 24 mg, Total Carbohydrate: 32.1 g, Dietary Fiber: 12 g, Total Sugars: 10.1 g, Protein: 3 g, Vitamin D: 0 mcg, Calcium: 163 mg, Iron: 3 mg, Potassium: 1166 mg

232)   QUINOA STUFFED EGGPLANT AND TAHINI SAUCE

Cooking Time: 30 Minutes   **Servings: 2**

Ingredients:

- ✓ 1 eggplant
- ✓ 2 tbsp olive oil, divided
- ✓ 1 medium shallot, diced, about 1/2 cup
- ✓ 1 cup chopped button mushrooms, about 2 cups whole
- ✓ 5-6 Tuttorosso whole plum tomatoes, chopped
- ✓ 1 tbsp tomato juice from the can
- ✓ 1 tbsp chopped fresh parsley, plus more to garnish
- ✓ 2 garlic cloves, minced
- ✓ 1/2 cup cooked quinoa
- ✓ 1/2 tsp ground cumin
- ✓ Salt, to taste
- ✓ Pepper, to taste
- ✓ 1 tbsp tahini
- ✓ 1 tsp lemon juice
- ✓ 1/2 tsp garlic powder
- ✓ Water to thin

Directions:

- ❖ Preheat the oven to 425 degrees F
- ❖ Prepare the eggplant by cutting it in half lengthwise and scoop out some of the flesh
- ❖ Place it on a baking sheet, drizzle with 1 tbsp of oil, sprinkle with salt
- ❖ Bake for 20 minutes
- ❖ In the meantime, add the remaining oil in a large skillet
- ❖ Once heated, add the shallots and mushrooms, sauté until mushrooms have softened, about 5 minutes Add in the tomatoes, quinoa and spices, cook until the liquid has evaporated
- ❖ Once the eggplant has cooked, reduce the oven temperature to 350 degrees F
- ❖ Stuff each half with the tomato-quinoa mixture
- ❖ Bake for another 10 minutes
- ❖ Allow to cool completely
- ❖ Distribute among the containers, store for 2 days
- ❖ To Serve: Reheat in the microwave for 1-2 minutes or until heated through. Quickly whisk together tahini, lemon, garlic, water and a sprinkle of salt and pepper, drizzle tahini over eggplants and sprinkle with parsley and enjoy.

Nutrition: Calories:345;Carbs: 38g;Total Fat: 19g;Protein: 9g

233)   POMODORO SOUP

Cooking Time: 30 Minutes   **Servings: 8**

Ingredients:

- ✓ 4 tbsp olive oil
- ✓ 2 medium yellow onions, thinly sliced
- ✓ 1 tsp salt (extra for taste if needed)
- ✓ 2 tsp curry powder
- ✓ 1 tsp red curry powder
- ✓ 1 tsp ground coriander
- ✓ 1 tsp ground cumin
- ✓ ¼-½ tsp red pepper flakes
- ✓ 1 15-ounce can diced tomatoes, undrained
- ✓ 1 28-ounce can diced or plum tomatoes, undrained
- ✓ 5½ cups water (vegetable broth or chicken broth also usable)
- ✓ 1 14-ounce can coconut milk
- ✓ optional add-ins: cooked brown rice, lemon wedges, fresh thyme, etc.

Directions:

- ❖ Heat oil in a medium-sized pot over medium heat.
- ❖ Add onions and salt and cook for about 10-1minutes until browned.
- ❖ Stir in curry powder, coriander, red pepper flakes, cumin, and cook for seconds, being sure to keep stirring well.
- ❖ Add tomatoes and water (or broth if you prefer).
- ❖ Simmer the mixture for 1minutes.
- ❖ Take an immersion blender and puree the mixture until a soupy consistency is achieved.
- ❖ Enjoy as it is, or add some extra add-ins for a more flavorful experience

Nutrition: Calories: 217, Total Fat: 19.3 g, Saturated Fat: 11.5 g, Cholesterol: 0 mg, Sodium: 40 mg, Total Carbohydrate: 12.1 g, Dietary Fiber: 3.g, Total Sugars: 7.1 g, Protein: 3 g, Vitamin D: 0 mcg, Calcium: 58 mg, Iron: 2 mg, Potassium: 570 mg

234) ONION CHEESE SOUP

Cooking Time: 25 Minutes   **Servings: 4**

Ingredients:

- ✓ 2 large onions, finely sliced
- ✓ 2 cups vegetable stock
- ✓ 1 tsp brown sugar
- ✓ 1 cup red wine
- ✓ 1 measure of brandy
- ✓ 1 tsp herbs de Provence
- ✓ 4 slices stale bread
- ✓ 4 ounces grated strong cheese
- ✓ 1-ounce grated parmesan
- ✓ 1 tbsp plain flour
- ✓ 2 tbsp olive oil
- ✓ 1-ounce butter
- ✓ salt
- ✓ pepper

Directions:

- ❖ Heat oil and butter in a pan over medium-high heat.
- ❖ Add onions and brown sugar.
- ❖ Cook until the onions are golden brown.
- ❖ Pour brandy and flambé, making sure to keep stirring until the flames are out.
- ❖ Add plain flour and herbs de Provence and keep stirring well.
- ❖ Slowly add the stock and red wine.
- ❖ Season well and simmer for 20 minutes, making sure to add water if the soup becomes too thick.
- ❖ Ladle the soup into jars.
- ❖ Before serving, place rounds of stale bread on top.
- ❖ Add strong cheese.
- ❖ Garnish with some parmesan.
- ❖ Place the bowls under a hot grill or in an oven until the cheese has melted.

Nutrition: Calories: 403, Total Fat: 22.4 g, Saturated Fat: 10.9 g, Cholesterol: 41 mg, Sodium: 886 mg, Total Carbohydrate: 24.9 g, Dietary Fiber: 3.6 g, Total Sugars: 7 g, Protein: 16.2 g, Vitamin D: 4 mcg, Calcium: 371 mg, Iron: 1 mg, Potassium: 242 mg

235) SOLE FISH WITH PISTACHIO

Cooking Time: 10 Minutes   **Servings: 4**

Ingredients:

- ✓ 4 (5 ounces boneless sole fillets
- ✓ Salt and pepper as needed
- ✓ ½ cup pistachios, finely chopped
- ✓ Zest of 1 lemon
- ✓ Juice of 1 lemon
- ✓ 1 tsp extra virgin olive oil

Directions:

- ❖ Pre-heat your oven to 350 degrees Fahrenheit
- ❖ Line a baking sheet with parchment paper and keep it on the side
- ❖ Pat fish dry with kitchen towels and lightly season with salt and pepper
- ❖ Take a small bowl and stir in pistachios and lemon zest
- ❖ Place sol on the prepped sheet and press 2 tbsp of pistachio mixture on top of each fillet
- ❖ Drizzle fish with lemon juice and olive oil
- ❖ Bake for 10 minutes until the top is golden and fish flakes with a fork
- ❖ Serve and enjoy!
- ❖ Meal Prep/Storage Options: Store in airtight containers in your fridge for 1-2 days.

Nutrition: Calories: 166;Fat: 6g;Carbohydrates: 2g;Protein: 26g

236) ITALIAN-STYLE LASAGNA

Cooking Time: 1 Hour 15 Minutes   **Servings: 8**

Ingredients:

- ✓ Lasagna noodles, oven-ready are the best, easiest, and quickest
- ✓ ⅓ cup flour
- ✓ 2 tbsp chives, divided and chopped
- ✓ ½ cup white wine
- ✓ 2 tbsp olive oil
- ✓ 1 ½ tbsp thyme
- ✓ 1 tsp salt
- ✓ 1 ¼ cups shallots, chopped
- ✓ 1 cup boiled water
- ✓ ½ cup Parmigiano-Reggiano cheese
- ✓ 3 cups milk, reduced-fat and divided
- ✓ 1 tbsp butter
- ✓ ⅓ cup cream cheese, less fat is the best choice
- ✓ 6 cloves of garlic, divided and minced
- ✓ ½ tsp ground black pepper, divided
- ✓ 4 ounces dried shiitake mushrooms, sliced
- ✓ 1 ounce dried porcini mushrooms, sliced
- ✓ 8 ounces cremini mushrooms, sliced

Directions:

- ❖ Keeping your mushrooms separated, drain them all and return them to separate containers.
- ❖ Bring 1 cup of water to a boil and cook your porcini mushrooms for a half hour.
- ❖ Preheat your oven to 0 degrees Fahrenheit.
- ❖ Set a large pan on your stove and turn the burner to medium-high heat.
- ❖ Add your butter and let it melt.
- ❖ Combine the olive oil and shallots. Stir the mixture and let it cook for 3 minutes.
- ❖ Pour half of the pepper, half of the salt, and mushrooms into the pan. Allow the mixture to cook for 6 to minutes.
- ❖ While stirring, add half of the garlic and thyme. Continue to stir for 1 minute.
- ❖ Pour the wine and turn your burner temperature to high. Let the mixture boil and watch the liquid evaporate for a couple of minutes to reduce it slightly.
- ❖ Turn off the burner and remove the pan from heat.
- ❖ Add the cream cheese and chives. Stir thoroughly.
- ❖ Set a medium-sized skillet on medium-high heat and add 1 tbsp of oil. Let the oil come to a simmer.
- ❖ Add the last of the garlic to the pan and saute for 30 seconds.
- ❖ Pour in 2 ⅓ cup milk and the liquid from the porcini mushrooms. Stir the mixture and allow it to boil.
- ❖ In a bowl, combine ¼ cup of milk and the flour. Add this mixture to the heated pan. Stir until the mixture starts to thicken.
- ❖ Grease a pan and add ½ cup of sauce along with a row of noodles.
- ❖ Spread half of the mushroom mixture on top of the noodles.
- ❖ Repeat the process, but make sure you top the lasagna with mushrooms and cheese.
- ❖ Turn your timer to 45 minutes and set the pan into the oven.
- ❖ Remember to garnish the lasagna with chives before enjoying!

Nutrition: calories: 268, fats: 12.6 grams, carbohydrates: 29 grams, protein: 10 grams.

237) CARROT SOUP AND PARMESAN CROUTONS

Cooking Time: 25 To 30 Minutes   **Servings: 4**

Ingredients:

- ✓ 2 cups vegetable broth, no salt added, and low sodium is best
- ✓ 1 tsp dried thyme
- ✓ ¼ tsp sea salt
- ✓ 1 ounce grated parmesan cheese
- ✓ 2 pounds of carrots, unpeeled
- ✓ 2 tbsp extra virgin olive oil
- ✓ ½ chopped onion
- ✓ 2 ½ cups water
- ✓ ¼ tsp crushed red pepper
- ✓ 4 slices of whole-grain bread

Directions:

- ❖ Cut your carrots into ½-inch slices
- ❖ Take one rack from your oven and place it four inches from the broiler heating element. One either rack, place two large-rimmed baking sheets and turn your oven to 450 degrees Fahrenheit.
- ❖ Add 1 tbsp of oil and carrots into a large bowl. Stir the carrots around so they become coated with the oil.
- ❖ Using oven mitts, remove the baking pans and distribute the carrots onto them.
- ❖ Place the pans back into the oven and turn your timer on for 20 minutes or until the carrots become tender.
- ❖ Take the carrots out of the oven.
- ❖ Turn your oven to broiler mode.
- ❖ Set a large stockpot on your stove and turn the range to medium-high.
- ❖ Pour in the remaining olive oil and the onion. Let it cook for 5 minutes while stirring occasionally.
- ❖ Pour in the broth, thyme, water, crushed red pepper, and sea salt. Stir well.
- ❖ Let the mixture cook until the ingredients come to a boil.
- ❖ Once the carrots are done in the oven, add them to the pot.
- ❖ Remove the pot from the heat and carefully pour the soup into a blender. You will want to pour it in batches and remember to hold the lid of the blender with a rag and release the steam after 30 seconds, so it doesn't explode.
- ❖ Once all the soup is mixed, add it all back into the pot and turn the range heat to medium. Cook until the soup is warm again.
- ❖ Spread a piece of parchment paper on top of a baking sheet, set the four pieces of bread on the paper.
- ❖ Sprinkle cheese across the slices and set them on the top rack in your oven.
- ❖ Turn your oven to broil and let the slices of bread roast for a couple of minutes. Once the cheese is melted, remove the bread from the oven so they don't burn.
- ❖ Chop the bread into croutons.
- ❖ Divide the soup into serving bowls, add the croutons, and enjoy!

Nutrition: Nutrition: calories: 272, fats: 10 grams, carbohydrates: 38 grams, protein: 10 grams.

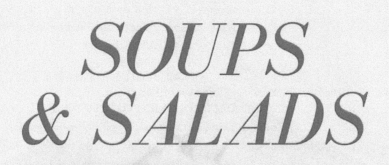

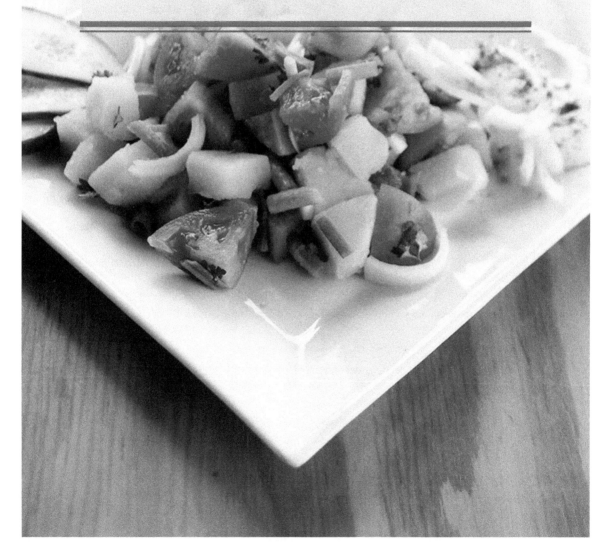

238) SPECIAL CHEESY BROCCOLI SOUP

Cooking Time: 30 Minutes   **Servings: 4**

Ingredients:

- ½ cup heavy whipping cream
- 1 cup broccoli
- ✓ 1 cup cheddar cheese
- ✓ Salt, to taste
- ✓ 1½ cups chicken broth

Directions:

- ❖ Heat chicken broth in a large pot and add broccoli.
- ❖ Bring to a boil and stir in the rest of the ingredients.
- ❖ Allow the soup to simmer on low heat for about 20 minutes.
- ❖ Ladle out into a bowl and serve hot.

Nutrition: Calories: 188;Carbs: 2.6g;Fats: 15g;Proteins: 9.8g;Sodium: 514mg;Sugar: 0.8g

239) DELICIOUS RICH POTATO SOUP

Cooking Time: 30 Minutes   **Servings: 4**

Ingredients:

- ✓ 1 tbsp butter
- ✓ 1 medium onion, diced
- ✓ 3 cloves garlic, minced
- ✓ 3 cups chicken broth
- ✓ 1 can/box cream of chicken soup
- ✓ 7-8 medium-sized russet potatoes, peeled and chopped
- ✓ 1 1/2 tsp salt
- ✓ Black pepper to taste
- ✓ 1 cup milk
- ✓ 1 tbsp flour
- ✓ 2 cups shredded cheddar cheese
- ✓ Garnish:
- ✓ 5-6 slices bacon, chopped
- ✓ Sliced green onions
- ✓ Shredded cheddar cheese

Directions:

- ❖ Heat butter in the insert of the Instant Pot on sauté mode.
- ❖ Add onions and sauté for 4 minutes until soft.
- ❖ Stir in garlic and sauté it for 1 minute.
- ❖ Add potatoes, cream of chicken, broth, salt, and pepper to the insert.
- ❖ Mix well then seal and lock the lid.
- ❖ Cook this mixture for 10 minutes at Manual Mode with high pressure.
- ❖ Meanwhile, mix flour with milk in a bowl and set it aside.
- ❖ Once the instant pot beeps, release the pressure completely.
- ❖ Remove the Instant Pot lid and switch the instant pot to Sauté mode.
- ❖ Pour in flour slurry and stir cook the mixture for 5 minutes until it thickens.
- ❖ Add 2 cups of cheddar cheese and let it melt.
- ❖ Garnish it as desired.
- ❖ Serve.

Nutrition: Calories: 784;Carbohydrate: 54.8g;Protein: 34g;Fat: 46.5g;Sugar: 7.5g;Sodium: 849mg

240) MEDITERRANEAN-STYLE LENTIL SOUP

Cooking Time: 20 Minutes   **Servings:** 4

Ingredients:

- ✓ 1 tbsp olive oil
- ✓ 1/2 cup red lentils
- ✓ 1 medium yellow or red onion
- ✓ 2 garlic cloves, chopped
- ✓ 1/2 tsp ground cumin
- ✓ 1/2 tsp ground coriander
- ✓ 1/2 tsp ground sumac
- ✓ 1/2 tsp red chili flakes
- ✓ 1/2 tsp dried parsley
- ✓ 3/4 tsp dried mint flakes
- ✓ pinch of sugar
- ✓ 2.5 cups water
- ✓ salt, to taste
- ✓ black pepper, to taste
- ✓ juice of 1/2 lime
- ✓ parsley or cilantro, to garnish

Directions:

- ❖ Preheat oil in the insert of your Instant Pot on Sauté mode.
- ❖ Add onion and sauté until it turns golden brown.
- ❖ Toss in the garlic, parsley sugar, mint flakes, red chili flakes, sumac, coriander, and cumin.
- ❖ Stir cook this mixture for 2 minutes.
- ❖ Add water, lentils, salt, and pepper. Stir gently.
- ❖ Seal and lock the Instant Pot lid and select Manual mode for 8 minutes at high pressure.
- ❖ Once done, release the pressure completely then remove the lid.
- ❖ Stir well then add lime juice.
- ❖ Serve warm.

Nutrition: Calories: 525;Carbohydrate: 59.8g;Protein: 30.1g;Fat: 19.3g;Sugar: 17.3g;Sodium: 897mg

241) DELICIOUS CREAMY KETO CUCUMBER SALAD

Cooking Time: 5 Minutes   **Servings:** 2

Ingredients:

- ✓ 2 tbsp mayonnaise
- ✓ Salt and black pepper, to taste
- ✓ 1 cucumber, sliced and quartered
- ✓ 2 tbsp lemon juice

Directions:

- ❖ Mix together the mayonnaise, cucumber slices, and lemon juice in a large bowl.
- ❖ Season with salt and black pepper and combine well.
- ❖ Dish out in a glass bowl and serve while it is cold.

Nutrition: Calories: 8Carbs: 9.3g;Fats: 5.2g;Proteins: 1.2g;Sodium: 111mg;Sugar: 3.8g

242) SAUSAGE KALE SOUP AND MUSHROOMS

Cooking Time: 1 Hour 10 Minutes   **Servings:** 6

Ingredients:

- ✓ 2 cups fresh kale, cut into bite sized pieces
- ✓ 6.5 ounces mushrooms, sliced
- ✓ 6 cups chicken bone broth
- ✓ 1 pound sausage, cooked and sliced
- ✓ Salt and black pepper, to taste

Directions:

- ❖ Heat chicken broth with two cans of water in a large pot and bring to a boil.
- ❖ Stir in the rest of the ingredients and allow the soup to simmer on low heat for about 1 hour.
- ❖ Dish out and serve hot.

Nutrition: Calories: 259;Carbs: ;Fats: 20g;Proteins: 14g;Sodium: 995mg;Sugar: 0.6g

243) CLASSIC MINESTRONE SOUP

Cooking Time: 25 Minutes   **Servings: 6**

Ingredients:

- ✓ 2 tbsp olive oil
- ✓ 3 cloves garlic, minced
- ✓ 1 onion, diced
- ✓ 2 carrots, peeled and diced
- ✓ 2 stalks celery, diced
- ✓ 1 1/2 tsp dried basil
- ✓ 1 tsp dried oregano
- ✓ 1/2 tsp fennel seed
- ✓ 6 cups low sodium chicken broth
- ✓ 1 (28-ounce can diced tomatoes
- ✓ 1 (16-ounce can kidney beans, drained and rinsed
- ✓ 1 zucchini, chopped
- ✓ 1 (3-inch Parmesan rind
- ✓ 1 bay leaf
- ✓ 1 bunch kale leaves, chopped
- ✓ 2 tsp red wine vinegar
- ✓ Kosher salt and black pepper, to taste
- ✓ 1/3 cup freshly grated Parmesan
- ✓ 2 tbsp chopped fresh parsley leaves

Directions:

- ❖ Preheat olive oil in the insert of the Instant Pot on Sauté mode.
- ❖ Add carrots, celery, and onion, sauté for 3 minutes.
- ❖ Stir in fennel seeds, oregano, and basil. Stir cook for 1 minute.
- ❖ Add stock, beans, tomatoes, parmesan, bay leaf, and zucchini.
- ❖ Secure and seal the Instant Pot lid then select Manual mode to cook for minutes at high pressure.
- ❖ Once done, release the pressure completely then remove the lid.
- ❖ Add kale and let it sit for 2 minutes in the hot soup.
- ❖ Stir in red wine, vinegar, pepper, and salt.
- ❖ Garnish with parsley and parmesan.
- ❖ Enjoy.

Nutrition: Calories: 805;Carbohydrate: 2.5g;Protein: 124.1g;Fat: 34g;Sugar: 1.4g;Sodium: 634mg

244) SPECIAL KOMBU SEAWEED SALAD

Cooking Time: 40 Minutes   **Servings: 6**

Ingredients:

- ✓ 4 garlic cloves, crushed
- ✓ 1 pound fresh kombu seaweed, boiled and cut into strips
- ✓ 2 tbsp apple cider vinegar
- ✓ Salt, to taste
- ✓ 2 tbsp coconut aminos

Directions:

- ❖ Mix together the kombu, garlic, apple cider vinegar, and coconut aminos in a large bowl.
- ❖ Season with salt and combine well.
- ❖ Dish out in a glass bowl and serve immediately.

Nutrition: Calories: 257;Carbs: 16.9g;Fats: 19.;Proteins: 6.5g;Sodium: 294mg;Sugar: 2.7g

245) LOVELY MINT AVOCADO CHILLED SOUP

Cooking Time: 5 Minutes   **Servings: 2**

Ingredients:

- ✓ 1 cup coconut milk, chilled
- ✓ 1 medium ripe avocado
- ✓ 1 tbsp lime juice
- ✓ Salt, to taste
- ✓ 20 fresh mint leaves

Directions:

- ❖ Put all the ingredients into an immersion blender and blend until a thick mixture is formed.
- ❖ Allow to cool in the fridge for about 10 minutes and serve chilled.

Nutrition: Calories: 286;Carbs: 12.6g;Fats: 26.9g;Proteins: 4.2g;Sodium: 70mg;Sugar: 4.6g

246) SPECIAL BUTTERNUT SQUASH SOUP

Cooking Time: 40 Minutes   **Servings:** 4

Ingredients:

- ✓ 1 tbsp olive oil
- ✓ 1 medium yellow onion chopped
- ✓ 1 large carrot chopped
- ✓ 1 celery rib chopped
- ✓ 3 cloves of garlic minced
- ✓ 2 lbs. butternut squash, peeled chopped
- ✓ 2 cups vegetable broth
- ✓ 1 green apple peeled, cored, and chopped
- ✓ 1/4 tsp ground cinnamon
- ✓ 1 sprig fresh thyme
- ✓ 1 sprig fresh rosemary
- ✓ 1 tsp kosher salt
- ✓ 1/2 tsp black pepper
- ✓ Pinch of nutmeg optional

Directions:

- ❖ Preheat olive oil in the insert of the Instant Pot on Sauté mode.
- ❖ Add celery, carrots, and garlic, sauté for 5 minutes.
- ❖ Stir in squash, broth, cinnamon, apple nutmeg, rosemary, thyme, salt, and pepper.
- ❖ Mix well gently then seal and secure the lid.
- ❖ Select Manual mode to cook for 10 minutes at high pressure.
- ❖ Once done, release the pressure completely then remove the lid.
- ❖ Puree the soup using an immersion blender.
- ❖ Serve warm.

Nutrition: Calories: 282;Carbohydrate: 50g;Protein: 13g;Fat: 4.7g;Sugar: 12.8g;Sodium: 213mg

247) LOVELY CREAMY CILANTRO LIME COLESLAW

Cooking Time: 10 Minutes   **Servings:** 2

Ingredients:

- ✓ ¾ avocado
- ✓ 1 lime, juiced
- ✓ 1/8 cup water
- ✓ Cilantro, to garnish
- ✓ 6 oz coleslaw, bagged
- ✓ 1/8 cup cilantro leaves
- ✓ 1 garlic clove
- ✓ ¼ tsp salt

Directions:

- ❖ Put garlic and cilantro in a food processor and process until chopped.
- ❖ Add lime juice, avocado and water and pulse until creamy.
- ❖ Put coleslaw in a large bowl and stir in the avocado mixture.
- ❖ Refrigerate for a few hours before serving.

Nutrition: Calories: 240;Carbs: 17.4g;Fats: 19.6g;Proteins: 2.8g;Sodium: 0mg;Sugar: 0.5g

248) CLASSIC SNAP PEA SALAD

Cooking Time: 15 Minutes   **Servings:** 2

Ingredients:

- ✓ 1/8 cup lemon juice
- ✓ ½ clove garlic, crushed
- ✓ 4 ounces cauliflower riced
- ✓ 1/8 cup olive oil
- ✓ ¼ tsp coarse grain Dijon mustard
- ✓ ½ tsp granulated stevia
- ✓ ¼ cup sugar snap peas, ends removed and each pod cut into three pieces
- ✓ 1/8 cup chives
- ✓ 1/8 cup red onions, minced
- ✓ Sea salt and black pepper, to taste
- ✓ ¼ cup almonds, sliced

Directions:

- ❖ Pour water in a pot fitted with a steamer basket and bring water to a boil.
- ❖ Place riced cauliflower in the steamer basket and season with sea salt.
- ❖ Cover the pot and steam for about 10 minutes until tender.
- ❖ Drain the cauliflower and dish out in a bowl to refrigerate for about 1 hour.
- ❖ Meanwhile, make a dressing by mixing olive oil, lemon juice, garlic, mustard, stevia, salt and black pepper in a bowl.
- ❖ Mix together chilled cauliflower, peas, chives, almonds and red onions in another bowl.
- ❖ Pour the dressing over this mixture and serve.

Nutrition: Calories: 203;Carbs: 7.6g;Fats: 18g;Proteins: 4.2g;Sodium: 28mg;Sugar: 2.9g

249) SPINACH AND BACON SALAD

Cooking Time: 15 Minutes   Servings: 4

Ingredients:

- ✓ 2 eggs, boiled, halved, and sliced
- ✓ 10 oz. organic baby spinach, rinsed, and dried
- ✓ 8 pieces thick bacon, cooked and sliced
- ✓ ½ cup plain mayonnaise
- ✓ ½ medium red onion, thinly sliced

Directions:

- ❖ Mix together the mayonnaise and spinach in a large bowl.
- ❖ Stir in the rest of the ingredients and combine well.
- ❖ Dish out in a glass bowl and serve well.

Nutrition: Calories: 373;Carbs: ;Fats: 34.5g;Proteins: 11g;Sodium: 707mg;Sugar: 1.1g

250) EGG, AVOCADO WITH TOMATO SALAD

Cooking Time: 40 Minutes   Servings: 4

Ingredients:

- ✓ 2 boiled eggs, chopped into chunks
- ✓ 1 ripe avocado, chopped into chunks
- ✓ 1 medium-sized tomato, chopped into chunks
- ✓ Salt and black pepper, to taste
- ✓ 1 lemon wedge, juiced

Directions:

- ❖ Mix together all the ingredients in a large bowl until well combined.
- ❖ Dish out in a glass bowl and serve immediately.

Nutrition: Calories: 140;Carbs: 5.9g;Fats: 12.1g;Proteins: 4g;Sodium: mg;Sugar: 1.3g

251) SPECIAL CREAMY LOW CARB BUTTERNUT SQUASH SOUP

Cooking Time: 1 Hour 10 Minutes   Servings: 8

Ingredients:

- ✓ 2 tbsp avocado oil, divided
- ✓ 2 pounds butternut squash, cut in half length-wise and seeds removed
- ✓ Sea salt and black pepper, to taste
- ✓ 1 (13.5-oz can coconut milk
- ✓ 4 cups chicken bone broth

Directions:

- ❖ Preheat the oven to 400 degrees F and grease a baking sheet.
- ❖ Arrange the butternut squash halves with open side up on the baking sheet.
- ❖ Drizzle with half of the avocado oil and season with sea salt and black pepper.
- ❖ Flip over and transfer into the oven.
- ❖ Roast the butternut squash for about minutes.
- ❖ Heat the remaining avocado oil over medium heat in a large pot and add the broth and coconut milk.
- ❖ Let it simmer for about 20 minutes and scoop the squash out of the shells to transfer into the soup.
- ❖ Puree this mixture in an immersion blender until smooth and serve immediately.

Nutrition: Calories: 185;Carbs: 12.6g;Fats: 12.6g;Proteins: 4.7g;Sodium: 3mg;Sugar: 4.5g

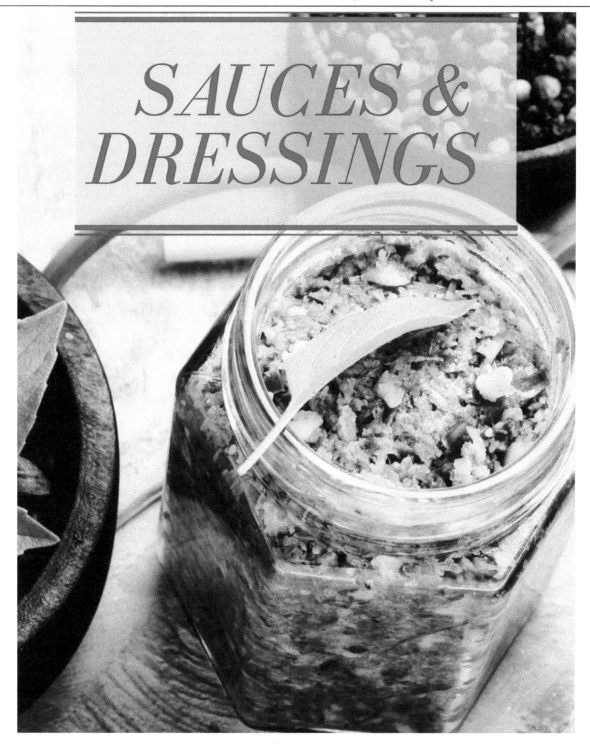

252) BULGUR PILAF AND ALMONDS

Cooking Time: 20 Minutes   **Servings:** 4

Ingredients:

- ✓ ⅔ cup uncooked bulgur
- ✓ 1⅓ cups water
- ✓ ¼ cup sliced almonds
- ✓ 1 cup small diced red bell pepper
- ✓ ⅓ cup chopped fresh cilantro
- ✓ 1 tbsp olive oil
- ✓ ¼ tsp salt

Directions:

- ❖ Place the bulgur and water in a saucepan and bring the water to a boil. Once the water is at a boil, cover the pot with a lid and turn off the heat. Let the covered pot stand for 20 minutes.
- ❖ Transfer the cooked bulgur to a large mixing bowl and add the almonds, peppers, cilantro, oil, and salt. Stir to combine.
- ❖ Place about 1 cup of bulgur in each of 4 containers.
- ❖ STORAGE: Store covered containers in the refrigerator for up to 5 days. Bulgur can be either reheated or eaten at room temperature.

Nutrition: Total calories: 17 Total fat: 7g; Saturated fat: 1g; Sodium: 152mg; Carbohydrates: 25g; Fiber: 6g; Protein: 4g

253) SPANISH GARLIC YOGURT SAUCE

Cooking Time: 5 Minutes   **Servings:** 1 Cup

Ingredients:

- ✓ 1 cup low-fat (2%) plain Greek yogurt
- ✓ ½ tsp garlic powder
- ✓ 1 tbsp freshly squeezed lemon juice
- ✓ 1 tbsp olive oil
- ✓ ¼ tsp kosher salt

Directions:

- ❖ Mix all the ingredients in a medium bowl until well combined.
- ❖ Spoon the yogurt sauce into a container and refrigerate.
- ❖ STORAGE: Store the covered container in the refrigerator for up to 7 days

Nutrition: (¼ cup): Total calories: 75; Total fat: 5g; Saturated fat: 1g; Sodium: 173mg; Carbohydrates: 3g; Fiber: 0g; Protein: 6g.

254) ORANGE WITH CINNAMON–SCENTED WHOLE-WHEAT COUSCOUS

Cooking Time: 10 Minutes   **Servings:** 4

Ingredients:

- ✓ 2 tsp olive oil
- ✓ ¼ cup minced shallot
- ✓ ½ cup freshly squeezed orange juice (from 2 oranges)
- ✓ ½ cup water
- ✓ ⅛ tsp ground cinnamon
- ✓ ¼ tsp kosher salt
- ✓ 1 cup whole-wheat couscous

Directions:

- ❖ Heat the oil in a saucepan over medium heat. Once the oil is shimmering, add the shallot and cook for 2 minutes, stirring frequently. Add the orange juice, water, cinnamon, and salt, and bring to a boil.
- ❖ Once the liquid is boiling, add the couscous, cover the pan, and turn off the heat. Leave the couscous covered for 5 minutes. When the couscous is done, fluff with a fork.
- ❖ Place ¾ cup of couscous in each of 4 containers.
- ❖ STORAGE: Store covered containers in the refrigerator for up to 5 days. Freeze for up to 2 months.

Nutrition: Total calories: 21 Total fat: 4g; Saturated fat: <1g; Sodium: 147mg; Carbohydrates: 41g; Fiber: 5g; Protein: 8g

255) CHUNKY ROASTED CHERRY TOMATO WITH BASIL SAUCE

Cooking Time: 40 Minutes   **Servings:** 1⅓ Cups

Ingredients:

- 2 pints cherry tomatoes (20 ounces total)
- 2 tsp olive oil, plus 3 tbsp
- ¼ tsp kosher salt
- ½ tsp chopped garlic
- ¼ cup fresh basil leaves

Directions:

- Preheat the oven to 350°F. Line a sheet pan with a silicone baking mat or parchment paper.
- Place the tomatoes on the lined sheet pan and toss with tsp of oil. Roast for 40 minutes, shaking the pan halfway through.
- While the tomatoes are still warm, place them in a medium mixing bowl and add the salt, the garlic, and the remaining tbsp of oil. Mash the tomatoes with the back of a fork. Stir in the fresh basil.
- Scoop the sauce into a container and refrigerate.
- STORAGE: Store the covered container in the refrigerator for up to days.

Nutrition: (⅓ cup): Total calories: 141; Total fat: 13g; Saturated fat: 2g; Sodium: 158mg; Carbohydrates: 7g; Fiber: 2g; Protein: 1g

256) CELERY HEART, BASIL, AND ALMOND PESTO

Cooking Time: 10 Minutes   **Servings: 1 Cup**

Ingredients:

- ½ cup raw, unsalted almonds
- 3 cups fresh basil leaves, (about 1½ ounces)
- ½ cup chopped celery hearts with leaves
- ¼ tsp kosher salt
- 1 tbsp freshly squeezed lemon juice
- ¼ cup olive oil
- 3 tbsp water

Directions:

- Place the almonds in the bowl of a food processor and process until they look like coarse sand.
- Add the basil, celery hearts, salt, lemon juice, oil and water and process until smooth. The sauce will be somewhat thick. If you would like a thinner sauce, add more water, oil, or lemon juice, depending on your taste preference.
- Scoop the pesto into a container and refrigerate.
- STORAGE: Store the covered container in the refrigerator for up to 2 weeks. Pesto may be frozen for up to 6 months.

Nutrition: (¼ cup): Total calories: 231; Total fat: 22g; Saturated fat: 3g; Sodium: 178mg; Carbohydrates: 6g; Fiber: 3g; Protein: 4g

257) SPECIAL POMEGRANATE VINAIGRETTE

Cooking Time: 5 Minutes   **Servings: ½ Cup**

Ingredients:

- ⅓ cup pomegranate juice
- 1 tsp Dijon mustard
- 1 tbsp apple cider vinegar
- ½ tsp dried mint
- 2 tbsp plus 2 tsp olive oil

Directions:

- Place the pomegranate juice, mustard, vinegar, and mint in a small bowl and whisk to combine.
- Whisk in the oil, pouring it into the bowl in a thin steam.
- Pour the vinaigrette into a container and refrigerate.
- STORAGE: Store the covered container in the refrigerator for up to 2 weeks. Bring the vinaigrette to room temperature and shake before serving.

Nutrition: (2 tbsp): Total calories: 94; Total fat: 10g; Saturated fat: 2g; Sodium: 30mg; Carbohydrates: 3g; Fiber: 0g; Protein: 0g

258)   GREEN OLIVE WITH SPINACH TAPENADE

Cooking Time: 20 Minutes   **Servings: 1½ Cups**

Ingredients:

- ✓ 1 cup pimento-stuffed green olives, drained
- ✓ 3 packed cups baby spinach
- ✓ 1 tsp chopped garlic
- ✓ ½ tsp dried oregano
- ✓ ⅓ cup packed fresh basil
- ✓ 2 tbsp olive oil
- ✓ 2 tsp red wine vinegar

Directions:

- ❖ Place all the ingredients in the bowl of a food processor and pulse until the mixture looks finely chopped but not puréed.
- ❖ Scoop the tapenade into a container and refrigerate.
- ❖ STORAGE: Store the covered container in the refrigerator for up to 5 days.

Nutrition: (¼ cup): Total calories: 80; Total fat: 8g; Saturated fat: 1g; Sodium: 6mg; Carbohydrates: 1g; Fiber: 1g; Protein: 1g

259)   SPANISH GARLIC YOGURT SAUCE

Cooking Time: 5 Minutes   **Servings: 1 Cup**

Ingredients:

- ✓ 1 cup low-fat (2%) plain Greek yogurt
- ✓ ½ tsp garlic powder
- ✓ 1 tbsp freshly squeezed lemon juice
- ✓ 1 tbsp olive oil
- ✓ ¼ tsp kosher salt

Directions:

- ❖ Mix all the ingredients in a medium bowl until well combined.
- ❖ Spoon the yogurt sauce into a container and refrigerate.
- ❖ STORAGE: Store the covered container in the refrigerator for up to 7 days

Nutrition: (¼ cup): Total calories: 75; Total fat: 5g; Saturated fat: 1g; Sodium: 173mg; Carbohydrates: 3g; Fiber: 0g; Protein: 6g.

260)   ORANGE WITH CINNAMON–SCENTED WHOLE-WHEAT COUSCOUS

Cooking Time: 10 Minutes   **Servings: 4**

Ingredients:

- ✓ 2 tsp olive oil
- ✓ ¼ cup minced shallot
- ✓ ½ cup freshly squeezed orange juice (from 2 oranges)
- ✓ ½ cup water
- ✓ ⅛ tsp ground cinnamon
- ✓ ¼ tsp kosher salt
- ✓ 1 cup whole-wheat couscous

Directions:

- ❖ Heat the oil in a saucepan over medium heat. Once the oil is shimmering, add the shallot and cook for 2 minutes, stirring frequently. Add the orange juice, water, cinnamon, and salt, and bring to a boil.
- ❖ Once the liquid is boiling, add the couscous, cover the pan, and turn off the heat. Leave the couscous covered for 5 minutes. When the couscous is done, fluff with a fork.
- ❖ Place ¾ cup of couscous in each of 4 containers.
- ❖ STORAGE: Store covered containers in the refrigerator for up to 5 days. Freeze for up to 2 months.

Nutrition: Total calories: 21 Total fat: 4g; Saturated fat: <1g; Sodium: 147mg; Carbohydrates: 41g; Fiber: 5g; Protein: 8g

261)   CHUNKY ROASTED CHERRY TOMATO WITH BASIL SAUCE

Cooking Time: 40 Minutes   **Servings: 1⅓ Cups**

Ingredients:

- ✓ 2 pints cherry tomatoes (20 ounces total)
- ✓ 2 tsp olive oil, plus 3 tbsp
- ✓ ¼ tsp kosher salt
- ✓ ½ tsp chopped garlic
- ✓ ¼ cup fresh basil leaves

Directions:

- ❖ Preheat the oven to 350°F. Line a sheet pan with a silicone baking mat or parchment paper.
- ❖ Place the tomatoes on the lined sheet pan and toss with tsp of oil. Roast for 40 minutes, shaking the pan halfway through.
- ❖ While the tomatoes are still warm, place them in a medium mixing bowl and add the salt, the garlic, and the remaining tbsp of oil. Mash the tomatoes with the back of a fork. Stir in the fresh basil.
- ❖ Scoop the sauce into a container and refrigerate.
- ❖ STORAGE: Store the covered container in the refrigerator for up to days.

Nutrition: (⅓ cup): Total calories: 141; Total fat: 13g; Saturated fat: 2g; Sodium: 158mg; Carbohydrates: 7g; Fiber: 2g; Protein: 1g

262)   CELERY HEART, BASIL, AND ALMOND PESTO

Cooking Time: 10 Minutes   **Servings: 1 Cup**

Ingredients:

- ✓ ½ cup raw, unsalted almonds
- ✓ 3 cups fresh basil leaves, (about 1½ ounces)
- ✓ ½ cup chopped celery hearts with leaves
- ✓ ¼ tsp kosher salt
- ✓ 1 tbsp freshly squeezed lemon juice
- ✓ ¼ cup olive oil
- ✓ 3 tbsp water

Directions:

- ❖ Place the almonds in the bowl of a food processor and process until they look like coarse sand.
- ❖ Add the basil, celery hearts, salt, lemon juice, oil and water and process until smooth. The sauce will be somewhat thick. If you would like a thinner sauce, add more water, oil, or lemon juice, depending on your taste preference.
- ❖ Scoop the pesto into a container and refrigerate.
- ❖ STORAGE: Store the covered container in the refrigerator for up to 2 weeks. Pesto may be frozen for up to 6 months.

Nutrition: (¼ cup): Total calories: 231; Total fat: 22g; Saturated fat: 3g; Sodium: 178mg; Carbohydrates: 6g; Fiber: 3g; Protein: 4g

263)   SAUTÉED KALE AND GARLIC WITH LEMON
Cooking Time: 7 Minutes   **Servings: 4**

Ingredients:

- ✓ 1 tbsp olive oil
- ✓ 3 bunches kale, stemmed and roughly chopped
- ✓ 2 tsp chopped garlic
- ✓ ¼ tsp kosher salt
- ✓ 1 tbsp freshly squeezed lemon juice

Directions:

- ❖ Heat the oil in a -inch skillet over medium-high heat. Once the oil is shimmering, add as much kale as will fit in the pan. You will probably only fit half the leaves into the pan at first. Mix the kale with tongs so that the leaves are coated with oil and start to wilt. As the kale wilts, keep adding more of the raw kale, continuing to use tongs to mix. Once all the kale is in the pan, add the garlic and salt and continue to cook until the kale is tender. Total cooking time from start to finish should be about 7 minutes.
- ❖ Mix the lemon juice into the kale. Add additional salt and/or lemon juice if necessary. Place 1 cup of kale in each of 4 containers and refrigerate.
- ❖ STORAGE: Store covered containers in the refrigerator for up to 5 days

Nutrition: Total calories: 8 Total fat: 1g; Saturated fat: <1g; Sodium: 214mg; Carbohydrates: 17g; Fiber: 6g; Protein: 6g

264)   CREAMY POLENTA AND CHIVES WITH PARMESAN
Cooking Time: 15 Minutes   **Servings: 5**

Ingredients:

- ✓ 1 tsp olive oil
- ✓ ¼ cup minced shallot
- ✓ ½ cup white wine
- ✓ 3¼ cups water
- ✓ ¾ cup cornmeal
- ✓ 3 tbsp grated Parmesan cheese
- ✓ ½ tsp kosher salt
- ✓ ¼ cup chopped chives

Directions:

- ❖ Heat the oil in a saucepan over medium heat. Once the oil is shimmering, add the shallot and sauté for 2 minutes. Add the wine and water and bring to a boil.
- ❖ Pour the cornmeal in a thin, even stream into the liquid, stirring continuously until the mixture starts to thicken.
- ❖ Reduce the heat to low and continue to cook for 10 to 12 minutes, whisking every 1 to 2 minutes.
- ❖ Turn the heat off and stir in the cheese, salt, and chives. Cool.
- ❖ Place about ¾ cup of polenta in each of containers.
- ❖ STORAGE: Store covered containers in the refrigerator for up to 5 days.

Nutrition: Total calories: 110; Total fat: 3g; Saturated fat: 1g; Sodium: 29g; Carbohydrates: 16g; Fiber: 1g; Protein: 3g

265) SPECIAL MOCHA-NUT STUFFED DATES

Cooking Time: 10 Minutes **Servings: 5**

Ingredients:

- ✓ 2 tbsp creamy, unsweetened, unsalted almond butter
- ✓ 1 tsp unsweetened cocoa powder
- ✓ 3 tbsp walnut pieces
- ✓ 2 tbsp water
- ✓ ¼ tsp honey
- ✓ ¾ tsp instant espresso powder
- ✓ 10 Medjool dates, pitted

Directions:

- ❖ In a small bowl, combine the almond butter, cocoa powder, and walnut pieces.
- ❖ Place the water in a small microwaveable mug and heat on high for 30 seconds. Add the honey and espresso powder to the water and stir to dissolve.
- ❖ Add the espresso water to the cocoa bowl and combine thoroughly until a creamy, thick paste forms.
- ❖ Stuff each pitted date with 1 tsp of mocha filling.
- ❖ Place 2 dates in each of small containers.
- ❖ STORAGE: Store covered containers in the refrigerator for up to 5 days.

Nutrition: Total calories: 205; Total fat: ; Saturated fat: 1g; Sodium: 1mg; Carbohydrates: 39g; Fiber: 4g; Protein: 3g

266) DELICIOUS HONEY-LEMON VINAIGRETTE

Cooking Time: 5 Minutes **Servings: ½ Cup**

Ingredients:

- ✓ ¼ cup freshly squeezed lemon juice
- ✓ 1 tsp honey
- ✓ 2 tsp Dijon mustard
- ✓ ⅛ tsp kosher salt
- ✓ ¼ cup olive oil

Directions:

- ❖ Place the lemon juice, honey, mustard, and salt in a small bowl and whisk to combine.
- ❖ Whisk in the oil, pouring it into the bowl in a thin steam.
- ❖ Pour the vinaigrette into a container and refrigerate.
- ❖ STORAGE: Store the covered container in the refrigerator for up to 2 weeks. Allow the vinaigrette to come to room temperature and shake before serving.

Nutrition: (2 tbsp): Total calories: 131; Total fat: 14g; Saturated fat: 2g; Sodium: 133mg; Carbohydrates: 3g; Fiber: <1g; Protein: <1g

267) SPANISH-STYLE ROMESCO SAUCE

Cooking Time: 10 Minutes **Servings: 1⅔ Cups**

Ingredients:

- ✓ ½ cup raw, unsalted almonds
- ✓ 4 medium garlic cloves (do not peel)
- ✓ 1 (12-ounce) jar of roasted red peppers, drained
- ✓ ½ cup canned diced fire-roasted tomatoes, drained
- ✓ 1 tsp smoked paprika
- ✓ ½ tsp kosher salt
- ✓ Pinch cayenne pepper
- ✓ 2 tsp red wine vinegar
- ✓ 2 tbsp olive oil

Directions:

- ❖ Preheat the oven to 350°F.
- ❖ Place the almonds and garlic cloves on a sheet pan and toast in the oven for 10 minutes. Remove from the oven and peel the garlic when cool enough to handle.
- ❖ Place the almonds in the bowl of a food processor. Process the almonds until they resemble coarse sand, to 45 seconds. Add the garlic, peppers, tomatoes, paprika, salt, and cayenne. Blend until smooth.
- ❖ Once the mixture is smooth, add the vinegar and oil and blend until well combined. Taste and add more vinegar or salt if needed.
- ❖ Scoop the romesco sauce into a container and refrigerate.
- ❖ STORAGE: Store the covered container in the refrigerator for up to 7 days.

Nutrition: (⅓ cup): Total calories: 158; Total fat: 13g; Saturated fat: 1g; Sodium: 292mg; Carbohydrates: 10g; Fiber: 3g; Protein: 4g

268) **CARDAMOM MASCARPONE AND STRAWBERRIES**

Cooking Time: 10 Minutes   **Servings:** 4

Ingredients:

- ✓ 1 (8-ounce) container mascarpone cheese
- ✓ 2 tsp honey
- ✓ ¼ tsp ground cardamom
- ✓ 2 tbsp milk
- ✓ 1 pound strawberries (should be 24 strawberries in the pack)

Directions:

- ❖ Combine the mascarpone, honey, cardamom, and milk in a medium mixing bowl.
- ❖ Mix the ingredients with a spoon until super creamy, about 30 seconds.
- ❖ Place 6 strawberries and 2 tbsp of the mascarpone mixture in each of 4 containers.
- ❖ STORAGE: Store covered containers in the refrigerator for up to 5 days.

Nutrition: Total calories: 289; Total fat: 2; Saturated fat: 10g; Sodium: 26mg; Carbohydrates: 11g; Fiber: 3g; Protein: 1g

269) **SWEET SPICY GREEN PUMPKIN SEEDS**

Cooking Time: 15 Minutes   **Servings:** 2 Cups

Ingredients:

- ✓ 2 cups raw green pumpkin seeds (pepitas)
- ✓ 1 egg white, beaten until frothy
- ✓ 3 tbsp honey
- ✓ 1 tbsp chili powder
- ✓ ¼ tsp cayenne pepper
- ✓ 1 tsp ground cinnamon
- ✓ ¼ tsp kosher salt

Directions:

- ❖ Preheat the oven to 350°F. Line a sheet pan with a silicone baking mat or parchment paper.
- ❖ In a medium bowl, mix all the ingredients until the seeds are well coated. Place on the lined sheet pan in a single, even layer.
- ❖ Bake for 15 minutes. Cool the seeds on the sheet pan, then peel clusters from the baking mat and break apart into small pieces.
- ❖ Place ¼ cup of seeds in each of 8 small containers or resealable sandwich bags.
- ❖ STORAGE: Store covered containers or resealable bags at room temperature for up to days.

Nutrition: (¼ cup): Total calories: 209; Total fat: 15g; Saturated fat: 3g; Sodium: 85mg; Carbohydrates: 11g; Fiber: 2g; Protein: 10g

270) **GREEK TZATZIKI SAUCE**

Cooking Time: 15 Minutes   **Servings:** 2½ Cups

Ingredients:

- ✓ 1 English cucumber
- ✓ 2 cups low-fat (2%) plain Greek yogurt
- ✓ 1 tbsp olive oil
- ✓ 2 tsp freshly squeezed lemon juice
- ✓ ½ tsp chopped garlic
- ✓ ½ tsp kosher salt
- ✓ ⅛ tsp freshly ground black pepper
- ✓ 2 tbsp chopped fresh dill
- ✓ 2 tbsp chopped fresh mint

Directions:

- ❖ Place a sieve over a medium bowl. Grate the cucumber, with the skin, over the sieve. Press the grated cucumber into the sieve with the flat surface of a spatula to press as much liquid out as possible.
- ❖ In a separate medium bowl, place the yogurt, oil, lemon juice, garlic, salt, pepper, dill, and mint and stir to combine.
- ❖ Press on the cucumber one last time, then add it to the yogurt mixture. Stir to combine. Taste and add more salt and lemon juice if necessary.
- ❖ Scoop the sauce into a container and refrigerate.
- ❖ STORAGE: Store the covered container in the refrigerator for up to days.

Nutrition: (¼ cup): Total calories: 51; Total fat: 2g; Saturated fat: 1g; Sodium: 137mg; Carbohydrates: 3g; Fiber: <1g; Protein: 5g

271) SPECIAL FRUIT SALAD WITH MINT AND ORANGE BLOSSOM WATER

Cooking Time: 10 Minutes   **Servings:** 5

Ingredients:

- ✓ 3 cups cantaloupe, cut into 1-inch cubes
- ✓ 2 cups hulled and halved strawberries
- ✓ ½ tsp orange blossom water
- ✓ 2 tbsp chopped fresh mint

Directions:

- ❖ In a large bowl, toss all the ingredients together.
- ❖ Place 1 cup of fruit salad in each of 5 containers.
- ❖ STORAGE: Store covered containers in the refrigerator for up to 5 days.

Nutrition: Total calories: 52; Total fat: 1g; Saturated fat: <1g; Sodium: 10mg; Carbohydrates: 12g; Fiber: 2g; Protein: 1g

272) ROASTED BROCCOLI WITH RED ONIONS AND POMEGRANATE SEEDS

Cooking Time: 20 Minutes   **Servings:** 5

Ingredients:

- ✓ 1 (12-ounce) package broccoli florets (about 6 cups)
- ✓ 1 small red onion, thinly sliced
- ✓ 2 tbsp olive oil
- ✓ ¼ tsp kosher salt
- ✓ 1 (5.3-ounce) container pomegranate seeds (1 cup)

Directions:

- ❖ Preheat the oven to 425°F and line 2 sheet pans with silicone baking mats or parchment paper.
- ❖ Place the broccoli and onion on the sheet pans and toss with the oil and salt. Place the pans in the oven and roast for minutes.
- ❖ After removing the pans from the oven, cool the veggies, then toss with the pomegranate seeds.
- ❖ Place 1 cup of veggies in each of 5 containers.
- ❖ STORAGE: Store covered containers in the refrigerator for up to days.

Nutrition: Total calories: 118; Total fat: ; Saturated fat: 1g; Sodium: 142mg; Carbohydrates: 12g; Fiber: 4g; Protein: 2g

273) DELICIOUS CHERMOULA SAUCE

Cooking Time: 10 Minutes   **Servings:** 1 Cup

Ingredients:

- ✓ 1 cup packed parsley leaves
- ✓ 1 cup cilantro leaves
- ✓ ½ cup mint leaves
- ✓ 1 tsp chopped garlic
- ✓ ½ tsp ground cumin
- ✓ ½ tsp ground coriander
- ✓ ½ tsp smoked paprika
- ✓ ⅛ tsp cayenne pepper
- ✓ ⅛ tsp kosher salt
- ✓ 3 tbsp freshly squeezed lemon juice
- ✓ 3 tbsp water
- ✓ ½ cup extra-virgin olive oil

Directions:

- ❖ Place all the ingredients in a blender or food processor and blend until smooth.
- ❖ Pour the chermoula into a container and refrigerate.
- ❖ STORAGE: Store the covered container in the refrigerator for up to 5 days.

Nutrition: (¼ cup): Total calories: 257; Total fat: 27g; Saturated fat: ; Sodium: 96mg; Carbohydrates: 4g; Fiber: 2g; Protein: 1g

274)   DEVILLED EGGS PESTO WITH SUN-DRIED TOMATOES

Cooking Time: 15 Minutes   **Servings: 5**

Ingredients:

- ✓ 5 large eggs
- ✓ 3 tbsp prepared pesto
- ✓ ¼ tsp white vinegar
- ✓ 2 tbsp low-fat (2%) plain Greek yogurt
- ✓ 5 tsp sliced sun-dried tomatoes

Directions:

- ❖ Place the eggs in a saucepan and cover with water. Bring the water to a boil. As soon as the water starts to boil, place a lid on the pan and turn the heat off. Set a timer for minutes.
- ❖ When the timer goes off, drain the hot water and run cold water over the eggs to cool.
- ❖ Peel the eggs, slice in half vertically, and scoop out the yolks. Place the yolks in a medium mixing bowl and add the pesto, vinegar, and yogurt. Mix well, until creamy.
- ❖ Scoop about 1 tbsp of the pesto-yolk mixture into each egg half. Top each with ½ tsp of sun-dried tomatoes.
- ❖ Place 2 stuffed egg halves in each of separate containers.
- ❖ STORAGE: Store covered containers in the refrigerator for up to 5 days.

Nutrition: Total calories: 124; Total fat: 9g; Saturated fat: 2g; Sodium: 204mg; Carbohydrates: 2g; Fiber: <1g; Protein: 8g

275)   WHITE BEAN WITH MUSHROOM DIP

Cooking Time: 8 Minutes   **Servings: 3 Cups**

Ingredients:

- ✓ 2 tsp olive oil, plus 2 tbsp
- ✓ 8 ounces button or cremini mushrooms, sliced
- ✓ 1 tsp chopped garlic
- ✓ 1 tbsp fresh thyme leaves
- ✓ 2 (15.5-ounce) cans cannellini beans, drained and rinsed
- ✓ 2 tbsp plus 1 tsp freshly squeezed lemon juice
- ✓ ½ tsp kosher salt

Directions:

- ❖ Heat 2 tsp of oil in a -inch skillet over medium-high heat. Once the oil is shimmering, add the mushrooms and sauté for 6 minutes. Add the garlic and thyme and continue cooking for 2 minutes.
- ❖ While the mushrooms are cooking, place the beans and lemon juice, the remaining tbsp of oil, and the salt in the bowl of a food processor. Add the mushrooms as soon as they are done cooking and blend everything until smooth. Scrape down the sides of the bowl if necessary and continue to process until smooth.
- ❖ Taste and adjust the seasoning with lemon juice or salt if needed.
- ❖ Scoop the dip into a container and refrigerate.
- ❖ STORAGE: Store the covered container in the refrigerator for up to days. Dip can be frozen for up to 3 months.

Nutrition: Total calories: 192; Total fat: ; Saturated fat: 1g; Sodium: 197mg; Carbohydrates: 25g; Fiber: 7g; Protein: 9g

276) NORTH AFRICAN-STYLE SPICED SAUTÉED CABBAGE

Cooking Time: 10 Minutes   **Servings:** 4

Ingredients:

- ✓ 2 tsp olive oil
- ✓ 1 small head green cabbage (about 1½ to 2 pounds), cored and thinly sliced
- ✓ 1 tsp ground coriander
- ✓ 1 tsp garlic powder
- ✓ ½ tsp caraway seeds
- ✓ ½ tsp ground cumin
- ✓ ¼ tsp kosher salt
- ✓ Pinch red chili flakes (optional—if you don't like heat, omit it)
- ✓ 1 tsp freshly squeezed lemon juice

Directions:

- ❖ Heat the oil in a -inch skillet over medium-high heat. Once the oil is hot, add the cabbage and cook down for 3 minutes. Add the coriander, garlic powder, caraway seeds, cumin, salt, and chili flakes (if using) and stir to combine. Continue cooking the cabbage for about 7 more minutes.
- ❖ Stir in the lemon juice and cool.
- ❖ Place 1 heaping cup of cabbage in each of 4 containers.
- ❖ STORAGE: Store covered containers in the refrigerator for up to 5 days.

Nutrition: Total calories: 69; Total fat: 3g; Saturated fat: <1g; Sodium: 178mg; Carbohydrates: 11g; Fiber: 4g; Protein: 3g

277) FLAX, BLUEBERRY, AND SUNFLOWER BUTTER BITES

Cooking Time: 10 Minutes   **Servings:** 6

Ingredients:

- ✓ ¼ cup ground flaxseed
- ✓ ½ cup unsweetened sunflower butter, preferably unsalted
- ✓ ⅓ cup dried blueberries
- ✓ 2 tbsp all-fruit blueberry preserves
- ✓ Zest of 1 lemon
- ✓ 2 tbsp unsalted sunflower seeds
- ✓ ⅓ cup rolled oats

Directions:

- ❖ Mix all the ingredients in a medium mixing bowl until well combined.
- ❖ Form 1balls, slightly smaller than a golf ball, from the mixture and place on a plate in the freezer for about 20 minutes to firm up.
- ❖ Place 2 bites in each of 6 containers and refrigerate.
- ❖ STORAGE: Store covered containers in the refrigerator for up to 5 days. Bites may also be stored in the freezer for up to 3 months.

Nutrition: Total calories: 229; Total fat: 14g; Saturated fat: 1g; Sodium: 1mg; Carbohydrates: 26g; Fiber: 3g; Protein: 7g

278) SPECIAL DIJON RED WINE VINAIGRETTE

Cooking Time: 5 Minutes   **Servings:** ½ Cup

Ingredients:

- ✓ 2 tsp Dijon mustard
- ✓ 3 tbsp red wine vinegar
- ✓ 1 tbsp water
- ✓ ¼ tsp dried oregano
- ✓ ¼ tsp chopped garlic
- ✓ ⅛ tsp kosher salt
- ✓ ¼ cup olive oil

Directions:

- ❖ Place the mustard, vinegar, water, oregano, garlic, and salt in a small bowl and whisk to combine.
- ❖ Whisk in the oil, pouring it into the mustard-vinegar mixture in a thin steam.
- ❖ Pour the vinaigrette into a container and refrigerate.
- ❖ STORAGE: Store the covered container in the refrigerator for up to 2 weeks. Allow the vinaigrette to come to room temperature and shake before serving.

Nutrition: (2 tbsp): Total calories: 123; Total fat: 14g; Saturated fat: 2g; Sodium: 133mg; Carbohydrates: 0g; Fiber: 0g; Protein: 0g

279) CLASSIC HUMMUS

Cooking Time: 5 Minutes   **Servings: 1½ Cups**

Ingredients:

- ✓ 1 (15-ounce) can low-sodium chickpeas, drained and rinsed
- ✓ ¼ cup unsalted tahini
- ✓ ½ tsp chopped garlic
- ✓ ¼ cup freshly squeezed lemon juice
- ✓ ¼ tsp kosher salt
- ✓ 3 tbsp olive oil
- ✓ 3 tbsp cold water

Directions:

- ❖ Place all the ingredients in a food processor or blender and blend until smooth.
- ❖ Taste and adjust the seasonings if needed.
- ❖ Scoop the hummus into a container and refrigerate.
- ❖ STORAGE: Store the covered container in the refrigerator for up to 5 days.

Nutrition: (¼ cup): Total calories: 192; Total fat: 13g; Saturated fat: 2g; Sodium: 109mg; Carbohydrates: 16g; Fiber: ; Protein: 5g

280) SPECIAL CANDIED MAPLE-CINNAMON WALNUTS

Cooking Time: 15 Minutes   **Servings: 4**

Ingredients:

- ✓ 1 cup walnut halves
- ✓ ½ tsp ground cinnamon
- ✓ 2 tbsp pure maple syrup

Directions:

- ❖ Preheat the oven to 325°F. Line a baking sheet with a silicone baking mat or parchment paper.
- ❖ In a small bowl, mix the walnuts, cinnamon, and maple syrup until the walnuts are coated.
- ❖ Pour the nuts onto the baking sheet, making sure to scrape out all the maple syrup. Bake for 15 minutes. Allow the nuts to cool completely.
- ❖ Place ¼ cup of nuts in each of containers or resealable sandwich bags.
- ❖ STORAGE: Store covered containers at room temperature for up to 7 days.

Nutrition: Total calories: 190; Total fat: 17g; Saturated fat: 2g; Sodium: 2mg; Carbohydrates: 10g; Fiber: 2g; Protein: 4g

281) DELICIOUS ARTICHOKE-OLIVE COMPOTE

Cooking Time: 15 Minutes   **Servings: 1⅓ Cups**

Ingredients:

- ✓ 1 (6-ounce) jar marinated artichoke hearts, chopped
- ✓ ⅓ cup chopped pitted green olives (8 to 9 olives)
- ✓ 3 tbsp chopped fresh basil
- ✓ ½ tsp freshly squeezed lemon juice
- ✓ 2 tsp olive oil

Directions:

- ❖ Place all the ingredients in a medium mixing bowl and stir to combine.
- ❖ Place the compote in a container and refrigerate.
- ❖ STORAGE: Store the covered container in the refrigerator for up to 7 days.

Nutrition: (⅓ cup): Total calories: 8 Total fat: 7g; Saturated fat: 1g; Sodium: 350mg; Carbohydrates: 5g; Fiber: <1g; Protein: <1g

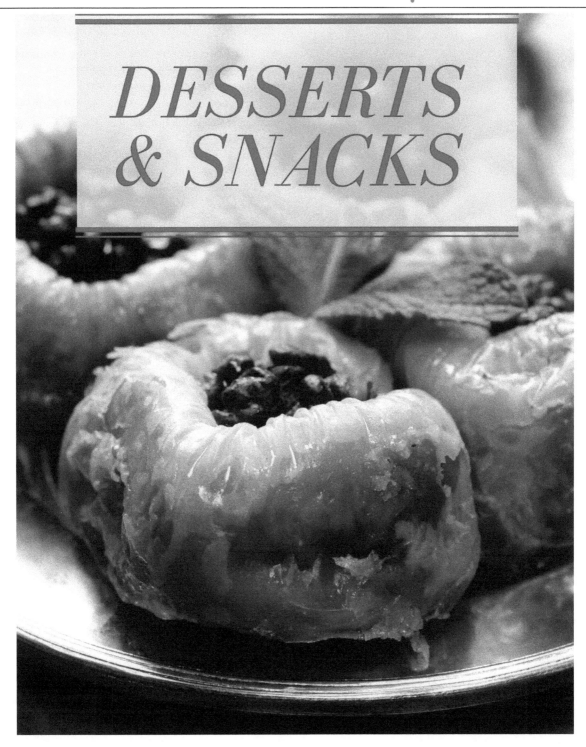

DESSERTS & SNACKS

282)   DELICIOUS LEMONY TREAT

Cooking Time: 30 Minutes   **Servings: 4**

Ingredients:

- ✓ 1 lemon, medium in size
- ✓ 1 ½ tsp cornstarch
- ✓ 1 cup Greek yogurt, plain is best
- ✓ Fresh fruit
- ✓ ¼ cup cold water
- ✓ ⅔ cup heavy whipped cream
- ✓ 3 tbsp honey
- ✓ Optional: mint leaves

Directions:

- ❖ Take a large glass bowl and your metal, electric mixer and set them in the refrigerator so they can chill.
- ❖ In a separate bowl, add the yogurt and set that in the fridge.
- ❖ Zest the lemon into a medium bowl that is microwavable.
- ❖ Cut the lemon in half and then squeeze 1 tbsp of lemon juice into the bowl.
- ❖ Combine the cornstarch and water. Mix the ingredients thoroughly.
- ❖ Pour in the honey and whisk the ingredients together.
- ❖ Put the mixture into the microwave for 1 minute on high.
- ❖ Once the microwave stops, remove the mixture and stir.
- ❖ Set it back into the microwave for 15 to 30 seconds or until the mixture starts to bubble and thicken.
- ❖ Take the bowl of yogurt from the fridge and pour in the warm mixture while whisking.
- ❖ Put the yogurt mixture back into the fridge.
- ❖ Take the large bowl and beaters out of the fridge.
- ❖ Put your electronic mixer together and pour the whipped cream into the chilled bowl.
- ❖ Beat the cream until soft peaks start to form. This can take up to 3 minutes, depending on how fresh your cream is.
- ❖ Remove the yogurt from the fridge.
- ❖ Fold the yogurt into the cream using a rubber spatula. Remember to lift and turn the mixture so it doesn't deflate.
- ❖ Place back into the fridge until you are serving the dessert or for 15 minutes. The dessert should not be in the fridge for longer than 1 hour.
- ❖ When you serve the lemony goodness, you will spoon it into four dessert dishes and drizzle with extra honey or even melt some chocolate to drizzle on top.
- ❖ Add a little fresh mint and enjoy!

Nutrition: calories: 241, fats: 16 grams, carbohydrates: 21 grams, protein: 7 grams

283)   MELON AND GINGER

Cooking Time: 10 To 15 Minutes   **Servings: 4**

Ingredients:

- ✓ ½ cantaloupe, cut into 1-inch chunks
- ✓ 2 cups of watermelon, cut into 1-inch chunks
- ✓ 2 cups honeydew melon, cut into 1-inch chunks
- ✓ 2 tbsp of raw honey
- ✓ Ginger, 2 inches in size, peeled, grated, and preserve the juice

Directions:

- ❖ In a large bowl, combine your cantaloupe, honeydew melon, and watermelon. Gently mix the ingredients.
- ❖ Combine the ginger juice and stir.
- ❖ Drizzle on the honey, serve, and enjoy! You can also chill the mixture for up to an hour before serving.

Nutrition: calories: 91, fats: 0 grams, carbohydrates: 23 grams, protein: 1 gram.

284)   CLASSIC CHOCOLATE FRUIT KEBABS

Cooking Time: 30 Minutes   **Servings:** 6

Ingredients:

- ✓ 24 blueberries
- ✓ 12 strawberries with the green leafy top part removed
- ✓ 12 green or red grapes, seedless
- ✓ 12 pitted cherries
- ✓ 8 ounces chocolate

Directions:

- ❖ Line a baking sheet with a piece of parchment paper and place 6, -inch long wooden skewers on top of the paper.
- ❖ Start by threading a piece of fruit onto the skewers. You can create and follow any pattern that you like with the ingredients. An example pattern is 1 strawberry, 1 cherry, blueberries, 2 grapes. Repeat the pattern until all of the fruit is on the skewers.
- ❖ In a saucepan on medium heat, melt the chocolate. Stir continuously until the chocolate has melted completely.
- ❖ Carefully scoop the chocolate into a plastic sandwich bag and twist the bag closed starting right above the chocolate.
- ❖ Snip the corner of the bag with scissors.
- ❖ Drizzle the chocolate onto the kebabs by squeezing it out of the bag.
- ❖ Put the baking pan into the freezer for 20 minutes.
- ❖ Serve and enjoy!

Nutrition: calories: 254, fats: 15 grams, carbohydrates: 28 grams, protein: 4 grams.

285)   PEACHES AND BLUE CHEESE CREAM

Cooking Time: 20 Hours 10 Minutes   **Servings:** 4

Ingredients:

- ✓ 4 peaches
- ✓ 1 cinnamon stick
- ✓ 4 ounces sliced blue cheese
- ✓ ⅓ cup orange juice, freshly squeezed is best
- ✓ 3 whole cloves
- ✓ 1 tsp of orange zest, taken from the orange peel
- ✓ ¼ tsp cardamom pods
- ✓ ⅔ cup red wine
- ✓ 2 tbsp honey, raw or your preferred variety
- ✓ 1 vanilla bean
- ✓ 1 tsp allspice berries
- ✓ 4 tbsp dried cherries

Directions:

- ❖ Set a saucepan on top of your stove range and add the cinnamon stick, cloves, orange juice, cardamom, vanilla, allspice, red wine, and orange zest. Whisk the ingredients well. Add your peaches to the mixture and poach them for hours or until they become soft.
- ❖ Take a spoon to remove the peaches and boil the rest of the liquid to make the syrup. You want the liquid to reduce itself by at least half.
- ❖ While the liquid is boiling, combine the dried cherries, blue cheese, and honey into a bowl. Once your peaches are cooled, slice them into halves.
- ❖ Top each peach with the blue cheese mixture and then drizzle the liquid onto the top. Serve and enjoy!

Nutrition: calories: 211, fats: 24 grams, carbohydrates: 15 grams, protein: 6 grams

286) **MEDITERRANEAN-STYLE BLACKBERRY ICE CREAM**

Cooking Time: 15 Minutes   **Servings:** 6

Ingredients:

- ✓ 3 egg yolks
- ✓ 1 container of Greek yogurt
- ✓ 1-pound mashed blackberries
- ✓ ½ tsp vanilla essence
- ✓ 1 tsp arrowroot powder
- ✓ ¼ tsp ground cloves
- ✓ 5 ounces sugar or sweetener substitute
- ✓ 1-pound heavy cream

Directions:

- ❖ In a small bowl, add the arrowroot powder and egg yolks. Whisk or beat them with an electronic mixture until they are well combined.
- ❖ Set a saucepan on top of your stove and turn your heat to medium.
- ❖ Add the heavy cream and bring it to a boil.
- ❖ Turn off the heat and add the egg mixture into the cream through folding.
- ❖ Turn the heat back on to medium and pour in the sugar. Cook the mixture for 10 minutes or until it starts to thicken.
- ❖ Remove the mixture from heat and place it in the fridge so it can completely cool. This should take about one hour.
- ❖ Once the mixture is cooled, add in the Greek yogurt, ground cloves, blackberries, and vanilla by folding in the ingredients.
- ❖ Transfer the ice cream into a container and place it in the freezer for at least two hours.
- ❖ Serve and enjoy!

Nutrition: calories: 402, fats: 20 grams, carbohydrates: 52 grams, protein: 8 grams

287) **CLASSIC STUFFED FIGS**

Cooking Time: 20 Minutes   **Servings:** 6

Ingredients:

- ✓ 10 halved fresh figs
- ✓ 20 chopped almonds
- ✓ 4 ounces goat cheese, divided
- ✓ 2 tbsp of raw honey

Directions:

- ❖ Turn your oven to broiler mode and set it to a high temperature.
- ❖ Place your figs, cut side up, on a baking sheet. If you like to place a piece of parchment paper on top you can do this, but it is not necessary.
- ❖ Sprinkle each fig with half of the goat cheese.
- ❖ Add a tbsp of chopped almonds to each fig.
- ❖ Broil the figs for 3 to 4 minutes.
- ❖ Take them out of the oven and let them cool for 5 to 7 minutes.
- ❖ Sprinkle with the remaining goat cheese and honey.

Nutrition: calories: 209, fats: 9 grams, carbohydrates: 26 grams, protein: grams.

288) CHIA PUDDING AND STRAWBERRIES

Cooking Time: 4 Hours 5 Minutes   **Servings:** 4

Ingredients:

- ✓ 2 cups unsweetened almond milk
- ✓ 1 tbsp vanilla extract
- ✓ 2 tbsp raw honey
- ✓ ¼ cup chia seeds
- ✓ 2 cups fresh and sliced strawberries

Directions:

- ❖ In a medium bowl, combine the honey, chia seeds, vanilla, and unsweetened almond milk. Mix well.
- ❖ Set the mixture in the refrigerator for at least 4 hours.
- ❖ When you serve the pudding, top it with strawberries. You can even create a design in a glass serving bowl or dessert dish by adding a little pudding on the bottom, a few strawberries, top the strawberries with some more pudding, and then top the dish with a few strawberries.

Nutrition: calories: 108, fats: grams, carbohydrates: 17 grams, protein: 3 grams

289) LOVELY STRAWBERRY POPSICLE

Cooking Time: 10 Minutes   **Servings:** 5

Ingredients:

- ✓ ½ cup almond milk
- ✓ 1 ½ cups fresh strawberries

Directions:

- ❖ Using a blender or hand mixer, combine the almond milk and strawberries thoroughly in a bowl.
- ❖ Using popsicle molds, pour the mixture into the molds and place the sticks into the mixture.
- ❖ Set in the freezer for at least 4 hours.
- ❖ Serve and enjoy—especially on a hot day!

Nutrition: calories: 3 fats: 0.5 grams, carbohydrates: 7 grams, protein: 0.6 grams.

290) SPECIAL FROZEN BLUEBERRY YOGURT

Cooking Time: 30 Minutes   **Servings:** 6

Ingredients:

- ✓ ⅔ cup honey
- ✓ 2 cups chilled yogurt
- ✓ 1 pint fresh blueberries
- ✓ 1 juiced and zested lime or lemon. You can even substitute an orange if your tastes prefer.

Directions:

- ❖ With a saucepan on your burner set to medium heat, add the honey, juiced fruit, zest, and blueberries.
- ❖ Stir the mixture continuously as it begins to simmer for 15 minutes.
- ❖ When the liquid is nearly gone, pour the contents into a bowl and place in the fridge for several minutes. You will want to stir the ingredients and check to see if they are chilled.
- ❖ Once the fruit is chilled, combine with the yogurt.
- ❖ Mix until the ingredients are well incorporated and enjoy.

Nutrition: calories: 233, fats: 3 grams, carbohydrates: 52 grams, protein: 3.5 grams

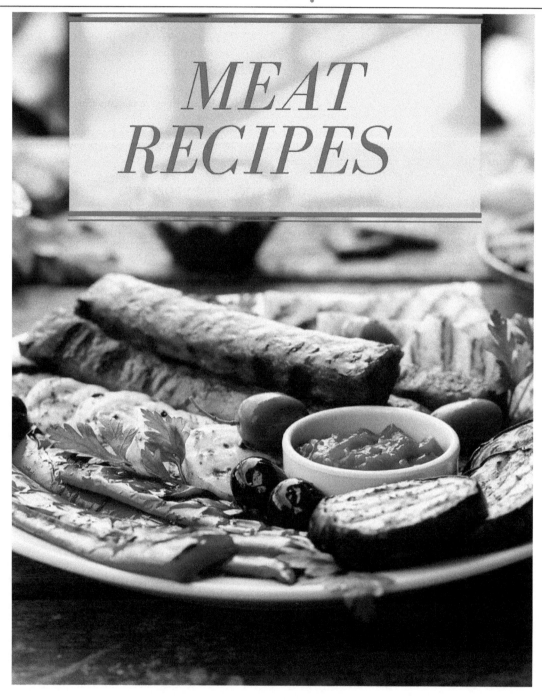

MEAT
RECIPES

291) SPECIAL SMOKED PORK SAUSAGE KETO BOMBS

Cooking Time: 15 Minutes   **Servings:** 6

Ingredients:

- ✓ 3/4 pound smoked pork sausage, ground
- ✓ 1 tsp ginger-garlic paste
- ✓ 2 tbsp scallions, minced
- ✓ 1 tbsp butter, room temperature
- ✓ 1 tomato, pureed
- ✓ 4 ounces mozzarella cheese, crumbled
- ✓ 2 tbsp flaxseed meal
- ✓ 8 ounces cream cheese, room temperature
- ✓ Sea salt and ground black pepper, to taste

Directions:

- ❖ Melt the butter in a frying pan over medium-high heat. Cook the sausage for about 4 minutes, crumbling with a spatula.
- ❖ Add in the ginger-garlic paste, scallions, and tomato; continue to cook over medium-low heat for a further 6 minutes. Stir in the remaining ingredients.
- ❖ Place the mixture in your refrigerator for 1 to 2 hours until firm. Roll the mixture into bite-sized balls.
- ❖ Storing
- ❖ Transfer the balls to the airtight containers and place in your refrigerator for up to 3 days.
- ❖ For freezing, place in a freezer safe containers and freeze up to 1 month. Enjoy!

Nutrition: 383 Calories; 32. Fat; 5.1g Carbs; 16.7g Protein; 1.7g Fiber

292) TURKEY MEATBALLS AND TANGY BASIL CHUTNEY

Cooking Time: 30 Minutes   **Servings:** 6

Ingredients:

- ✓ 2 tbsp sesame oil
- ✓ For the Meatballs:
- ✓ 1/2 cup Romano cheese, grated
- ✓ 1 tsp garlic, minced
- ✓ 1/2 tsp shallot powder
- ✓ 1/4 tsp dried thyme
- ✓ 1/2 tsp mustard seeds
- ✓ 2 small-sized eggs, lightly beaten
- ✓ 1 ½ pounds ground turkey
- ✓ 1/2 tsp sea salt
- ✓ 1/4 tsp ground black pepper, or more to taste
- ✓ 3 tbsp almond meal
- ✓ For the Basil Chutney:
- ✓ 2 tbsp fresh lime juice
- ✓ 1/4 cup fresh basil leaves
- ✓ 1/4 cup fresh parsley
- ✓ 1/2 cup cilantro leaves
- ✓ 1 tsp fresh ginger root, grated
- ✓ 2 tbsp olive oil
- ✓ 2 tbsp water
- ✓ 1 tbsp habanero chili pepper, deveined and minced

Directions:

- ❖ In a mixing bowl, combine all ingredients for the meatballs. Roll the mixture into meatballs and reserve.
- ❖ Heat the sesame oil in a frying pan over a moderate flame. Sear the meatballs for about 8 minutes until browned on all sides.
- ❖ Make the chutney by mixing all the ingredients in your blender or food processor.
- ❖ Storing
- ❖ Place the meatballs in airtight containers or Ziploc bags; keep in your refrigerator for up to 3 to 4 days.
- ❖ Freeze the meatballs in airtight containers or heavy-duty freezer bags. Freeze up to 3 to 4 months. To defrost, slowly reheat in a frying pan.
- ❖ Store the basil chutney in the refrigerator for up to a week. Bon appétit!

Nutrition: 390 Calories; 27.2g Fat; 1. Carbs; 37.4g Protein; 0.3g Fiber

293) ROASTED CHICKEN AND CASHEW PESTO

Cooking Time: 35 Minutes   **Servings:** 4

Ingredients:

- 1 cup leeks, chopped
- 1 pound chicken legs, skinless
- Salt and ground black pepper, to taste
- 1/2 tsp red pepper flakes
- For the Cashew-Basil Pesto:
- 1/2 cup cashews
- 2 garlic cloves, minced
- 1/2 cup fresh basil leaves
- 1/2 cup Parmigiano-Reggiano cheese, preferably freshly grated
- 1/2 cup olive oil

Directions:

- Place the chicken legs in a parchment-lined baking pan. Season with salt and pepper, Then, scatter the leeks around the chicken legs.
- Roast in the preheated oven at 390 degrees F for 30 to 35 minutes, rotating the pan occasionally.
- Pulse the cashews, basil, garlic, and cheese in your blender until pieces are small. Continue blending while adding olive oil to the mixture. Mix until the desired consistency is reached.
- Storing
- Place the chicken in airtight containers or Ziploc bags; keep in your refrigerator for up 3 to 4 days.
- To freeze the chicken legs, place them in airtight containers or heavy-duty freezer bags. Freeze up to 3 months. Once thawed in the refrigerator, heat in the preheated oven at 375 degrees F for 20 to 25 minutes.
- Store your pesto in the refrigerator for up to a week. Bon appétit!

Nutrition: 5 Calories; 44.8g Fat; 5g Carbs; 38.7g Protein; 1g Fiber

294) TARO LEAF WITH CHICKEN SOUP

Cooking Time: 45 Minutes   **Servings:** 4

Ingredients:

- 1 pound whole chicken, boneless and chopped into small chunks
- 1/2 cup onions, chopped
- 1/2 cup rutabaga, cubed
- 2 carrots, peeled
- 2 celery stalks
- Salt and black pepper, to taste
- 1 cup chicken bone broth
- 1/2 tsp ginger-garlic paste
- 1/2 cup taro leaves, roughly chopped
- 1 tbsp fresh coriander, chopped
- 3 cups water
- 1 tsp paprika

Directions:

- Place all ingredients in a heavy-bottomed pot. Bring to a boil over the highest heat.
- Turn the heat to simmer. Continue to cook, partially covered, an additional 40 minutes.
- Storing
- Spoon the soup into four airtight containers or Ziploc bags; keep in your refrigerator for up to 3 to days.
- For freezing, place the soup in airtight containers. It will maintain the best quality for about to 6 months. Defrost in the refrigerator. Bon appétit!

Nutrition: 25Calories; 12.9g Fat; 3.2g Carbs; 35.1g Protein; 2.2g Fiber

295) CREAMY GREEK-STYLE SOUP

Cooking Time: 30 Minutes   **Servings: 4**

Ingredients:

- ✓ 1/2 stick butter
- ✓ 1/2 cup zucchini, diced
- ✓ 2 garlic cloves, minced
- ✓ 4 ½ cups roasted vegetable broth
- ✓ Sea salt and ground black pepper, to season
- ✓ 1 ½ cups leftover turkey, shredded
- ✓ 1/3 cup double cream
- ✓ 1/2 cup Greek-style yogurt

Directions:

- ❖ In a heavy-bottomed pot, melt the butter over medium-high heat. Once hot, cook the zucchini and garlic for 2 minutes until they are fragrant.
- ❖ Add in the broth, salt, black pepper, and leftover turkey. Cover and cook for minutes, stirring periodically.
- ❖ Then, fold in the cream and yogurt. Continue to cook for 5 minutes more or until thoroughly warmed.
- ❖ Storing
- ❖ Spoon the soup into four airtight containers or Ziploc bags; keep in your refrigerator for up to 3 to 4 days.
- ❖ For freezing, place the soup in airtight containers. It will maintain the best quality for about 4 to months. Defrost in the refrigerator. Enjoy!

Nutrition: 256 Calories; 18.8g Fat; 5.4g Carbs; 15.8g Protein; 0.2g Fiber

296) LOW-CARB PORK WRAPS

Cooking Time: 15 Minutes   **Servings: 4**

Ingredients:

- ✓ 1 pound ground pork
- ✓ 2 garlic cloves, finely minced
- ✓ 1 chili pepper, deveined and finely minced
- ✓ 1 tsp mustard powder
- ✓ 1 tbsp sunflower seeds
- ✓ 2 tbsp champagne vinegar
- ✓ 1 tbsp coconut aminos
- ✓ Celery salt and ground black pepper, to taste
- ✓ 2 scallion stalks, sliced
- ✓ 1 head lettuce

Directions:

- ❖ Sear the ground pork in the preheated pan for about 8 minutes. Stir in the garlic, chili pepper, mustard seeds, and sunflower seeds; continue to sauté for minute longer or until aromatic.
- ❖ Add in the vinegar, coconut aminos, salt, black pepper, and scallions. Stir to combine well.
- ❖ Storing
- ❖ Place the ground pork mixture in airtight containers or Ziploc bags; keep in your refrigerator for up to 3 to days.
- ❖ For freezing, place the ground pork mixture it in airtight containers or heavy-duty freezer bags. Freeze up to 2 to 3 months. Defrost in the refrigerator and reheat in the skillet.
- ❖ Add spoonfuls of the pork mixture to the lettuce leaves, wrap them and serve.

Nutrition: 281 Calories; 19.4g Fat; 5.1g Carbs; 22.1g Protein; 1.3g Fiber

297) MISSISSIPPI-STYLE PULLED PORK

Cooking Time: 6 Hours   **Servings:** 4

Ingredients:

- ✓ 1 ½ pounds pork shoulder
- ✓ 1 tbsp liquid smoke sauce
- ✓ 1 tsp chipotle powder
- ✓ Au Jus gravy seasoning packet
- ✓ 2 onions, cut into wedges
- ✓ Kosher salt and freshly ground black pepper, taste

Directions:

- ❖ Mix the liquid smoke sauce, chipotle powder, Au Jus gravy seasoning packet, salt and pepper. Rub the spice mixture into the pork on all sides.
- ❖ Wrap in plastic wrap and let it marinate in your refrigerator for 3 hours.
- ❖ Prepare your grill for indirect heat. Place the pork butt roast on the grate over a drip pan and top with onions; cover the grill and cook for about 6 hours.
- ❖ Transfer the pork to a cutting board. Now, shred the meat into bite-sized pieces using two forks.
- ❖ Storing
- ❖ Divide the pork between four airtight containers or Ziploc bags; keep in your refrigerator for up to 3 to 5 days.
- ❖ For freezing, place the pork in airtight containers or heavy-duty freezer bags. Freeze up to 4 months. Defrost in the refrigerator. Bon appétit!

Nutrition: 350 Calories; 11g Fat; 5g Carbs; 53.6g Protein; 2.2g Fiber

298) SPICY WITH CHEESY TURKEY DIP

Cooking Time: 25 Minutes   **Servings:** 4

Ingredients:

- ✓ 1 Fresno chili pepper, deveined and minced
- ✓ 1 ½ cups Ricotta cheese, creamed, 4% fat, softened
- ✓ 1/4 cup sour cream
- ✓ 1 tbsp butter, room temperature
- ✓ 1 shallot, chopped
- ✓ 1 tsp garlic, pressed
- ✓ 1 pound ground turkey
- ✓ 1/2 cup goat cheese, shredded
- ✓ Salt and black pepper, to taste
- ✓ 1 ½ cups Gruyère, shredded

Directions:

- ❖ Melt the butter in a frying pan over a moderately high flame. Now, sauté the onion and garlic until they have softened.
- ❖ Stir in the ground turkey and continue to cook until it is no longer pink.
- ❖ Transfer the sautéed mixture to a lightly greased baking dish. Add in Ricotta, sour cream, goat cheese, salt, pepper, and chili pepper.
- ❖ Top with the shredded Gruyère cheese. Bake in the preheated oven at 350 degrees F for about 20 minutes or until hot and bubbly in top.
- ❖ Storing
- ❖ Place your dip in an airtight container; keep in your refrigerator for up 3 to 4 days. Enjoy!

Nutrition: 284 Calories; 19g Fat; 3.2g Carbs; 26. Protein; 1.6g Fiber

299) TURKEY CHORIZO AND BOK CHOY

Cooking Time: 50 Minutes   **Servings:** 4

Ingredients:

- ✓ 4 mild turkey Chorizo, sliced
- ✓ 1/2 cup full-fat milk
- ✓ 6 ounces Gruyère cheese, preferably freshly grated
- ✓ 1 yellow onion, chopped
- ✓ Coarse salt and ground black pepper, to taste
- ✓ 1 pound Bok choy, tough stem ends trimmed
- ✓ 1 cup cream of mushroom soup
- ✓ 1 tbsp lard, room temperature

Directions:

- ❖ Melt the lard in a nonstick skillet over a moderate flame; cook the Chorizo sausage for about 5 minutes, stirring occasionally to ensure even cooking; reserve.
- ❖ Add in the onion, salt, pepper, Bok choy, and cream of mushroom soup. Continue to cook for 4 minutes longer or until the vegetables have softened.
- ❖ Spoon the mixture into a lightly oiled casserole dish. Top with the reserved Chorizo.
- ❖ In a mixing bowl, thoroughly combine the milk and cheese. Pour the cheese mixture over the sausage.
- ❖ Cover with foil and bake at 36degrees F for about 35 minutes.
- ❖ Storing
- ❖ Cut your casserole into four portions. Place each portion in an airtight container; keep in your refrigerator for 3 to 4 days.
- ❖ For freezing, wrap your portions tightly with heavy-duty aluminum foil or freezer wrap. Freeze up to 1 to 2 months. Defrost in the refrigerator. Enjoy!

Nutrition: 18Calories; 12g Fat; 2.6g Carbs; 9.4g Protein; 1g Fiber

300) DELICIOUS SAUCY BOSTON BUTT

Cooking Time: 1 Hour 20 Minutes   **Servings:** 8

Ingredients:

- ✓ 1 tbsp lard, room temperature
- ✓ 2 pounds Boston butt, cubed
- ✓ Salt and freshly ground pepper
- ✓ 1/2 tsp mustard powder
- ✓ A bunch of spring onions, chopped
- ✓ 2 garlic cloves, minced
- ✓ 1/2 tbsp ground cardamom
- ✓ 2 tomatoes, pureed
- ✓ 1 bell pepper, deveined and chopped
- ✓ 1 jalapeno pepper, deveined and finely chopped
- ✓ 1/2 cup unsweetened coconut milk
- ✓ 2 cups chicken bone broth

Directions:

- ❖ In a wok, melt the lard over moderate heat. Season the pork belly with salt, pepper and mustard powder.
- ❖ Sear the pork for 8 to 10 minutes, stirring periodically to ensure even cooking; set aside, keeping it warm.
- ❖ In the same wok, sauté the spring onions, garlic, and cardamom. Spoon the sautéed vegetables along with the reserved pork into the slow cooker.
- ❖ Add in the remaining ingredients, cover with the lid and cook for 1 hour 10 minutes over low heat.
- ❖ Storing
- ❖ Divide the pork and vegetables between airtight containers or Ziploc bags; keep in your refrigerator for up to 3 to 5 days.
- ❖ For freezing, place the pork and vegetables in airtight containers or heavy-duty freezer bags. Freeze up to 4 months. Defrost in the refrigerator. Bon appétit!

Nutrition: 369 Calories; 20.2g Fat; 2.9g Carbs; 41.3g Protein; 0.7g Fiber

301) FLATBREAD AND CHICKEN LIVER PÂTÉ

Cooking Time: 2 Hours 15 Minutes   **Servings: 4**

Ingredients:

- ✓ 1 yellow onion, finely chopped
- ✓ 10 ounces chicken livers
- ✓ 1/2 tsp Mediterranean seasoning blend
- ✓ 4 tbsp olive oil
- ✓ 1 garlic clove, minced

- ✓ For Flatbread:
- ✓ 1 cup lukewarm water
- ✓ 1/2 stick butter
- ✓ 1/2 cup flax meal
- ✓ 1 ½ tbsp psyllium husks
- ✓ 1 ¼ cups almond flour

Directions:

- ❖ Pulse the chicken livers along with the seasoning blend, olive oil, onion and garlic in your food processor; reserve.
- ❖ Mix the dry ingredients for the flatbread. Mix in all the wet ingredients. Whisk to combine well.
- ❖ Let it stand at room temperature for 2 hours. Divide the dough into 8 balls and roll them out on a flat surface.
- ❖ In a lightly greased pan, cook your flatbread for 1 minute on each side or until golden.
- ❖ Storing
- ❖ Wrap the chicken liver pate in foil before packing it into airtight containers; keep in your refrigerator for up to 7 days.
- ❖ For freezing, place the chicken liver pate in airtight containers or heavy-duty freezer bags. Freeze up to 2 months. Defrost overnight in the refrigerator.
- ❖ As for the keto flatbread, wrap them in foil before packing them into airtight containers; keep in your refrigerator for up to 4 days.
- ❖ Bon appétit!

Nutrition: 395 Calories; 30.2g Fat; 3.6g Carbs; 17.9g Protein; 0.5g Fiber

302) SATURDAY CHICKEN WITH CAULIFLOWER SALAD

Cooking Time: 20 Minutes   **Servings: 2**

Ingredients:

- ✓ 1 tsp hot paprika
- ✓ 2 tbsp fresh basil, snipped
- ✓ 1/2 cup mayonnaise
- ✓ 1 tsp mustard
- ✓ 2 tsp butter
- ✓ 2 chicken wings

- ✓ 1/2 cup cheddar cheese, shredded
- ✓ Sea salt and ground black pepper, to taste
- ✓ 2 tbsp dry sherry
- ✓ 1 shallot, finely minced
- ✓ 1/2 head of cauliflower

Directions:

- ❖ Boil the cauliflower in a pot of salted water until it has softened; cut into small florets and place in a salad bowl.
- ❖ Melt the butter in a saucepan over medium-high heat. Cook the chicken for about 8 minutes or until the skin is crisp and browned. Season with hot paprika salt, and black pepper.
- ❖ Whisk the mayonnaise, mustard, dry sherry, and shallot and dress your salad. Top with cheddar cheese and fresh basil.
- ❖ Storing
- ❖ Place the chicken wings in airtight containers or Ziploc bags; keep in your refrigerator for up 3 to 4 days.
- ❖ Keep the cauliflower salad in your refrigerator for up 3 days.
- ❖ For freezing, place the chicken wings in airtight containers or heavy-duty freezer bags. Freeze up to 3 months. Once thawed in the refrigerator, reheat in a saucepan until thoroughly warmed.

Nutrition: 444 Calories; 36g Fat; 5.7g Carbs; 20.6g Protein; 4.3g Fiber

303) SPECIAL KANSAS-STYLE MEATLOAF

Cooking Time: 1 Hour 10 Minutes   **Servings:** 8

Ingredients:

- ✓ 2 pounds ground pork
- ✓ 2 eggs, beaten
- ✓ 1/2 cup onions, chopped
- ✓ 1/2 cup marinara sauce, bottled
- ✓ 8 ounces Colby cheese, shredded
- ✓ 1 tsp granulated garlic
- ✓ Sea salt and freshly ground black pepper, to taste
- ✓ 1 tsp lime zest
- ✓ 1 tsp mustard seeds
- ✓ 1/2 cup tomato puree
- ✓ 1 tbsp Erythritol

Directions:

- ❖ Mix the ground pork with the eggs, onions, marinara salsa, cheese, granulated garlic, salt, pepper, lime zest, and mustard seeds; mix to combine.
- ❖ Press the mixture into a lightly-greased loaf pan. Mix the tomato paste with the Erythritol and spread the mixture over the top of your meatloaf.
- ❖ Bake in the preheated oven at 5 degrees F for about 1 hour 10 minutes, rotating the pan halfway through the cook time. Storing Wrap your meatloaf tightly with heavy-duty aluminum foil or plastic wrap. Then, keep in your refrigerator for up to 3 to 4 days.
- ❖ For freezing, wrap your meatloaf tightly to prevent freezer burn. Freeze up to 3 to 4 months. Defrost in the refrigerator. Bon appétit!

Nutrition: 318 Calories; 14. Fat; 6.2g Carbs; 39.3g Protein; 0.3g Fiber

304) ORIGINAL TURKEY KEBABS

Cooking Time: 30 Minutes   **Servings:** 6

Ingredients:

- ✓ 1 ½ pounds turkey breast, cubed
- ✓ 3 Spanish peppers, sliced
- ✓ 2 zucchinis, cut into thick slices
- ✓ 1 onion, cut into wedges
- ✓ 2 tbsp olive oil, room temperature
- ✓ 1 tbsp dry ranch seasoning

Directions:

- ❖ Thread the turkey pieces and vegetables onto bamboo skewers. Sprinkle the skewers with dry ranch seasoning and olive oil.
- ❖ Grill your kebabs for about 10 minutes, turning them periodically to ensure even cooking.
- ❖ Storing
- ❖ Wrap your kebabs in foil before packing them into airtight containers; keep in your refrigerator for up to 3 to days.
- ❖ For freezing, place your kebabs in airtight containers or heavy-duty freezer bags. Freeze up to 2-3 months. Defrost in the refrigerator. Bon appétit!

Nutrition: 2 Calories; 13.8g Fat; 6.7g Carbs; 25.8g Protein; 1.2g Fiber

305) ORIGINAL MEXICAN-STYLE TURKEY BACON BITES

Cooking Time: 5 Minutes   **Servings:** 4

- ✓ 1 jalapeno pepper, deveined and minced
- ✓ 1 tsp Mexican oregano
- ✓ 2 tbsp scallions, finely chopped

Directions:

- ❖ Thoroughly combine all ingredients in a mixing bowl.
- ❖ Roll the mixture into 8 balls.
- ❖ Storing
- ❖ Divide the turkey bacon bites between two airtight containers or Ziploc bags; keep in your refrigerator for up 3 to days.

Nutrition: 19Calories; 16.7g Fat; 2.2g Carbs; 8.8g Protein; 0.3g Fiber

306) TYPICAL MEDITERRANEAN-STYLE CHEESY PORK LOIN

Cooking Time: 25 Minutes   **Servings: 4**

Ingredients:

- ✓ 1 pound pork loin, cut into 1-inch-thick pieces
- ✓ 1 tsp Mediterranean seasoning mix
- ✓ Salt and pepper, to taste
- ✓ 1 onion, sliced
- ✓ 1 tsp fresh garlic, smashed
- ✓ 2 tbsp black olives, pitted and sliced
- ✓ 2 tbsp balsamic vinegar
- ✓ 1/2 cup Romano cheese, grated
- ✓ 2 tbsp butter, room temperature
- ✓ 1 tbsp curry paste
- ✓ 1 cup roasted vegetable broth
- ✓ 1 tbsp oyster sauce

Directions:

- ❖ In a frying pan, melt the butter over a moderately high heat. Once hot, cook the pork until browned on all sides; season with salt and black pepper and set aside.
- ❖ In the pan drippings, cook the onion and garlic for 4 to 5 minutes or until they've softened.
- ❖ Add in the Mediterranean seasoning mix, curry paste, and vegetable broth. Continue to cook until the sauce has thickened and reduced slightly or about 10 minutes. Add in the remaining ingredients along with the reserved pork.
- ❖ Top with cheese and cook for 10 minutes longer or until cooked through.
- ❖ Storing
- ❖ Divide the pork loin between four airtight containers; keep in your refrigerator for 3 to 5 days.
- ❖ For freezing, place the pork loin in airtight containers or heavy-duty freezer bags. Freeze up to 4 to 6 months. Defrost in the refrigerator. Enjoy!

Nutrition: 476 Calories; 35.3g Fat; 6.2g Carbs; 31.1g Protein; 1.4g Fiber

307) OVEN-ROASTED SPARE RIBS

Cooking Time: 3 Hour 40 Minutes   **Servings: 6**

Ingredients:

- ✓ 2 pounds spare ribs
- ✓ 1 garlic clove, minced
- ✓ 1 tsp dried marjoram
- ✓ 1 lime, halved
- ✓ Salt and ground black pepper, to taste

Directions:

- ❖ Toss all ingredients in a ceramic dish.
- ❖ Cover and let it refrigerate for 5 to 6 hours.
- ❖ Roast the foil-wrapped ribs in the preheated oven at 275 degrees F degrees for about hours 30 minutes.
- ❖ Storing
- ❖ Divide the ribs into six portions. Place each portion of ribs in an airtight container; keep in your refrigerator for 3 to days.
- ❖ For freezing, place the ribs in airtight containers or heavy-duty freezer bags. Freeze up to 4 to months. Defrost in the refrigerator and reheat in the preheated oven. Bon appétit!

Nutrition: 385 Calories; 29g Fat; 1.8g Carbs; 28.3g Protein; 0.1g Fiber

308) HEALTHY PARMESAN CHICKEN SALAD

Cooking Time: 20 Minutes   **Servings:** 6

Ingredients:

- ✓ 2 romaine hearts, leaves separated
- ✓ Flaky sea salt and ground black pepper, to taste
- ✓ 1/4 tsp chili pepper flakes
- ✓ 1 tsp dried basil
- ✓ 1/4 cup Parmesan, finely grated
- ✓ 2 chicken breasts
- ✓ 2 Lebanese cucumbers, sliced
- ✓ For the dressing:
- ✓ 2 large egg yolks
- ✓ 1 tsp Dijon mustard
- ✓ 1 tbsp fresh lemon juice
- ✓ 1/4 cup olive oil
- ✓ 2 garlic cloves, minced

Directions:

- ❖ In a grilling pan, cook the chicken breast until no longer pink or until a meat thermometer registers 5 degrees F. Slice the chicken into strips.
- ❖ Storing
- ❖ Place the chicken breasts in airtight containers or Ziploc bags; keep in your refrigerator for to 4 days.
- ❖ For freezing, place the chicken breasts in airtight containers or heavy-duty freezer bags. It will maintain the best quality for about months. Defrost in the refrigerator.
- ❖ Toss the chicken with the other ingredients. Prepare the dressing by whisking all the ingredients.
- ❖ Dress the salad and enjoy! Keep the salad in your refrigerator for 3 to 5 days.

Nutrition: 183 Calories; 12.5g Fat; 1. Carbs; 16.3g Protein; 0.9g Fiber

309) GRILL-STYLE CHICKEN SALAD WITH AVOCADO

Cooking Time: 20 Minutes   **Servings:** 4

Ingredients:

- ✓ 1/3 cup olive oil
- ✓ 2 chicken breasts
- ✓ Sea salt and crushed red pepper flakes
- ✓ 2 egg yolks
- ✓ 1 tbsp fresh lemon juice
- ✓ 1/2 tsp celery seeds
- ✓ 1 tbsp coconut aminos
- ✓ 1 large-sized avocado, pitted and sliced

Directions:

- ❖ Grill the chicken breasts for about 4 minutes per side. Season with salt and pepper, to taste.
- ❖ Slice the grilled chicken into bite-sized strips.
- ❖ To make the dressing, whisk the egg yolks, lemon juice, celery seeds, olive oil and coconut aminos in a measuring cup.
- ❖ Storing
- ❖ Place the chicken breasts in airtight containers or Ziploc bags; keep in your refrigerator for 3 to 4 days.
- ❖ For freezing, place the chicken breasts in airtight containers or heavy-duty freezer bags. It will maintain the best quality for about 4 months. Defrost in the refrigerator.
- ❖ Store dressing in your refrigerator for 3 to 4 days. Dress the salad and garnish with fresh avocado. Bon appétit!

Nutrition: 40Calories; 34.2g Fat; 4.8g Carbs; 22.7g Protein; 3.1g Fiber

310) **EASY-COOKING FALL-OFF-THE-BONE RIBS**

Cooking Time: 8 Hours   **Servings:** 4

Ingredients:

- ✓ 1 pound baby back ribs
- ✓ 4 tbsp coconut aminos
- ✓ 1/4 cup dry red wine
- ✓ 1/2 tsp cayenne pepper
- ✓ 1 garlic clove, crushed
- ✓ 1 tsp Italian herb mix
- ✓ 1 tbsp butter
- ✓ 1 tsp Serrano pepper, minced
- ✓ 1 Italian pepper, thinly sliced
- ✓ 1 tsp grated lemon zest

Directions:

- ❖ Butter the sides and bottom of your Crock pot. Place the pork and peppers on the bottom.
- ❖ Add in the remaining ingredients.
- ❖ Slow cook for 9 hours on Low heat setting.
- ❖ Storing
- ❖ Divide the baby back ribs into four portions. Place each portion of the ribs along with the peppers in an airtight container; keep in your refrigerator for 3 to days.
- ❖ For freezing, place the ribs in airtight containers or heavy-duty freezer bags. Freeze up to 4 to months. Defrost in the refrigerator. Reheat in your oven at 250 degrees F until heated through.

Nutrition: 192 Calories; 6.9g Fat; 0.9g Carbs; 29.8g Protein; 0.5g Fiber

311) **CLASSIC BRIE-STUFFED MEATBALLS**

Cooking Time: 25 Minutes   **Servings:** 5

Ingredients:

- ✓ 2 eggs, beaten
- ✓ 1 pound ground pork
- ✓ 1/3 cup double cream
- ✓ 1 tbsp fresh parsley
- ✓ Kosher salt and ground black pepper
- ✓ 1 tsp dried rosemary
- ✓ 10 (1-inch cubes of brie cheese
- ✓ 2 tbsp scallions, minced
- ✓ 2 cloves garlic, minced

Directions:

- ❖ Mix all ingredients, except for the brie cheese, until everything is well incorporated.
- ❖ Roll the mixture into 10 patties; place a piece of cheese in the center of each patty and roll into a ball.
- ❖ Roast in the preheated oven at 0 degrees F for about 20 minutes.
- ❖ Storing
- ❖ Place the meatballs in airtight containers or Ziploc bags; keep in your refrigerator for up to 3 to 4 days.
- ❖ Freeze the meatballs in airtight containers or heavy-duty freezer bags. Freeze up to 3 to 4 months. To defrost, slowly reheat in a saucepan. Bon appétit!

Nutrition: 302 Calories; 13g Fat; 1.9g Carbs; 33.4g Protein; 0.3g Fiber

312) SPECIAL SPICY AND TANGY CHICKEN DRUMSTICKS

Cooking Time: 55 Minutes   **Servings:** 6

Ingredients:

- ✓ 3 chicken drumsticks, cut into chunks
- ✓ 1/2 stick butter
- ✓ 2 eggs
- ✓ 1/4 cup hemp seeds, ground
- ✓ Salt and cayenne pepper, to taste
- ✓ 2 tbsp coconut aminos
- ✓ 3 tsp red wine vinegar
- ✓ 2 tbsp salsa
- ✓ 2 cloves garlic, minced

Directions:

- ❖ Rub the chicken with the butter, salt, and cayenne pepper.
- ❖ Drizzle the chicken with the coconut aminos, vinegar, salsa, and garlic. Allow it to stand for 30 minutes in your refrigerator.
- ❖ Whisk the eggs with the hemp seeds. Dip each chicken strip in the egg mixture. Place the chicken chunks in a parchment-lined baking pan.
- ❖ Roast in the preheated oven at 390 degrees F for 25 minutes.
- ❖ Storing
- ❖ Divide the roasted chicken between airtight containers; keep in your refrigerator for up 3 to 4 days.
- ❖ For freezing, place the roasted chicken in airtight containers or heavy-duty freezer bags. Freeze up to 3 months. Defrost in the refrigerator and reheat in a pan. Enjoy!

Nutrition: 420 Calories; 22g Fat; 5g Carbs; 35.3g Protein; 0.8g Fiber

313) ORIGINAL ITALIAN-STYLE CHICKEN MEATBALLS WITH PARMESAN

Cooking Time: 20 Minutes   **Servings:** 6

Ingredients:

- ✓ For the Meatballs:
- ✓ 1 ¼ pounds chicken, ground
- ✓ 1 tbsp sage leaves, chopped
- ✓ 1 tsp shallot powder
- ✓ 1 tsp porcini powder
- ✓ 2 garlic cloves, finely minced
- ✓ 1/3 tsp dried basil
- ✓ 3/4 cup Parmesan cheese, grated
- ✓ 2 eggs, lightly beaten
- ✓ Salt and ground black pepper, to your liking
- ✓ 1/2 tsp cayenne pepper
- ✓ For the sauce:
- ✓ 2 tomatoes, pureed
- ✓ 1 cup chicken consommé
- ✓ 2 ½ tbsp lard, room temperature
- ✓ 1 onion, peeled and finely chopped

Directions:

- ❖ In a mixing bowl, combine all ingredients for the meatballs. Roll the mixture into bite-sized balls.
- ❖ Melt 1 tbsp of lard in a skillet over a moderately high heat. Sear the meatballs for about 3 minutes or until they are thoroughly cooked; reserve.
- ❖ Melt the remaining lard and cook the onions until tender and translucent. Add in pureed tomatoes and chicken consommé and continue to cook for 4 minutes longer.
- ❖ Add in the reserved meatballs, turn the heat to simmer and continue to cook for 6 to 7 minutes.
- ❖ Storing
- ❖ Place the meatballs in airtight containers or Ziploc bags; keep in your refrigerator for up to 3 to 4 days.
- ❖ Freeze the meatballs in airtight containers or heavy-duty freezer bags. Freeze up to 3 to 4 months. To defrost, slowly reheat in a saucepan. Bon appétit!

Nutrition: 252 Calories; 9.7g Fat; 5.3g Carbs; 34.2g Protein; 1.4g Fiber

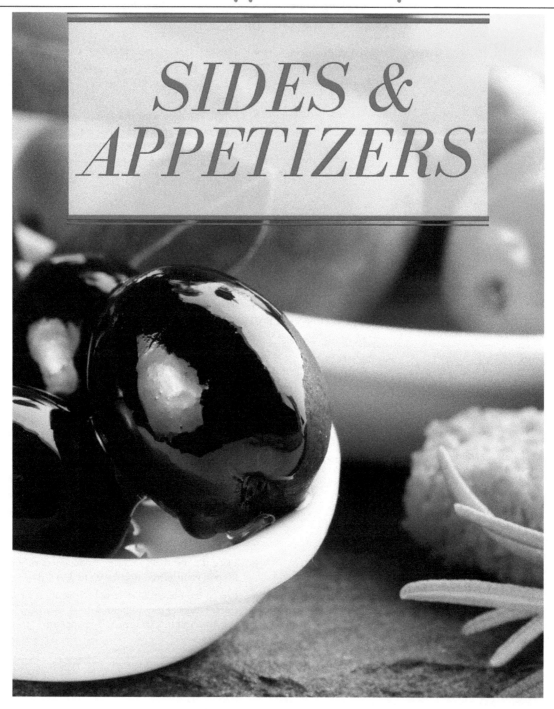

SIDES & APPETIZERS

314) ORIGINAL LEMON GARLIC SARDINE FETTUCCINE

Cooking Time: 15 Minutes   **Servings:** 4

Ingredients:

- ✓ 8 ounces whole-wheat fettuccine
- ✓ 4 tbsp extra-virgin olive oil, divided
- ✓ 4 cloves garlic, minced
- ✓ 1 cup fresh breadcrumbs
- ✓ ¼ cup lemon juice
- ✓ 1 tsp freshly ground pepper
- ✓ ½ tsp of salt
- ✓ 2 4-ounce cans boneless and skinless sardines, dipped in tomato sauce
- ✓ ½ cup fresh parsley, chopped
- ✓ ¼ cup finely shredded parmesan cheese

Directions:

- ❖ Fill a large pot with water and bring to a boil.
- ❖ Cook pasta according to package instructions until tender (about 10 minutes).
- ❖ In a small skillet, heat 2 tbsp of oil over medium heat.
- ❖ Add garlic and cook for about 20 seconds, until sizzling and fragrant.
- ❖ Transfer the garlic to a large bowl.
- ❖ Add the remaining 2 tbsp of oil to skillet and heat over medium heat.
- ❖ Add breadcrumbs and cook for 5-6 minutes until golden and crispy.
- ❖ Whisk lemon juice, salt, and pepper into the garlic bowl.
- ❖ Add pasta to the garlic bowl, along with garlic, sardines, parmesan, and parsley; give it a gentle stir.
- ❖ Cool and spread over the containers.
- ❖ Before eating, sprinkle with breadcrumbs.
- ❖ Enjoy!

Nutrition: 633, Total Fat: 27.7 g, Saturated Fat: 6.4 g, Cholesterol: 40 mg, Sodium: 771 mg, Total Carbohydrate: 55.9 g, Dietary Fiber: 7.7 g, Total Sugars: 2.1 g, Protein: 38.6 g, Vitamin D: 0 mcg, Calcium: 274 mg, Iron: 7 mg, Potassium: mg

315) DELICIOUS SPINACH ALMOND STIR-FRY

Cooking Time: 10 Minutes   **Servings:** 2

Ingredients:

- ✓ 2 ounces spinach
- ✓ 1 tbsp coconut oil
- ✓ 3 tbsp almond, slices
- ✓ sea salt or plain salt
- ✓ freshly ground black pepper

Directions:

- ❖ Start by heating a skillet with coconut oil; add spinach and let it cook.
- ❖ Then, add salt and pepper as the spinach is cooking.
- ❖ Finally, add in the almond slices.
- ❖ Serve warm.

Nutrition: 117, Total Fat: 11.4 g, Saturated Fat: 6.2 g, Cholesterol: 0 mg, Sodium: 23 mg, Total Carbohydrate: 2.9 g, Dietary Fiber: 1.7 g, Total Sugars: 0.g, Protein: 2.7 g, Vitamin D: 0 mcg, Calcium: 52 mg, Iron: 1 mg, Potassium: 224 mg

316) ITALIAN BBQ CARROTS

Cooking Time: 30 Minutes   **Servings:** 8

Ingredients:

- ✓ 2 pounds baby carrots (organic)
- ✓ 1 tbsp olive oil
- ✓ 1 tbsp garlic powder
- ✓ 1 tbsp onion powder
- ✓ sea salt or plain salt
- ✓ freshly ground black pepper

Directions:

- ❖ Mix all the Ingredients: in a plastic bag so that the carrots are well coated with the mixture.
- ❖ Then, on the BBQ grill place a piece of aluminum foil and spread the carrots in a single layer.
- ❖ Finally, grill for 30 minutes or until tender.
- ❖ Serve warm.

Nutrition: 388, Total Fat: 1.9 g, Saturated Fat: 0.3 g, Cholesterol: 0 mg, Sodium: 89 mg, Total Carbohydrate: 10.8 g, Dietary Fiber: 3.4 g, Total Sugars: 6 g, Protein: 1 g, Vitamin D: 0 mcg, Calcium: 40 mg, Iron: 1 mg, Potassium: 288 mg

317) MEDITERRANEAN-STYLE BAKED ZUCCHINI STICKS

Cooking Time: 20 Minutes   **Servings:** 8

Ingredients:

- ✓ ¼ cup feta cheese, crumbled
- ✓ 4 zucchini
- ✓ ¼ cup parsley, chopped
- ✓ ½ cup tomatoes, minced
- ✓ ½ cup kalamata olives, pitted and minced
- ✓ 1 cup red bell pepper, minced
- ✓ 1 tbsp oregano
- ✓ ¼ cup garlic, minced
- ✓ 1 tbsp basil
- ✓ sea salt or plain salt
- ✓ freshly ground black pepper

Directions:

- ❖ Start by cutting zucchini in half (lengthwise) and scoop out the middle.
- ❖ Then, combine garlic, black pepper, bell pepper, oregano, basil, tomatoes, and olives in a bowl.
- ❖ Now, fill in the middle of each zucchini with this mixture. Place these on a prepared baking dish and bake the dish at 0 degrees F for about 15 minutes.
- ❖ Finally, top with feta cheese and broil on high for 3 minutes or until done. Garnish with parsley.
- ❖ Serve warm.

Nutrition: 53, Total Fat: 2.2 g, Saturated Fat: 0.9 g, Cholesterol: 4 mg, Sodium: 138 mg, Total Carbohydrate: 7.5 g, Dietary Fiber: 2.1 g, Total Sugars: 3 g, Protein: 2.g, Vitamin D: 0 mcg, Calcium: 67 mg, Iron: 1 mg, Potassium: 353 mg

318) ARTICHOKE OLIVE PASTA

Cooking Time: 25 Minutes   **Servings:** 4

Ingredients:

- ✓ salt
- ✓ pepper
- ✓ 2 tbsp olive oil, divided
- ✓ 2 garlic cloves, thinly sliced
- ✓ 1 can artichoke hearts, drained, rinsed, and quartered lengthwise
- ✓ 1-pint grape tomatoes, halved lengthwise, divided
- ✓ ½ cup fresh basil leaves, torn apart
- ✓ 12 ounces whole-wheat spaghetti
- ✓ ½ medium onion, thinly sliced
- ✓ ½ cup dry white wine
- ✓ 1/3 cup pitted Kalamata olives, quartered lengthwise
- ✓ ¼ cup grated Parmesan cheese, plus extra for serving

Directions:

- ❖ Fill a large pot with salted water.
- ❖ Pour the water to a boil and cook your pasta according to package instructions until al dente.
- ❖ Drain the pasta and reserve 1 cup of the cooking water.
- ❖ Return the pasta to the pot and set aside.
- ❖ Heat 1 tbsp of olive oil in a large skillet over medium-high heat.
- ❖ Add onion and garlic, season with pepper and salt, and cook well for about 3-4 minutes until nicely browned.
- ❖ Add wine and cook for 2 minutes until evaporated.
- ❖ Stir in artichokes and keep cooking 2-3 minutes until brown.
- ❖ Add olives and half of your tomatoes.
- ❖ Cook well for 1-2 minutes until the tomatoes start to break down.
- ❖ Add pasta to the skillet.
- ❖ Stir in the rest of the tomatoes, cheese, basil, and remaining oil.
- ❖ Thin the mixture with the reserved pasta water if needed.
- ❖ Place in containers and sprinkle with extra cheese.
- ❖ Enjoy!

Nutrition: 340, Total Fat: 11.9 g, Saturated Fat: 3.3 g, Cholesterol: 10 mg, Sodium: 278 mg, Total Carbohydrate: 35.8 g, Dietary Fiber: 7.8 g, Total Sugars: 4.8 g, Protein: 11.6 g, Vitamin D: 0 mcg, Calcium: 193 mg, Iron: 3 mg, Potassium: 524 mg

319)   VEGGIE MEDITERRANEAN-STYLE PASTA

Cooking Time: 2 Hours   **Servings:** 4

Ingredients:

- ✓ 1 tbsp olive oil
- ✓ 1 small onion, finely chopped
- ✓ 2 small garlic cloves, finely chopped
- ✓ 2 14-ounce cans diced tomatoes
- ✓ 1 tbsp sun-dried tomato paste
- ✓ 1 bay leaf
- ✓ 1 tsp dried thyme
- ✓ 1 tsp dried basil
- ✓ 1 tsp oregano
- ✓ 1 tsp dried parsley
- ✓ bread of your choice

- ✓ ½ tsp salt
- ✓ ½ tsp brown sugar
- ✓ freshly ground black pepper
- ✓ 1 piece aubergine
- ✓ 2 pieces courgettes
- ✓ 2 pieces red peppers, de-seeded
- ✓ 2 garlic cloves, peeled
- ✓ 2-3 tbsp olive oil
- ✓ 12 small vine-ripened tomatoes
- ✓ 16 ounces of pasta of your preferred shape, such as Gigli, conchiglie, etc.
- ✓ 3½ ounces parmesan cheese

Directions:

- ❖ Heat oil in a pan over medium heat.
- ❖ Add onions and fry them until tender.
- ❖ Add garlic and stir-fry for 1 minute.
- ❖ Add the remaining Ingredients: listed under the sauce and bring to a boil.
- ❖ Reduce the heat, cover, and simmer for 60 minutes.
- ❖ Season with black pepper and salt as needed. Set aside.
- ❖ Preheat oven to 350 degrees F.
- ❖ Chop up courgettes, aubergine and red peppers into 1-inch pieces.
- ❖ Place them on a roasting pan along with whole garlic cloves.
- ❖ Drizzle with olive oil and season with salt and black pepper.
- ❖ Mix the veggies well and roast in the oven for 45 minutes until they are tender.
- ❖ Add tomatoes just before 20 minutes to end time.
- ❖ Cook your pasta according to package instructions.
- ❖ Drain well and stir into the sauce.
- ❖ Divide the pasta sauce between 4 containers and top with vegetables.
- ❖ Grate some parmesan cheese on top and serve with bread.
- ❖ Enjoy!

Nutrition: Calories: 211, Total Fat: 14.9 g, Saturated Fat: 2.1 g, Cholesterol: 0 mg, Sodium: 317 mg, Total Carbohydrate: 20.1 g, Dietary Fiber: 5.7 g, Total Sugars: 11.7 g, Protein: 4.2 g, Vitamin D: 0 mcg, Calcium: 66 mg, Iron: 2 mg, Potassium: 955 mg

320)   TUSCAN BAKED MUSHROOMS

Cooking Time: 20 Minutes   **Servings:** 2

Ingredients:

- ✓ ½ pound mushrooms (sliced)
- ✓ 2 tbsp olive oil (onion and garlic flavored)
- ✓ 1 can tomatoes
- ✓ 1 cup Parmesan cheese

- ✓ ½ tsp oregano
- ✓ 1 tbsp basil
- ✓ sea salt or plain salt
- ✓ freshly ground black pepper

Directions:

- ❖ Heat the olive oil in the pan and add the mushrooms, salt, and pepper. Cook for about 2 minutes.
- ❖ Then, transfer the mushrooms into a baking dish.
- ❖ Now, in a separate bowl mix the tomatoes, basil, oregano, salt, and pepper, and layer it on the mushrooms. Top it with Parmesan cheese.
- ❖ Finally, bake the dish at 0 degrees F for about 18-22 minutes or until done.
- ❖ Serve warm.

Nutrition: Calories: 358, Total Fat: 27 g, Saturated Fat: 10.2 g, Cholesterol: 40 mg, Sodium: 535 mg, Total Carbohydrate: 13 g, Dietary Fiber: 3.5 g, Total Sugars: 6.7 g, Protein: 23.2 g, Vitamin D: 408 mcg, Calcium: 526 mg, Iron: 4 mg, Potassium: 797 mg

321) CLASSIC BASIL PASTA

Cooking Time: 40 Minutes   **Servings:** 4

Ingredients:

- ✓ 2 red peppers, de-seeded and cut into chunks
- ✓ 2 red onions cut into wedges
- ✓ 2 mild red chilies, de-seeded and diced
- ✓ 3 garlic cloves, coarsely chopped
- ✓ 1 tsp golden caster sugar
- ✓ 2 tbsp olive oil, plus extra for serving
- ✓ 2 pounds small ripe tomatoes, quartered
- ✓ 12 ounces pasta
- ✓ a handful of basil leaves, torn
- ✓ 2 tbsp grated parmesan
- ✓ salt
- ✓ pepper

Directions:

- ❖ Preheat oven to 390 degrees F.
- ❖ On a large roasting pan, spread peppers, red onion, garlic, and chilies.
- ❖ Sprinkle sugar on top.
- ❖ Drizzle olive oil and season with salt and pepper.
- ❖ Roast the veggies for 1minutes.
- ❖ Add tomatoes and roast for another 15 minutes.
- ❖ In a large pot, cook your pasta in salted boiling water according to instructions.
- ❖ Once ready, drain pasta.
- ❖ Remove the veggies from the oven and carefully add pasta.
- ❖ Toss everything well and let it cool.
- ❖ Spread over the containers.
- ❖ Before eating, place torn basil leaves on top, and sprinkle with parmesan.
- ❖ Enjoy!

Nutrition: Calories: 384, Total Fat: 10.8 g, Saturated Fat: 2.3 g, Cholesterol: 67 mg, Sodium: 133 mg, Total Carbohydrate: 59.4 g, Dietary Fiber: 2.3 g, Total Sugars: 5.7 g, Protein: 1 g, Vitamin D: 0 mcg, Calcium: 105 mg, Iron: 4 mg, Potassium: 422 mg

322) TYPICAL MINT TABBOULEH

Cooking Time: 15 Minutes   **Servings:** 6

Ingredients:

- ✓ ¼ cup fine bulgur
- ✓ 1/3 cup water, boiling
- ✓ 3 tbsp lemon juice
- ✓ ¼ tsp honey
- ✓ 1 1/3 cups pistachios, finely chopped
- ✓ 1 cup curly parsley, finely chopped
- ✓ 1 small cucumber, finely chopped
- ✓ 1 medium tomato, finely chopped
- ✓ 4 green onions, finely chopped
- ✓ 1/3 cup fresh mint, finely chopped
- ✓ 3 tbsp olive oil

Directions:

- ❖ Take a large bowl and add bulgur and 3 cup of boiling water.
- ❖ Allow it to stand for about 5 minutes.
- ❖ Stir in honey and lemon juice and allow it to stand for 5 minutes more.
- ❖ Fluff up the bulgur with a fork and stir in the rest of the Ingredients.
- ❖ Season with salt and pepper.
- ❖ Enjoy!

Nutrition: Calories: 15 Total Fat: 13.5 g, Saturated Fat: 1.8 g, Cholesterol: 0 mg, Sodium: 78 mg, Total Carbohydrate: 9.2 g, Dietary Fiber: 2.8 g, Total Sugars: 2.9 g, Protein: 3.8 g, Vitamin D: 0 mcg, Calcium: 46 mg, Iron: 2 mg, Potassium: 359 mg

323) ORIGINAL RED ONION KALE PASTA

Cooking Time: 25 Minutes   **Servings: 4**

Ingredients:

- ✓ 2½ cups vegetable broth
- ✓ ¾ cup dry lentils
- ✓ ½ tsp of salt
- ✓ 1 bay leaf
- ✓ ¼ cup olive oil
- ✓ 1 large red onion, chopped
- ✓ 1 tsp fresh thyme, chopped
- ✓ ½ tsp fresh oregano, chopped
- ✓ 1 tsp salt, divided
- ✓ ½ tsp black pepper
- ✓ 8 ounces vegan sausage, sliced into ¼-inch slices
- ✓ 1 bunch kale, stems removed and coarsely chopped
- ✓ 1 pack rotini

Directions:

- ❖ Add vegetable broth, ½ tsp of salt, bay leaf, and lentils to a saucepan over high heat and bring to a boil.
- ❖ Reduce the heat to medium-low and allow to cook for about minutes until tender.
- ❖ Discard the bay leaf.
- ❖ Take another skillet and heat olive oil over medium-high heat.
- ❖ Stir in thyme, onions, oregano, ½ a tsp of salt, and pepper; cook for 1 minute.
- ❖ Add sausage and reduce heat to medium-low.
- ❖ Cook for 10 minutes until the onions are tender.
- ❖ Bring water to a boil in a large pot, and then add rotini pasta and kale.
- ❖ Cook for about 8 minutes until al dente.
- ❖ Remove a bit of the cooking water and put it to the side.
- ❖ Drain the pasta and kale and return to the pot.
- ❖ Stir in both the lentils mixture and the onions mixture.
- ❖ Add the reserved cooking liquid to add just a bit of moistness.
- ❖ Spread over containers.

Nutrition: Calories: 508, Total Fat: 17 g, Saturated Fat: 3 g, Cholesterol: 0 mg, Sodium: 2431 mg, Total Carbohydrate: 59.3 g, Dietary Fiber: 6 g, Total Sugars: 4.8 g, Protein: 30.9 g, Vitamin D: 0 mcg, Calcium: 256 mg, Iron: 8 mg, Potassium: 1686 mg

324) SPECIAL BRAISED ARTICHOKES

Cooking Time: 30 Minutes   **Servings: 6**

Ingredients:

- ✓ 6 tbsp olive oil
- ✓ 2 pounds baby artichokes, trimmed
- ✓ ½ cup lemon juice
- ✓ 4 garlic cloves, thinly sliced
- ✓ ½ tsp salt
- ✓ 1½ pounds tomatoes, seeded and diced
- ✓ ½ cup almonds, toasted and sliced

Directions:

- ❖ Heat oil in a skillet over medium heat.
- ❖ Add artichokes, garlic, and lemon juice, and allow the garlic to sizzle.
- ❖ Season with salt.
- ❖ Reduce heat to medium-low, cover, and simmer for about 15 minutes.
- ❖ Uncover, add tomatoes, and simmer for another 10 minutes until the tomato liquid has mostly evaporated.
- ❖ Season with more salt and pepper.
- ❖ Sprinkle with toasted almonds.
- ❖ Enjoy!

Nutrition: Calories: 265, Total Fat: 1g, Saturated Fat: 2.6 g, Cholesterol: 0 mg, Sodium: 265 mg, Total Carbohydrate: 23 g, Dietary Fiber: 8.1 g, Total Sugars: 12.4 g, Protein: 7 g, Vitamin D: 0 mcg, Calcium: 81 mg, Iron: 2 mg, Potassium: 1077 mg

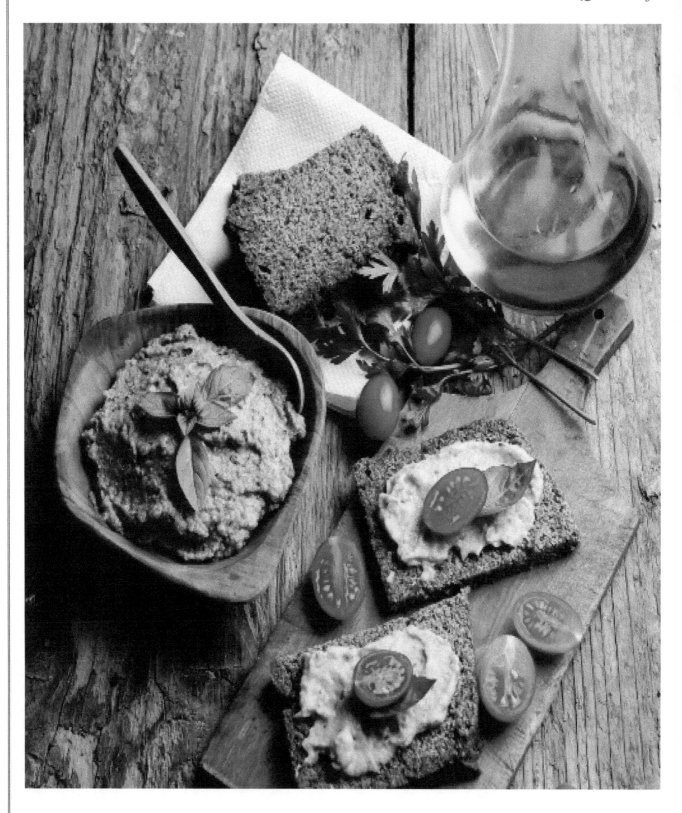

PART III-INTRODUCTION

The Mediterranean diet does not explicitly exclude any food group; it simply promotes better food choices such as replacing bad fats with good fats, red meat with seafood, etc. It encourages foods that are as close to their natural state as possible. The Mediterranean diet is one the easiest diets to follow and one of the best diets for a wide range of chronic diseases. Mediterranean diet has been shown to lower the risk of diabetes, cardiovascular disease, and cancer. The Mediterranean diet can help you shed unwanted pounds and slow the aging process by five to ten years. And you know, what makes the eating habits of the Italians and Greeks such a brilliant diet plan is that it's not just about the food, but an entire lifestyle! Over the decades, the Mediterranean diet has seen a slow rise in the Western world. Many Western countries were slow to pick it up, but they realized they had discovered the key to the Elixir of Life once they did. Not only has the Mediterranean diet helped people rely on a healthy, wholesome diet, but it has helped them lose weight, boost their immune systems, improve their vitality, and even contribute to healthy skin. In other words, the Mediterranean diet helped people feel good and look good. The combination of benefits changed people's perceptions of what they should eat and challenged their eating habits.

For example, many people often skip breakfast because they think having a meal in the morning adds more weight to their bodies. However, the Mediterranean diet does not skip breakfast. On the contrary, it considers breakfasting the most important meal of the day. Countries that have relied on the Mediterranean diet had seen its benefits long before scientific research was conducted. They did not have any study conducted to guide them to a particular dietary pattern or food content. Essentially, the diet has been refined over the millennia as new cooking methods were introduced. But adherence to a healthy form of the diet has remained, regardless of the diet's age.

This diet is the typical diet of the people of the Mediterranean area. It has been proven to be healthier than typical American and British diets. This diet contains lots of fresh fruits, vegetables, and fish. It also allows you to consume whole grains instead of refined white rice like other diets. The Mediterranean diet is considered a low-glycemic eating pattern, which means it does not raise blood sugar levels. It has many vitamins and minerals that help support a healthy heart and robust immune system.

This book was written specifically for people who want to get into this healthy way of eating. It will teach you how the Mediterranean diet can change your life forever!

For centuries, people have been cutting back on unhealthy foods and adding more healthy foods to their diets. Yet, for some reason, this good habit seems to have stopped before it even began. Not anymore. In "Mediterranean Diet Meal Preparation," you'll learn the secrets to losing belly fat: and getting your body in better shape.

This book will help you on how you can:

Get healthy with new food choices. Get more energy.

Lose belly fat: without diets; by taking advantage of homemade meal preparation methods. Find healthy alternatives for traditional desserts. We are getting the proper nutrients.

The Mediterranean could be considered a decorative and beautiful plant. In the Mediterranean region, there are so many palm trees that give the area a resort-like atmosphere. However, the plant has gained popularity in recent years because it has several health benefits. This diet emphasizes foods that are fresh, whole, unprocessed, and minimally altered. Benefits of eating the Mediterranean way include a lower risk of heart disease, cancer, stroke, depression, obesity, and diabetes.

MEDITERRANEAN DIET AND IT'S THE BENEFITS

In this nutrition and health-conscious world, medical scientists, nutritionists, and health scientists continue to search for healthy options and lifestyle changes that can ensure health and longevity along with agility. There is an emerging consensus among health experts that a diet with fiber and a balanced amount of protein, healthy fats, and minerals can lead to optimal health and healthy living. It can control cardiovascular disease, diabetes, cancer, and stroke and help maintain a healthy weight. The Mediterranean diet has all of these attributes. Its ingredients are rich in plants, healthy fats, fruits, whole grains, healthy meats, and more. It has all the elements that are essential for a healthy diet. There have been claims about its positive effect on health and physical well-being.

A study conducted on 25,000 women over 12 years determined that those who consume the Mediterranean diet have a 25% lower chance of having cardiovascular disease. This positive change is decreased inflammation and blood glucose levels and a better body mass index.

There is little saturated fat with a high amount of monounsaturated fat, protein, and dietary fiber. Olive oil has an important health element which is oleic acid. It is highly beneficial for human heart health. It has the European Food Safety Authority Panel's approval on Dietetic Products, Nutrition, and Allergies. It has been said that its polyphenols protect against the oxidation of blood lipids. This happens because of the priority given to olive oil, which has oleic acid that helps maintain normal LDL in the blood and control cardiovascular disease. The American Heart Association has also stated that consuming olive oil can help maintain cardiovascular health. If you follow this diet, your refined bread, processed foods, and unhealthy meats will be reduced. The diet also recommends replacing hard liquor with red wine. It is scientifically already proven that the Mediterranean diet can reduce the risk of cardiovascular disease.

This diet has a high fiber content. This reduces the blood glucose level and controls the causes that develop type 2 diabetes. This fiber makes you feel full and keeps cravings under control. This also helps in keeping weight under control and reduces constipation and helps in regulating bowel movement.

Maintaining a healthy weight is the main point in good health. It becomes easy to maintain an ideal weight when you follow a diet rich in fruits and vegetables. When combined with a physical routine, it becomes easy to maintain a healthy weight. This can help reduce obesity as well. Besides, maintaining an ideal weight can give us multiple health benefits.

Through comprehensive research, it has been found that regular, monitored consumption of the Mediterranean diet can minimize the risk of death from cancer by five to six percent. This was confirmed in a study conducted on cancer patients in 2017. It was also found that the Mediterranean diet can decrease the chances of cancer.

Stress is the key factor that negatively affects life today. The Mediterranean diet can be a relaxant in this case. In various studies, a sincere adherence to the Mediterranean diet can control the deterioration of cognitive abilities. It does this by improving good cholesterol, blood sugar levels, and overall blood vessel health. This, as a result, reduces the risk of dementia or Alzheimer's disease.

With whole vegetables, fruits, and nuts, the Mediterranean diet is rich in antioxidants, vitamins, and other nutrients. This protects cells from damage that would otherwise occur from oxidative stress. As a result, it reduces the risk of Parkinson's disease by fifty percent. Adhering to this diet can also lower the causes of depression and give you a healthier state of mind.

A study conducted by food scientists on women who had chances of stroke in the UK noted that when they followed the Mediterranean diet very strictly, it reduced their chances of getting a stroke by twenty percent. By the way, this was not the case in men. Clinical research is underway to observe its effect on the male gender as well.

The National Institute on Aging funded a small study on aging that was published in 2018. The review showed that brain scans of 70 people showed that people who adhered strictly to the Mediterranean diet showed no signs of aging, while those who had a preference for other forms of diet had a pattern of plaques that added to the adverse effect of aging. This shows that the Mediterranean diet adds longevity to human life and gives lasting health. The lungs play an important role in oxygenating our bodies, but their ability to inhale deteriorates as we age. Whole grains, dairy products, and fish can improve the lungs' ability to function better. Besides, those who remain disciplined and consistent in following the Mediterranean diet have a 22-29% lower chance of losing their hearing.

It is an obvious fact that the Mediterranean diet has ample amounts of nutrients. If we consume this diet, it helps prevent muscle damage, increases muscle strength, and improves agility. This improves the efficiency of the brain. This means that this diet's consumers have better thinking and learning abilities, better memory, and concentration.

This diet is very beneficial for kidney patients and those who have had a kidney transplant. In some studies, it has been found that diet can reduce the risk of kidney dysfunction. It can also minimize graft failure by 32 percent and graft loss by 26 percent in kidney transplant patients.

If a person develops inflammatory bowel disease such as hemorrhoids, the Mediterranean diet can cause a cure. After studies and case studies, it has been found that consumers of this diet are 57% less likely to develop Crohn's disease. The benefits are manifold, and nutritionists are still counting.

HOW TO START

The best way to cause change is to initiate it. But the bigger question is how to get started. The situation is much better if what we need to begin has multiple benefits. The Mediterranean diet falls into this category, where the benefits outweigh the limitations it can impose on our lifestyle.

If you feel that it is challenging to change your diet, you can choose alternatives that work well and switch to a healthier option. Here are some ways that can help you make the switch to the Mediterranean diet.

It's good to start by keeping vegetables and fruits at the top of the priority list and putting sausage and pepperoni on the back burner in your salad dressing. You can start by giving a plate of tomato slices a try. You should give it just a drizzle of olive oil and some crushed feta cheese. Soups, crudité dishes, and salads can be great starters.

Skipping breakfast may seem effective, but it can put an extra load on your system to keep you going. On the other hand, whole grains, fruits, and other fiber-rich foods can be an effective way to start your day. Plus, they'll keep you full and your cravings at bay.

Replace the usual calorie-laden sweets like cakes, ice cream, pastries, etc., with fruits like apples, grapes, fresh figs, or strawberries. This will make you digest better and stay lighter. A refreshing feeling will work as motivation and keep you adhering to this magical diet.

If you pop in for a change, it may never happen. There is a famous saying, "A journey of a thousand miles begins with a single step." This is quite applicable to switching to the Mediterranean diet. You can start with small steps like skipping with olive oil and eating more vegetables and fruits in your salad. Replace your snacks with fruit. Similarly, other heavy dishes can be replaced with vegetables.

Choose skim milk or milk with 2% fat instead of whole milk. This will make you feel lighter and healthier. As a result, it will work as a motivating factor to opt for the Mediterranean diet. The change in energy level and diet will work as a trigger and driving force.

It is said that if it is easy, it is doable. The most affordable thing is to use whole grains instead of refined grains. Your choice should be whole-grain bread and not white bread that is made from refined flour. Similarly, brown rice or wild rice should replace white rice. Sometimes it is difficult to choose authentic whole grains. However, it's easy because the Oldways Whole Grain Council has developed a black and gold stamp to select quality over pasta.

Ancient grains or whole grains are an essential part of the Mediterranean diet. There is a huge variety of these grains. These are amaranth, faro, millet, spelled, and the credible Egyptian Kamut; another is teff, which is similar in size to poppy seeds. You can try one seed at a time. Slowly and steadily, you can move on to more options. Each seed has its flavor and texture. The good news is that these whole grains have become quite popular and are pretty standard. In fact, they are now available in mainstream restaurants as well. This means that you can try them and then make them part of your diet.

If you decide to do so, you should have at least six servings a day. Half should be whole grains. It may be worrisome for some because of the carbs, but you can throw your caution to the wind because it will indeed cause long-term benefits. You shouldn't overlook the fact that rapid weight loss may not be healthy. So, whole wheat in the Mediterranean diet is the best option.

You may not be able to change your current diet with the Mediterranean diet at once. So, try a meal of vegetables, whole grains, and beans. Use spices and herbs to add a palatable punch.

If you are protein-conscious and remain preoccupied with your diet, your dependence on meat could end by making room for lentils in your diet. Lentils are high sources of protein and also have a lot of fiber. Beans have an advantage because they have a lot of antioxidants. What motivation!

Fill your pantry with beneficial ingredients. These ingredients should be easy to use. Some of them can be popular protein sources like lentils, chickpeas, and beans. Lentils require only 25 minutes of cooking time, with no overnight soaking required. As for canned chickpeas and beans, just rinse them; then, you can put them in soups, burgers, salads, sandwiches, and more.

Giving up meat altogether can be a challenge, but you can give it a start by taking meat in small proportions. Use cut pieces of chicken or slices of lean meat. You can fry your dish and avoid frying. This will keep it less impregnated with oil and more nutritious. This is good news for fish eaters, as when they are on the Mediterranean diet, they can eat two servings of salmon, sardines, and tuna, which are essential to the Mediterranean diet. There may be a risk of mercury, but in the opinion of American nutritionists, the benefits outweigh the risk. The variety of fish mentioned here has relatively less mercury.

Dairy products can be a great source of protein. A Greek yogurt is a great option, but it should be consumed in moderation.

In short, the Mediterranean diet is a healthy option with a wide range of tasty choices. If you start with a simple approach, taking small steps at a time, making minor changes to your eating plan, you can go a long way.

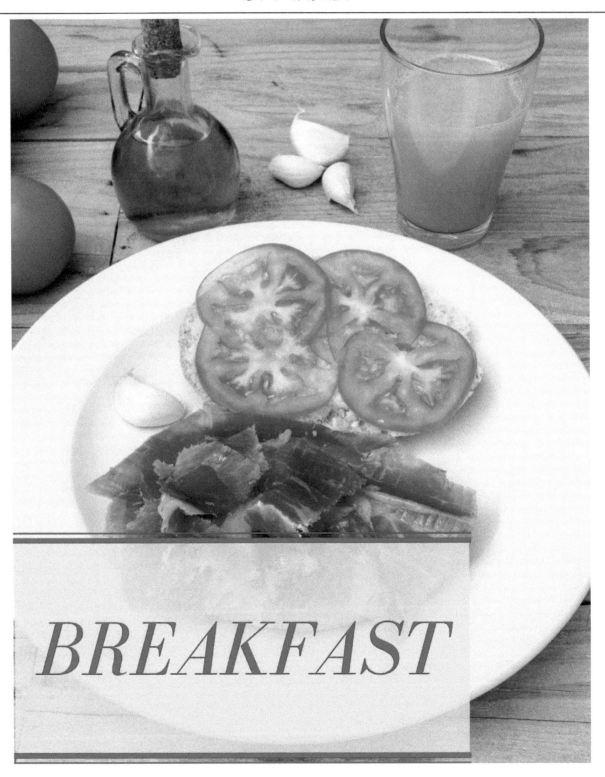

BREAKFAST

325) COUSCOUS PEARL SALAD

Cooking Time: 10 Minutes   **Servings:** 6

Ingredients:

- lemon juice, 1 large lemon
- 1/3 cup extra-virgin olive oil
- 1 tsp dill weed
- 1 tsp garlic powder
- salt
- pepper
- 2 cups Pearl Couscous
- 2 tbsp extra virgin olive oil
- 2 cups grape tomatoes, halved
- water as needed
- 1/3 cup red onions, finely chopped
- ½ English cucumber, finely chopped
- 1 15-ounce can chickpeas
- 1 14-ounce can artichoke hearts, roughly chopped
- ½ cup pitted Kalamata olives
- 15-20 pieces fresh basil leaves, roughly torn and chopped
- 3 ounces fresh mozzarella

Directions:

- Start by preparing the vinaigrette by mixing all Ingredients: in a bowl. Set aside.
- Heat olive oil in a medium-sized heavy pot over medium heat.
- Add couscous and cook until golden brown.
- Add 3 cups of boiling water and cook the couscous according to package instructions.
- Once done, drain in a colander and put it to the side.
- In a large mixing bowl, add the rest of the Ingredients: except the cheese and basil.
- Add the cooked couscous, basil, and mix everything well.
- Give the vinaigrette a gentle stir and whisk it into the couscous salad. Mix well.
- Adjust/add seasoning as desired.
- Add mozzarella cheese.
- Garnish with some basil.
- Enjoy!

Nutrition: Calories: 578, Total Fat: 25.3g, Saturated Fat: 4.6, Cholesterol: 8 mg, Sodium: 268 mg, Total Carbohydrate: 70.1g, Dietary Fiber: 17.5 g, Total Sugars: 10.8 g, Protein: 23.4 g, Vitamin D: 0 mcg, Calcium: 150 mg, Iron: 6 mg, Potassium: 1093 mg

326) TOMATO MUSHROOM EGG CUPS

Cooking Time: 5 Minutes   **Servings:** 4

Ingredients:

- 4 eggs
- 1/2 cup tomatoes, chopped
- 1/2 cup mushrooms, chopped
- 2 tbsp fresh parsley, chopped
- 1/4 cup half and half
- 1/2 cup cheddar cheese, shredded
- Pepper
- Salt

Directions:

- In a bowl, whisk the egg with half and half, pepper, and salt.
- Add tomato, mushrooms, parsley, and cheese and stir well.
- Pour egg mixture into the four small jars and seal jars with lid.
- Pour 1 1/2 cups of water into the instant pot then place steamer rack in the pot.
- Place jars on top of the steamer rack.
- Seal pot with lid and cook on high for 5 minutes.
- Once done, release pressure using quick release. Remove lid.
- Serve and enjoy.

Nutrition: Calories: 146;Fat: 10.g;Carbohydrates: 2.5 g;Sugar: 1.2 g;Protein: 10 g;Cholesterol: 184 mg

327) BREAKFAST MEDITERRANEAN-STYLE SALAD

Cooking Time: 10 Minutes   **Servings:** 2

Ingredients:

- 4 eggs (optional)
- 10 cups arugula
- 1/2 seedless cucumber, chopped
- 1 cup cooked quinoa, cooled
- 1 large avocado
- 1 cup natural almonds, chopped
- 1/2 cup mixed herbs like mint and dill, chopped
- 2 cups halved cherry tomatoes and/or heirloom tomatoes cut into wedges
- Extra virgin olive oil
- 1 lemon
- Sea salt, to taste
- Freshly ground black pepper, to taste

Directions:

- Cook the eggs by soft-boiling them - Bring a pot of water to a boil, then reduce heat to a simmer. Gently lower all the eggs into water and allow them to simmer for 6 minutes. Remove the eggs from water and run cold water on top to stop the cooking, process set aside and peel when ready to use
- In a large bowl, combine the arugula, tomatoes, cucumber, and quinoa
- Divide the salad among 2 containers, store in the fridge for 2 days
- To Serve: Garnish with the sliced avocado and halved egg, sprinkle herbs and almonds over top. Drizzle with olive oil, season with salt and pepper, toss to combine. Season with more salt and pepper to taste, a squeeze of lemon juice, and a drizzle of olive oil

Nutrition: Calories:2;Carbs: 18g;Total Fat: 16g;Protein: 10g

328)   CARROT OATMEAL BREAKFAST

Cooking Time: 10 Minutes   **Servings: 2**

Ingredients:

- ✓ 1 cup steel-cut oats
- ✓ 1/2 cup raisins
- ✓ 1/2 tsp ground nutmeg
- ✓ 1/2 tsp ground cinnamon
- ✓ 2 carrots, grated
- ✓ 2 cups of water
- ✓ 2 cups unsweetened almond milk
- ✓ 1 tbsp honey

Directions:

- ❖ Spray instant pot from inside with cooking spray.
- ❖ Add all ingredients into the instant pot and stir well.
- ❖ Seal pot with lid and cook on high for 10 minutes.
- ❖ Once done, release pressure using quick release. Remove lid.
- ❖ Stir and serve.

Nutrition: Calories: 3;Fat: 6.6 g;Carbohydrates: 73.8 g;Sugar: 33.7 g;Protein: 8.1 g;Cholesterol: 0 mg

329)   ARBORIO RICE RUM-RAISIN PUDDING

Cooking Time: 4 Hours   **Servings: 2**

Ingredients:

- ✓ ¾ cup Arborio rice
- ✓ 1 can evaporated milk
- ✓ ½ cup raisins
- ✓ ¼ tsp nutmeg, grated
- ✓ 1½ cups water
- ✓ 1/3 cup sugar
- ✓ ¼ cup dark rum
- ✓ sea salt or plain salt

Directions:

- ❖ Start by mixing rum and raisins in a bowl and set aside.
- ❖ Then, heat the evaporated milk and water in a saucepan and then simmer.
- ❖ Now, add sugar and stir until dissolved.
- ❖ Finally, convert this milk mixture into a slow cooker and stir in rice and salt. Cook on low heat for hours.
- ❖ Now, stir in the raisin mixture and nutmeg and let sit for 10 minutes.
- ❖ Serve warm.

Nutrition: Calories: 3, Total Fat: 10.1g, Saturated Fat: 5.9, Cholesterol: 36 mg, Sodium: 161 mg, Total Carbohydrate: 131.5 g, Dietary Fiber: 3.3 g, Total Sugars: 54.8 g, Protein: 14.4 g, Vitamin D: 0 mcg, Calcium: 372 mg, Iron: 2 mg, Potassium: 712 mg

330)   MEDITERRANEAN-STYLE QUINOA WITH FETA EGG MUFFINS

Cooking Time: 30 Minutes   **Servings: 12**

Ingredients:

- ✓ 8 eggs
- ✓ 1 cup cooked quinoa
- ✓ 1 cup crumbled feta cheese
- ✓ 1/4 tsp salt
- ✓ 2 cups baby spinach finely chopped
- ✓ 1/2 cup finely chopped onion
- ✓ 1 cup chopped or sliced tomatoes, cherry or grape tomatoes
- ✓ 1/2 cup chopped and pitted Kalamata olives
- ✓ 1 tbsp chopped fresh oregano
- ✓ 2 tsp high oleic sunflower oil plus optional extra for greasing muffin tins

Directions:

- ❖ Pre-heat oven to 350 degrees F
- ❖ Prepare 1silicone muffin holders on a baking sheet, or grease a 12-cup muffin tin with oil, set aside
- ❖ In a skillet over medium heat, add the vegetable oil and onions, sauté for 2 minutes
- ❖ Add tomatoes, sauté for another minute, then add spinach and sauté until wilted, about 1 minute
- ❖ Remove from heat and stir in olives and oregano, set aside
- ❖ Place the eggs in a blender or mixing bowl and blend or mix until well combined
- ❖ Pour the eggs in to a mixing bowl (if you used a blender) then add quinoa, feta cheese, veggie mixture, and salt, and stir until well combined
- ❖ Pour mixture in to silicone cups or greased muffin tins, dividing equally, and bake for 30 minutes, or until eggs have set and muffins are a light golden brown
- ❖ Allow to cool completely
- ❖ Distribute among the containers, store in fridge for 2-3 days
- ❖ To Serve: Heat in the microwave for 30 seconds or until slightly heated through
- ❖ Recipe Notes: Muffins can also be eaten cold. For the quinoa, I recommend making a large batch \'7b2 cups water per each cup of dry, rinsed quinoa\'7d and saving the extra for leftovers.

Nutrition: Calories:1Total Carbohydrates: 5g;Total Fat: 7g;Protein: 6g

331) GREEK YOGURT BLUEBERRY PANCAKES

Cooking Time: 15 Minutes   **Servings:** 6

Ingredients:

- ✓ 1 1/4 cup all-purpose flour
- ✓ 2 tsp baking powder
- ✓ 1 tsp baking soda
- ✓ 1/4 tsp salt
- ✓ 1/4 cup sugar
- ✓ 3 eggs
- ✓ 3 tbsp vegan butter unsalted, melted
- ✓ 1/2 cup milk
- ✓ 1 1/2 cups Greek yogurt plain, non-fat
- ✓ 1/2 cup blueberries optional
- ✓ Toppings:
- ✓ Greek yogurt
- ✓ Mixed berries – blueberries, raspberries and blackberries

Directions:

- ❖ In a large bowl, whisk together the flour, salt, baking powder and baking soda
- ❖ In a separate bowl, whisk together butter, sugar, eggs, Greek yogurt, and milk until the mixture is smooth
- ❖ Then add in the Greek yogurt mixture from step to the dry mixture in step 1, mix to combine, allow the patter to sit for 20 minutes to get a smooth texture – if using blueberries fold them into the pancake batter
- ❖ Heat the pancake griddle, spray with non-stick butter spray or just brush with butter
- ❖ Pour the batter, in 1/4 cupful's, onto the griddle
- ❖ Cook until the bubbles on top burst and create small holes, lift up the corners of the pancake to see if they're golden browned on the bottom
- ❖ With a wide spatula, flip the pancake and cook on the other side until lightly browned
- ❖ Distribute the pancakes in among the storage containers, store in the fridge for 3 day or in the freezer for 2 months
- ❖ To Serve: Reheat microwave for 1 minute (until 80% heated through) or on the stove top, drizzle warm syrup on top, scoop of Greek yogurt, and mixed berries (including blueberries, raspberries, blackberries)

Nutrition: Calories:258;Total Carbohydrates: 33g;Total Fat: 8g;Protein: 11g

332) BREAKFAST VEGETABLE BOWL

Cooking Time: 5 Minutes   **Servings:** 2

Ingredients:

- ✓ Breakfast Bowl:
- ✓ 1 ½ cups cooked quinoa
- ✓ 1 lb asparagus[1], cut into bite-sized pieces, ends trimmed and discarded
- ✓ 1 tbsp avocado oil or olive oil
- ✓ 3 cups shredded kale leaves
- ✓ 1 batch lemony dressing
- ✓ 3 cups shredded, uncooked Brussels sprouts
- ✓ 1 avocado, peeled, pitted and thinly-sliced
- ✓ 4 eggs, cooked to your preference (optional)
- ✓ Garnishes:
- ✓ Toasted sesame seeds
- ✓ Crushed red pepper
- ✓ Sunflower seeds
- ✓ Sliced almonds
- ✓ Hummus
- ✓ Lemon Dressing:
- ✓ 2 tsp Dijon mustard
- ✓ 1 garlic clove, minced
- ✓ 2 tbsp avocado oil or olive oil
- ✓ 2 tbsp freshly-squeezed lemon juice
- ✓ Salt, to taste
- ✓ Freshly-cracked black pepper, to taste

Directions:

- ❖ In a large sauté pan over medium-high heat, add the oil
- ❖ Once heated, add the asparagus and sauté for 4-5 minutes, stirring occasionally, until tender. Remove from heat and set side
- ❖ Add the Brussels sprouts, quinoa, and cooked asparagus, and toss until combined
- ❖ Distribute among the container, store in fridge for 2-3 days
- ❖ To serve: In a large, mixing bowl combine the kale and lemony dressing. Use your fingers to massage the dressing into the kale for 2-3 minutes, or until the leaves are dark and softened, set aside. In a small mixing bowl, combine the avocado, lemon juice, dijon mustard, garlic clove, salt, and pepper. Assemble the bowls by smearing a spoonful of hummus along the side of each bowl, then portion the kale salad evenly between the four bowls. Top with the avocado slices, egg, and your desired garnishes
- ❖ Recipe Note: Feel free to sub the asparagus with your favorite vegetable(s), sautéing or roasting them until cooked

Nutrition: Calories:632;Carbs: 52g;Total Fat: 39g;Protein: 24g

333) BREAKFAST EGG-ARTICHOKE CASSEROLE

Cooking Time: 30 To 35 Minutes   **Servings: 8**

Ingredients:

- ✓ 14 ounces artichoke hearts, if using canned remember to drain them
- ✓ 16 eggs
- ✓ 1 cup shredded cheddar cheese
- ✓ 10 ounces chopped spinach, if frozen make sure it is thawed and well-drained
- ✓ 1 clove of minced garlic
- ✓ ½ cup ricotta cheese
- ✓ ½ cup parmesan cheese
- ✓ ½ tsp crushed red pepper
- ✓ 1 tsp sea salt
- ✓ ½ tsp dried thyme
- ✓ ¼ cup onion, shaved
- ✓ ¼ cup milk

Directions:

- ❖ Grease a 9 x -inch baking pan or place a piece of parchment paper inside of it.
- ❖ Turn the temperature on your oven to 350 degrees Fahrenheit.
- ❖ Crack the eggs into a bowl and whisk them well.
- ❖ Pour in the milk and whisk the two ingredients together.
- ❖ Squeeze any excess moisture from the spinach with a paper towel.
- ❖ Toss the spinach and leafless artichoke hearts into the bowl. Stir until well combined.
- ❖ Add the cheddar cheese, minced garlic, parmesan cheese, red pepper, sea salt, thyme, and onion into the bowl. Mix until all the ingredients are fully incorporated.
- ❖ Pour the eggs into the baking pan.
- ❖ Add the ricotta cheese in even dollops before placing the casserole in the oven.
- ❖ Set your timer for 30 minutes, but watch the casserole carefully after about 20 minutes. Once the eggs stop jiggling and are cooked, remove the meal from the oven. Let the casserole cool down a bit and enjoy!

Nutrition: calories: 302, fats: 18 grams, carbohydrates: grams, protein: 22 grams.

334) CAULIFLOWER RICE BOWL BREAKFAST

Cooking Time: 12 Minutes   **Servings: 6**

Ingredients:

- ✓ 1 cup cauliflower rice
- ✓ 1/2 tsp red pepper flakes
- ✓ 1 1/2 tsp curry powder
- ✓ 1/2 tbsp ginger, grated
- ✓ 1 cup vegetable stock
- ✓ 4 tomatoes, chopped
- ✓ 3 cups broccoli, chopped
- ✓ Pepper
- ✓ Salt

Directions:

- ❖ Spray instant pot from inside with cooking spray.
- ❖ Add all ingredients into the instant pot and stir well.
- ❖ Seal pot with lid and cook on high for 12 minutes.
- ❖ Once done, allow to release pressure naturally for 10 minutes then release remaining using quick release. Remove lid.
- ❖ Stir and serve.

Nutrition: Calories: 44;Fat: 0.8 g;Carbohydrates: 8.2 g;Sugar: 3.8 g;Protein: 2.8 g;Cholesterol: 0 mg

335) CUCUMBER-DILL SAVORY YOGURT

Cooking Time: 10 Minutes   **Servings: 4**

Ingredients:

- ✓ 2 cups low-fat (2%) plain Greek yogurt
- ✓ 4 tsp minced shallot
- ✓ 4 tsp freshly squeezed lemon juice
- ✓ ¼ cup chopped fresh dill
- ✓ 2 tsp olive oil
- ✓ ¼ tsp kosher salt
- ✓ Pinch freshly ground black pepper
- ✓ 2 cups chopped Persian cucumbers (about 4 medium cucumbers)

Directions:

- ❖ Combine the yogurt, shallot, lemon juice, dill, oil, salt, and pepper in a large bowl. Taste the mixture and add another pinch of salt if needed.
- ❖ Scoop ½ cup of yogurt into each of 4 containers. Place ½ cup of chopped cucumbers in each of 4 separate small containers or resealable sandwich bags.
- ❖ STORAGE: Store covered containers in the refrigerator for up to 5 days.

Nutrition: Total calories: 127; Total fat: 5g; Saturated fat: 2g; Sodium: 200mg; Carbohydrates: 9g; Fiber: 2g; Protein: 11g

336) SPICE CRANBERRY TEA

Cooking Time: 18 Minutes   **Servings:** 2

Ingredients:

- ✓ 1-ounce cranberries
- ✓ ½ lemon, juice, and zest
- ✓ 1 cinnamon stick
- ✓ 2 teabags
- ✓ ½ inch ginger, peeled and grated
- ✓ raw honey to taste
- ✓ 3 cups water

Directions:

- ❖ Start by adding all the Ingredients: except honey into a pot or saucepan.
- ❖ Bring to a boil and then simmer for about 115 minutes.
- ❖ Strain and serve the tea.
- ❖ Add honey or any other sweetener of your preference.
- ❖ Enjoy.

Nutrition: Calories: 38, Total Fat: 0.3g, Saturated Fat: 0.1, Cholesterol: 0 mg, Sodium: 2 mg, Total Carbohydrate: 10 g, Dietary Fiber: 4.9 g, Total Sugars: 1.1 g, Protein: 0.7 g, Vitamin D: 0 mcg, Calcium: 77 mg, Iron: 1 mg, Potassium: 110 mg

337) ZUCCHINI PUDDING

Cooking Time: 10 Minutes   **Servings:** 4

Ingredients:

- ✓ 2 cups zucchini, grated
- ✓ 1/2 tsp ground cardamom
- ✓ 1/4 cup swerve
- ✓ 5 oz half and half
- ✓ 5 oz unsweetened almond milk
- ✓ Pinch of salt

Directions:

- ❖ Spray instant pot from inside with cooking spray.
- ❖ Add all ingredients into the instant pot and stir well.
- ❖ Seal pot with lid and cook on high for 10 minutes.
- ❖ Once done, allow to release pressure naturally for 10 minutes then release remaining using quick release. Remove lid.
- ❖ Stir well and serve.

Nutrition: Calories: ;Fat: 4.7 g;Carbohydrates: 18.9 g;Sugar: 16 g;Protein: 1.9 g;Cholesterol: 13 mg

338) MEDITERRANEAN-STYLE BREAKFAST BURRITO

Cooking Time: 20 Minutes   **Servings:** 6

Ingredients:

- ✓ 9 eggs
- ✓ 3 tbsp chopped sun-dried tomatoes
- ✓ 6 tortillas that are 10 inches
- ✓ 2 cups baby spinach
- ✓ ½ cup feta cheese
- ✓ ¾ cups of canned refried beans
- ✓ 3 tbsp sliced black olives
- ✓ Salsa, sour cream, or any other toppings you desire

Directions:

- ❖ Wash and dry your spinach.
- ❖ Grease a medium frying pan with oil or nonstick cooking spray.
- ❖ Add the eggs into the pan and cook for about 5 minutes. Make sure you stir the eggs well, so they become scrambled.
- ❖ Combine the black olives, spinach, and sun-dried tomatoes with the eggs. Stir until the ingredients are fully incorporated.
- ❖ Add the feta cheese and then set the lid on the pan so the cheese will melt quickly.
- ❖ Spoon a bit of egg mixture into the tortilla.
- ❖ Wrap the tortillas tightly.
- ❖ Wash your pan or get a new skillet. Remember to grease the pan.
- ❖ Set each tortilla into the pan and cook each side for a couple of minutes. Once they are lightly brown, remove them from the pan and allow the burritos to cool on a serving plate. Top with your favorite condiments and enjoy!
- ❖ To store the burritos, wrap them in aluminum foil and place them in the fridge. They can be stored for up to two days.

Nutrition: calories: 252, fats: grams, carbohydrates: 21 grams, protein: 14 grams

339) DRY FRUIT HEALTHY PORRIDGE

Cooking Time: 8 Hours   **Servings: 6**

Ingredients:

- ✓ 2 cups steel-cut oats
- ✓ 1/8 tsp ground nutmeg
- ✓ 1 tsp vanilla
- ✓ 1 1/2 tsp cinnamon
- ✓ 1/2 cup dry apricots, chopped
- ✓ 1/2 cup dry cranberries, chopped
- ✓ 1/2 cup dates, chopped
- ✓ 1/2 cup raisins
- ✓ 8 cups of water
- ✓ Pinch of salt

Directions:

- ❖ Spray instant pot from inside with cooking spray.
- ❖ Add all ingredients into the instant pot and stir well.
- ❖ Seal the pot with a lid and select slow cook mode and cook on low for 8 hours.
- ❖ Stir well and serve.

Nutrition: Calories: 196;Fat: 2 g;Carbohydrates: 42 g;Sugar: 18.4 g;Protein: 4.g;Cholesterol: 0 mg

340) SCRAMBLED EGGS PESTO

Cooking Time: 10 Minutes   **Servings: 2**

Ingredients:

- ✓ 5 eggs
- ✓ 2 tbsp butter
- ✓ 2 tbsp pesto
- ✓ 4 tbsp milk
- ✓ salt to taste
- ✓ pepper to taste

Directions:

- ❖ Beat the eggs into a bowl and add salt and pepper as per your taste.
- ❖ Then, heat a pan and add the butter, then the eggs, stirring continuously.
- ❖ While stirring continuously, add the pesto.
- ❖ Switch off the heat and quickly add the creamed milk and mix it well with eggs.
- ❖ Serve hot.

Nutrition: Calories: 342, Total Fat: 29.8g, Saturated Fat: 12.3, Cholesterol: 44mg, Sodium: 345 mg, Total Carbohydrate: 3.4g, Dietary Fiber: 0.3 g, Total Sugars: 3.2 g, Protein: 16.8 g, Vitamin D: 47 mcg, Calcium: 148 mg, Iron: 2 mg, Potassium: 168 mg

341) SWEET POTATOES AND SPICED MAPLE YOGURT WITH WALNUTS BREAKFAST

Cooking Time: 45 Minutes   **Servings: 4**

Ingredients:

- ✓ 4 red garnet sweet potatoes, about 6 inches long and 2 inches in diameter
- ✓ 2 cups low-fat (2%) plain Greek yogurt
- ✓ ¼ tsp pumpkin pie spice
- ✓ 1 tbsp pure maple syrup
- ✓ ½ cup walnut pieces

Directions:

- ❖ Preheat the oven to 425°F. Line a sheet pan with a silicone baking mat or parchment paper.
- ❖ Prick the sweet potatoes in multiple places with a fork and place on the sheet pan. Bake until tender when pricked with a paring knife, 40 to 45 minutes.
- ❖ While the potatoes are baking, mix the yogurt, pumpkin pie spice, and maple syrup until well combined in a medium bowl.
- ❖ When the potatoes are cool, slice the skin down the middle vertically to open up each potato. If you'd like to eat the sweet potatoes warm, place 1 potato in each of containers and ½ cup of spiced yogurt plus 2 tbsp of walnut pieces in each of 4 other containers. If you want to eat the potatoes cold, place ½ cup of yogurt and 2 tbsp of walnuts directly on top of each of the 4 potatoes in the 4 containers.
- ❖ STORAGE: Store covered containers in the refrigerator for up to days.

Nutrition: Total calories: 350; Total fat: 13g; Saturated fat: 3g; Sodium: 72mg; Carbohydrates: 4; Fiber: 5g; Protein: 16g

342) BLUEBERRY PEACH OATMEAL

Cooking Time: 4 Hours   **Servings: 4**

Ingredients:

- ✓ 1 cup steel-cut oats
- ✓ 1/2 cup blueberries
- ✓ 3 1/2 cups unsweetened almond milk
- ✓ 7 oz can peach
- ✓ Pinch of salt

Directions:

- ❖ Spray instant pot from inside with cooking spray.
- ❖ Add all ingredients into the instant pot and stir well.
- ❖ Seal the pot with a lid and select slow cook mode and cook on low for 4 hours.
- ❖ Stir well and serve.

Nutrition: 1;Fat: 4.5 g;Carbohydrates: 25.4 g;Sugar: 8.6 g;Protein: 3.9 g;Cholesterol: 0 mg

343) **MEDITERRANEAN-STYLE VEGGIE QUICHE**

Cooking Time: 55 Minutes   **Servings:** 8

Ingredients:

- ✓ 1/2 cup sundried tomatoes - dry or in olive oil*
- ✓ Boiling water
- ✓ 1 prepared pie crust
- ✓ 2 tbsp vegan butter
- ✓ 1 onion, diced
- ✓ 2 cloves garlic, minced
- ✓ 1 red pepper, diced
- ✓ 1/4 cup sliced Kalamata olives
- ✓ 1 tsp dried oregano
- ✓ 1 tsp dried parsley
- ✓ 1/3 cup crumbled feta cheese
- ✓ 4 large eggs
- ✓ 1 1/4 cup milk
- ✓ 2 cups fresh spinach or 1/2 cup frozen spinach, thawed and squeezed dry
- ✓ Salt, to taste
- ✓ Pepper, to taste
- ✓ 1 cup shredded cheddar cheese, divided

Directions:

- ❖ If you're using dry sundried tomatoes - In a measure cup, add the sundried tomatoes and pour the boiling water over until just covered, allow to sit for 5 minutes or until the tomatoes are soft. The drain and chop tomatoes, set aside
- ❖ Preheat oven to 375 degrees F
- ❖ Fit a 9-inch pie plate with the prepared pie crust, then flute edges, and set aside
- ❖ In a skillet over medium high heat, melt the butter
- ❖ Add in the onion and garlic, and cook until fragrant and tender, about 3 minutes
- ❖ Add in the red pepper, cook for an additional 3 minutes, or until the peppers are just tender
- ❖ Add in the spinach, olives, oregano, and parsley, cook until the spinach is wilted (if you're using fresh) or heated through (if you're using frozen), about 5 minutes
- ❖ Remove the pan from heat, stir in the feta cheese and tomatoes, spoon the mixture into the prepared pie crust, spreading out evenly, set aside
- ❖ In a medium-sized mixing bowl, whisk together the eggs, 1/2 cup of the cheddar cheese, milk, salt, and pepper
- ❖ Pour this egg and cheese mixture evenly over the spinach mixture in the pie crust
- ❖ Sprinkle top with the remaining cheddar cheese
- ❖ Bake for 50-55 minutes, or until the crust is golden brown and the egg is set
- ❖ Allow to cool completely before slicing
- ❖ Wrap the slices in plastic wrap and then aluminum foil and place in the freezer.
- ❖ To Serve: Remove the aluminum foil and plastic wrap, and microwave for 2 minutes, then allow to rest for 30 seconds, enjoy!
- ❖ Recipe Notes: You'll find two types of sundried tomatoes available in your local grocery store—dry ones and ones packed in olive oil. Both will work for this recipe.
- ❖ If you decide to use dry ones, follow the directions in the recipe to reconstitute them. If you're using oil-packed sundried tomatoes, skip the first step and just remove them from the oil, chop them, and continue with the recipe.
- ❖ Season carefully! Between the feta, cheddar, and olives, this recipe is naturally salty.

Nutrition: Calories:239;Carbs: ;Total Fat: 15g;Protein: 7g

344) SCRAMBLED EGGS MEDITERRANEAN-STYLE

Cooking Time: 10 Minutes   **Servings: 2**

Ingredients:

- ✓ 1 tbsp oil
- ✓ 1 yellow pepper, diced
- ✓ 2 spring onions, sliced
- ✓ 8 cherry tomatoes, quartered
- ✓ 2 tbsp sliced black olives
- ✓ 1 tbsp capers
- ✓ 4 eggs
- ✓ 1/4 tsp dried oregano
- ✓ Black pepper
- ✓ Topping:
- ✓ Fresh parsley, to serve

Directions:

- ❖ In a frying pan over medium heat, add the oil
- ❖ Once heated, add the diced pepper and chopped spring onions, cook for a few minutes, until slightly soft
- ❖ Add in the quartered tomatoes, olives and capers, and cook for 1 more minute
- ❖ Crack the eggs into the pan, immediately scramble with a spoon or spatula
- ❖ Sprinkle with oregano and plenty of black pepper, and stir until the eggs are fully cooked
- ❖ Distribute the eggs evenly into the containers, store in the fridge for 2-3 days
- ❖ To Serve: Reheat in the microwave for 30 seconds or in a toaster oven until warmed through

Nutrition: Calories:249;Carbs: 13g;Total Fat: 17g;Protein: 14g

345) PUDDING WITH CHIA

Cooking Time: 15 Minutes   **Servings: 2**

Ingredients:

- ✓ ½ cup chia seeds
- ✓ 2 cups milk
- ✓ 1 tbsp honey

Directions:

- ❖ Combine and mix the chia seeds, milk, and honey in a bowl.
- ❖ Put the mixture in the freezer and let it set.
- ❖ Take the pudding out of the freezer only when you see that the pudding has thickened.
- ❖ Serve chilled.

Nutrition: Calories: 429, Total Fat: 22.4g, Saturated Fat: 4.9, Cholesterol: 20 mg, Sodium: 124 mg, Total Carbohydrate: 44.g, Dietary Fiber: 19.5 g, Total Sugars: 19.6 g, Protein: 17.4 g, Vitamin D: 1 mcg, Calcium: 648 mg, Iron: 4 mg, Potassium: 376 mg

346) RICE BOWLS FOR BREAKFAST

Cooking Time: 8 Minutes   **Servings: 4**

Ingredients:

- ✓ 1 cup of brown rice
- ✓ 1 tsp ground cinnamon
- ✓ 1/4 cup almonds, sliced
- ✓ 2 tbsp sunflower seeds
- ✓ 1/4 cup pecans, chopped
- ✓ 1/4 cup walnuts, chopped
- ✓ 2 cup unsweetened almond milk
- ✓ Pinch of salt

Directions:

- ❖ Spray instant pot from inside with cooking spray.
- ❖ Add all ingredients into the instant pot and stir well.
- ❖ Seal pot with lid and cook on high for 8 minutes.
- ❖ Once done, allow to release pressure naturally for 5 minutes then release remaining using quick release. Remove lid.
- ❖ Stir well and serve.

Nutrition: Calories: 291;Fat: 12 g;Carbohydrates: 40.1 g;Sugar: 0.4 g;Protein: 7.g;Cholesterol: 0 mg

Lunch and Dinner

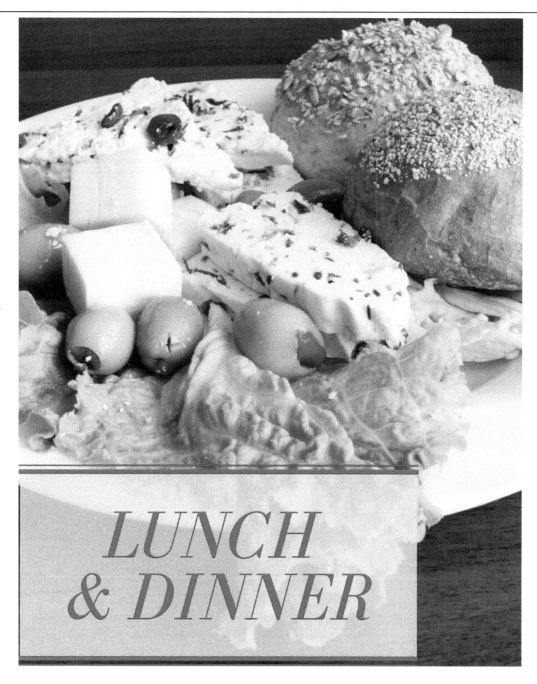

LUNCH
& DINNER

347) MEDITERRANEAN-STYLE PEARL COUSCOUS

Cooking Time: 10 Minutes   **Servings:** 6

Ingredients:

- ✓ For the Lemon Dill Vinaigrette:
- ✓ 1 large lemon, juice of
- ✓ 1/3 cup Extra virgin olive oil
- ✓ 1 tsp dill weed
- ✓ 1 tsp garlic powder
- ✓ Salt and pepper
- ✓ For the Israeli Couscous:
- ✓ 2 cups Pearl Couscous, Israeli Couscous
- ✓ Extra virgin olive oil

- ✓ 2 cups grape tomatoes, halved
- ✓ 1/3 cup finely chopped red onions
- ✓ 1/2 English cucumber, finely chopped
- ✓ 15 oz can chickpeas
- ✓ 14 oz can good quality artichoke hearts, roughly chopped if needed
- ✓ 1/2 cup good pitted kalamata olives
- ✓ 15–20 fresh basil leaves, roughly chopped or torn; more for garnish
- ✓ 3 oz fresh baby mozzarella or feta cheese, optional
- ✓ Water

Directions:

- ❖ Make the lemon-dill vinaigrette, place the lemon juice, olive oil, dill weed, garlic powder, salt and pepper in a bowl, whisk together to combine and set aside
- ❖ In a medium-sized heavy pot, heat two tbsp of olive oil
- ❖ Sauté the couscous in the olive oil briefly until golden brown, then add cups of boiling water (or follow the instructed on the package), and cook according to package
- ❖ Once done, drain in a colander, set aside in a bowl and allow to cool
- ❖ In a large mixing bowl, combine the extra virgin olive oil, grape tomatoes, red onions, cucumber, chickpeas, artichoke hearts, and kalamata olives
- ❖ Then add in the couscous and the basil, mix together gently
- ❖ Now, give the lemon-dill vinaigrette a quick whisk and add to the couscous salad, mix to combine
- ❖ Taste and adjust salt, if needed
- ❖ Distribute among the containers, store for 2-3 days
- ❖ To Serve: Add in the mozzarella cheese, garnish with more fresh basil and enjoy

Nutrition: Calories:393;Carbs: 57g;Total Fat: 13g;Protein: 13g

348) POTATO WITH TUNA SALAD

Cooking Time: Nil   **Servings:** 4

Ingredients:

- ✓ 1-pound baby potatoes, scrubbed, boiled
- ✓ 1 cup tuna chunks, drained
- ✓ 1 cup cherry tomatoes, halved
- ✓ 1 cup medium onion, thinly sliced
- ✓ 8 pitted black olives
- ✓ 2 medium hard-boiled eggs, sliced

- ✓ 1 head Romaine lettuce
- ✓ Honey lemon mustard dressing
- ✓ ¼ cup olive oil
- ✓ 2 tbsp lemon juice
- ✓ 1 tbsp Dijon mustard
- ✓ 1 tsp dill weed, chopped
- ✓ Salt as needed
- ✓ Pepper as needed

Directions:

- ❖ Take a small glass bowl and mix in your olive oil, honey, lemon juice, Dijon mustard and dill
- ❖ Season the mix with pepper and salt
- ❖ Add in the tuna, baby potatoes, cherry tomatoes, red onion, green beans, black olives and toss everything nicely
- ❖ Arrange your lettuce leaves on a beautiful serving dish to make the base of your salad
- ❖ Top them up with your salad mixture and place the egg slices
- ❖ Drizzle it with the previously prepared Salad Dressing
- ❖ Serve hot
- ❖ Meal Prep/Storage Options: Store in airtight containers in your fridge for 1-2 days. Keep the fish and salad ingredients separated, mix together before serving!

Nutrition: Calories: 406;Fat: 22g;Carbohydrates: 28g;Protein: 26g

349)   MEDITERRANEAN-STYLE PASTA SALAD

Cooking Time: 25 Minutes   **Servings: 8**

Ingredients:

- ✓ Salad:
- ✓ 8 oz pasta, I used farfalle, any smallish pasta works great!
- ✓ 1 cup rotisserie chicken, chopped
- ✓ 1/2 cup sun-dried tomatoes packed in oil, drained and coarsely chopped
- ✓ 1/2 cup jarred marinated artichoke hearts, drained and coarsely chopped
- ✓ 1/2 of 1 full English cucumber, chopped
- ✓ 1/3 cup kalamata olives, coarsely chopped
- ✓ 2 cups lightly packed fresh arugula
- ✓ 1/4 cup fresh flat leaf Italian parsley, coarsely chopped
- ✓ 1 small avocado, pit removed and coarsely chopped
- ✓ 1/3 cup feta cheese

- ✓ Dressing:
- ✓ 4 tbsp red wine vinegar
- ✓ 1 ½ tbsp
- ✓ dijon mustard, do not use regular mustard
- ✓ 1/2 tsp dried oregano
- ✓ 1 tsp dried basil
- ✓ 1 clove garlic, minced
- ✓ 1-2 tsp honey
- ✓ 1/2 cup olive oil
- ✓ 3 tbsp freshly squeezed lemon juice
- ✓ Fine sea salt, to taste
- ✓ Freshly cracked pepper, to taste

Directions:

- ❖ Prepare the pasta according to package directions until al dente, drain the pasta and allow it to completely cool to room temperature, then add it to a large bowl
- ❖ Add in the chopped rotisserie chicken, chopped cucumber, coarsely chopped kalamata olives, coarsely chopped sun-dried tomatoes, coarsely chopped artichoke hearts, arugula, and parsley, toss
- ❖ Distribute the salad among the containers, store for 2-days
- ❖ Prepare the dressing - In a mason jar with a lid, combine the red wine vinegar, Dijon mustard, garlic, 1/2 tsp salt (or to taste), dried oregano, dried basil and 1/tsp pepper (or to taste, honey (add to sweetness preference), olive oil, and freshly squeezed lemon juice, place the lid on the mason jar and shake to combine, store in fridge
- ❖ To Serve: Add in the avocado and feta cheese to the salad, drizzle with the dressing, adjust any seasonings salt and pepper to taste, serve

Nutrition: Calories:32Carbs: 24g;Total Fat: 21g;Protein: 8g

350)   AVOCADO LEMON HERB CHICKEN SALAD

Cooking Time: 15 Minutes   **Servings: 4**

Ingredients:

- ✓ Marinade/ Dressing:
- ✓ 2 tbsp olive oil
- ✓ 1/4 cup fresh lemon juice
- ✓ 2 tbsp water
- ✓ 2 tbsp fresh chopped parsley
- ✓ 2 tsp garlic, minced
- ✓ 1 tsp each dried thyme and dried rosemary
- ✓ 1 tsp salt
- ✓ 1/4 tsp cracked pepper, or to taste

- ✓ 1 pound skinless & boneless chicken thigh fillets or chicken breasts
- ✓ Salad:
- ✓ 4 cups Romaine lettuce leaves, washed and dried
- ✓ 1 large avocado, pitted, peeled and sliced
- ✓ 8 oz feta cheese
- ✓ 1 cup grape tomatoes, halved
- ✓ 1/4 of a red onion, sliced, optional
- ✓ 1/4 cup diced bacon, trimmed of rind and fat (optional)
- ✓ Lemon wedges, to serve

Directions:

- ❖ In a large jug, whisk together the olive oil, lemon juice, water, chopped parsley, garlic, thyme, rosemary, salt, and pepper
- ❖ Pour half of the marinade into a large, shallow dish and refrigerate the remaining marinade to use as the dressing
- ❖ Add the chicken to the marinade in the bowl, allow the chicken to marinade for 15- minutes (or up to two hours in the refrigerator if you can)
- ❖ In the meantime,
- ❖ Once the chicken is ready, place a skillet or grill over medium-high heat add 1 tbsp of oil in, sear the chicken on both sides until browned and cooked through about 7 minutes per side, depending on thickness, and discard of the marinade
- ❖ Allow the chicken to rest for 5 minutes, slice and then allow the chicken to cool
- ❖ Distribute among the containers, and keep in the refrigerator
- ❖ To Serve: Reheat the chicken in the microwave for 30 seconds to 1 minutes. In a bowl, add the romaine lettuce, avocado, feta cheese, grape tomatoes, red onion and bacon, mix to combine. Arrange the chicken over salad. Drizzle the salad with the Untouched dressing. Serve with lemon wedges and enjoy!

Nutrition: Calories:378;Carbs: 6g;Total Fat: 22g;Protein: 31g

351) LEEKS, GREENS, AND POTATOES IN GREEK-STYLE BRAISED PORK

Cooking Time: 1 Hour 40 Minutes   **Servings:** 4

Ingredients:

- ✓ 1 tbsp olive oil, plus 2 tsp
- ✓ 1¼ pounds boneless pork loin chops, fat cap removed and cut into 1-inch pieces
- ✓ 2 leeks, white and light green parts quartered vertically and thinly sliced
- ✓ 1 bulb fennel, quartered and thinly sliced
- ✓ 1 cup chopped onion
- ✓ 1 tsp chopped garlic
- ✓ 2 cups reduced-sodium chicken broth
- ✓ 1 tsp fennel seed
- ✓ 1 tsp dried oregano
- ✓ ½ tsp kosher salt
- ✓ 1 pound baby red potatoes, halved
- ✓ 1 bunch chard, including stems, chopped
- ✓ 2 tbsp freshly squeezed lemon juice

Directions:

- ❖ Heat tbsp of oil in a soup pot or Dutch oven over medium-high heat. When the oil is shimmering, add the pork cubes and brown for about 6 minutes, turning the cubes over after 3 minutes. Remove the pork to a plate.
- ❖ Add the remaining tsp of oil to the same pot and add the leeks, fennel, onion, and garlic. Cook for 3 minutes.
- ❖ Pour the broth into the pan, scraping up any browned bits on the bottom. Add the fennel seed, oregano, and salt, and add the pork, plus any juices that may have accumulated on the plate. Make sure the pork is submerged in the liquid. Place the potatoes on top, then place the chard on top of the potatoes.
- ❖ Cover, turn down the heat to low, and simmer for 1½ hours, until the pork is tender. When the pork is done cooking, add the lemon juice. Taste and add more salt if needed. Cool.
- ❖ Scoop 2 cups of the mixture into each of 4 containers.
- ❖ STORAGE: Store covered containers in the refrigerator for up to 5 days.

Nutrition: Total calories: 3; Total fat: 13g; Saturated fat: 3g; Sodium: 1,607mg; Carbohydrates: 33g; Fiber: 8g; Protein: 34g

352) DELIZIOSA BROCCOLI TORTELLINI SALAD

Cooking Time: 20 To 25 Minutes   **Servings:** 12

Ingredients:

- ✓ 1 cup sunflower seeds, or any of your favorite seeds
- ✓ 3 heads of broccoli, fresh is best!
- ✓ ½ cup sugar
- ✓ 20 ounces cheese-filled tortellini
- ✓ 1 onion
- ✓ 2 tsp cider vinegar
- ✓ ½ cup mayonnaise
- ✓ 1 cup raisins-optional

Directions:

- ❖ Cut your broccoli into florets and chop the onion.
- ❖ Follow the directions to make the cheese-filled tortellini. Once they are cooked, drain and rinse them with cold water.
- ❖ In a bowl, combine your mayonnaise, sugar, and vinegar. Whisk well to give the ingredients a dressing consistency.
- ❖ In a separate large bowl, toss in your seeds, onion, tortellini, raisins, and broccoli.
- ❖ Pour the salad dressing into the large bowl and toss the ingredients together. You will want to ensure everything is thoroughly mixed as you'll want a taste of the salad dressing with every bite!

Nutrition: calories: 272, fats: 8.1 grams, carbohydrates: 38.grams, protein: 5 grams.

353) AVOCADO ARUGULA SALAD

Cooking Time: 15 Minutes   **Servings:** 4

Ingredients:

- ✓ 4 cups packed baby arugula
- ✓ 4 green onions, tops trimmed, chopped
- ✓ 1½ cups shelled fava beans
- ✓ 3 Persian cucumbers, chopped
- ✓ 2 cups grape tomatoes, halved
- ✓ 1 jalapeno pepper, sliced
- ✓ 1 avocado, cored, peeled, and roughly chopped
- ✓ lemon juice, 1½ lemons
- ✓ ½ cup extra virgin olive oil
- ✓ salt
- ✓ pepper
- ✓ 1 garlic clove, finely chopped
- ✓ 2 tbsp fresh cilantro, finely chopped
- ✓ 2 tbsp fresh mint, finely chopped

Directions:

- ❖ Place the lemon-honey vinaigrette Ingredients: in a small bowl and whisk them well.
- ❖ In a large mixing bowl, add baby arugula, fava beans, green onions, tomatoes, cucumbers, and jalapeno.
- ❖ Divide the whole salad among four containers.
- ❖ Before serving, dress the salad with the vinaigrette and toss.
- ❖ Add the avocado to the salad.
- ❖ Enjoy!

Nutrition: Calories: 229, Total Fat: 11.1 g, Saturated Fat: 2.5 g, Cholesterol: 0 mg, Sodium: 24 mg, Total Carbohydrate: 32.1 g, Dietary Fiber: 12 g, Total Sugars: 10.1 g, Protein: 3 g, Vitamin D: 0 mcg, Calcium: 163 mg, Iron: 3 mg, Potassium: 1166 mg

354) QUINOA STUFFED EGGPLANT AND TAHINI SAUCE

Cooking Time: 30 Minutes   **Servings: 2**

Ingredients:

- ✓ 1 eggplant
- ✓ 2 tbsp olive oil, divided
- ✓ 1 medium shallot, diced, about 1/2 cup
- ✓ 1 cup chopped button mushrooms, about 2 cups whole
- ✓ 5-6 Tuttorosso whole plum tomatoes, chopped
- ✓ 1 tbsp tomato juice from the can
- ✓ 1 tbsp chopped fresh parsley, plus more to garnish
- ✓ 2 garlic cloves, minced
- ✓ 1/2 cup cooked quinoa
- ✓ 1/2 tsp ground cumin
- ✓ Salt, to taste
- ✓ Pepper, to taste
- ✓ 1 tbsp tahini
- ✓ 1 tsp lemon juice
- ✓ 1/2 tsp garlic powder
- ✓ Water to thin

Directions:

- ❖ Preheat the oven to 425 degrees F
- ❖ Prepare the eggplant by cutting it in half lengthwise and scoop out some of the flesh
- ❖ Place it on a baking sheet, drizzle with 1 tbsp of oil, sprinkle with salt
- ❖ Bake for 20 minutes
- ❖ In the meantime, add the remaining oil in a large skillet
- ❖ Once heated, add the shallots and mushrooms, sauté until mushrooms have softened, about 5 minutes Add in the tomatoes, quinoa and spices, cook until the liquid has evaporated
- ❖ Once the eggplant has cooked, reduce the oven temperature to 350 degrees F
- ❖ Stuff each half with the tomato-quinoa mixture
- ❖ Bake for another 10 minutes
- ❖ Allow to cool completely
- ❖ Distribute among the containers, store for 2 days
- ❖ To Serve: Reheat in the microwave for 1-2 minutes or until heated through. Quickly whisk together tahini, lemon, garlic, water and a sprinkle of salt and pepper, drizzle tahini over eggplants and sprinkle with parsley and enjoy.

Nutrition: Calories:345;Carbs: 38g;Total Fat: 19g;Protein: 9g

355) ITALIAN-STYLE LASAGNA

Cooking Time: 1 Hour 15 Minutes   **Servings: 8**

Ingredients:

- ✓ Lasagna noodles, oven-ready are the best, easiest, and quickest
- ✓ 1/3 cup flour
- ✓ 2 tbsp chives, divided and chopped
- ✓ 1/2 cup white wine
- ✓ 2 tbsp olive oil
- ✓ 1 1/2 tbsp thyme
- ✓ 1 tsp salt
- ✓ 1 1/4 cups shallots, chopped
- ✓ 1 cup boiled water
- ✓ 1/2 cup Parmigiano-Reggiano cheese
- ✓ 3 cups milk, reduced-fat and divided
- ✓ 1 tbsp butter
- ✓ 1/3 cup cream cheese, less fat is the best choice
- ✓ 6 cloves of garlic, divided and minced
- ✓ 1/2 tsp ground black pepper, divided
- ✓ 4 ounces dried shiitake mushrooms, sliced
- ✓ 1 ounce dried porcini mushrooms, sliced
- ✓ 8 ounces cremini mushrooms, sliced

Directions:

- ❖ Keeping your mushrooms separated, drain them all and return them to separate containers.
- ❖ Bring 1 cup of water to a boil and cook your porcini mushrooms for a half hour.
- ❖ Preheat your oven to 0 degrees Fahrenheit.
- ❖ Set a large pan on your stove and turn the burner to medium-high heat.
- ❖ Add your butter and let it melt.
- ❖ Combine the olive oil and shallots. Stir the mixture and let it cook for 3 minutes.
- ❖ Pour half of the pepper, half of the salt, and mushrooms into the pan. Allow the mixture to cook for 6 to minutes.
- ❖ While stirring, add half of the garlic and thyme. Continue to stir for 1 minute.
- ❖ Pour the wine and turn your burner temperature to high. Let the mixture boil and watch the liquid evaporate for a couple of minutes to reduce it slightly.
- ❖ Turn off the burner and remove the pan from heat.
- ❖ Add the cream cheese and chives. Stir thoroughly.
- ❖ Set a medium-sized skillet on medium-high heat and add 1 tbsp of oil. Let the oil come to a simmer.
- ❖ Add the last of the garlic to the pan and saute for 30 seconds.
- ❖ Pour in 2 1/3 cup milk and the liquid from the porcini mushrooms. Stir the mixture and allow it to boil.
- ❖ In a bowl, combine 1/4 cup of milk and the flour. Add this mixture to the heated pan. Stir until the mixture starts to thicken.
- ❖ Grease a pan and add 1/2 cup of sauce along with a row of noodles.
- ❖ Spread half of the mushroom mixture on top of the noodles.
- ❖ Repeat the process, but make sure you top the lasagna with mushrooms and cheese.
- ❖ Turn your timer to 45 minutes and set the pan into the oven.
- ❖ Remember to garnish the lasagna with chives before enjoying!

Nutrition: calories: 268, fats: 12.6 grams, carbohydrates: 29 grams, protein: 10 grams.

356) TUNA AND VEGETABLE MIX

Cooking Time: 15 Minutes **Servings:** 4

Ingredients:

- ✓ ¼ cup extra-virgin olive oil, divided
- ✓ 1 tbsp rice vinegar
- ✓ 1 tsp kosher salt, divided
- ✓ ¾ tsp Dijon mustard
- ✓ ¾ tsp honey
- ✓ 4 ounces baby gold beets, thinly sliced
- ✓ 4 ounces fennel bulb, trimmed and thinly sliced
- ✓ 4 ounces baby turnips, thinly sliced
- ✓ 6 ounces Granny Smith apple, very thinly sliced
- ✓ 2 tsp sesame seeds, toasted
- ✓ 6 ounces tuna steaks
- ✓ ½ tsp black pepper
- ✓ 1 tbsp fennel fronds, torn

Directions:

- ❖ In a large bowl, add 2 tbsp of oil, ½ a tsp of salt, honey, vinegar, and mustard.
- ❖ Give the mixture a nice mix.
- ❖ Add fennel, beets, apple, and turnips; mix and toss until everything is evenly coated.
- ❖ Sprinkle with sesame seeds and toss well.
- ❖ In a cast-iron skillet, heat 2 tbsp of oil over high heat.
- ❖ Carefully season the tuna with ½ a tsp of salt and pepper
- ❖ Place the tuna in the skillet and cook for about 3 minutes total, giving 1½ minutes per side.
- ❖ Remove the tuna and slice it up.
- ❖ Place in containers with the vegetable mix.
- ❖ Serve with the fennel mix, and enjoy!

Nutrition: Calories: 443, Total Fat: 17.1 g, Saturated Fat: 2.6 g, Cholesterol: 21 mg, Sodium: 728 mg, Total Carbohydrate: 62.5 g, Dietary Fiber: 12.3 g, Total Sugars: 45 g, Protein: 16.5 g, Vitamin D: 0 mcg, Calcium: 79 mg, Iron: 4 mg, Potassium: 1008 mg

357) SPICY BURGERS

Cooking Time: 25-30 Minutes **Servings:** 6/2 Chops Each

Ingredients:

- ✓ Medium onion (1)
- ✓ Fresh parsley (3 tbsp.)
- ✓ Clove of garlic (1)
- ✓ Ground allspice (.75 tsp.)
- ✓ Pepper (.75 tsp.)
- ✓ Ground nutmeg (.25 tsp.)
- ✓ Cinnamon (.5 tsp.)
- ✓ Salt (.5 tsp.)
- ✓ Fresh mint (2 tbsp.)
- ✓ 90% lean ground beef (1.5 lb.)
- ✓ Optional: Cold Tzatziki sauce

Directions:

- ❖ Finely chop/mince the parsley, mint, garlic, and onions.
- ❖ Whisk the nutmeg, salt, cinnamon, pepper, allspice, garlic, mint, parsley, and onion.
- ❖ Add the beef and prepare six (6 2x4-inch oblong patties.
- ❖ Use the medium temperature setting to grill the patties or broil them four inches from the heat source for four to six minutes per side.
- ❖ When they're done, the meat thermometer will register 160° Fahrenheit. Serve with the sauce if desired.

Nutrition: Calories: 231;Protein: 32 grams;Fat: 9 grams

358) TUNA BOWL AND KALE

Cooking Time: 15 To 20 Minutes **Servings:** 6

Ingredients:

- ✓ 3 tbsp extra virgin olive oil
- ✓ 1 ½ tsp minced garlic
- ✓ ¼ cup of capers
- ✓ 2 tsp sugar
- ✓ 15 ounce can of drained and rinsed great northern beans
- ✓ 1 pound chopped kale with the center ribs removed
- ✓ ½ tsp ground black pepper
- ✓ 1 cup chopped onion
- ✓ 2 ½ ounces of drained sliced olives
- ✓ ¼ tsp sea salt
- ✓ ¼ tsp crushed red pepper
- ✓ 6 ounces of tuna in olive oil, do not drain

Directions:

- ❖ Place a large pot, like a stockpot, on your stove and turn the burner to high heat.
- ❖ Fill the pot about 3-quarters of the way full with water and let it come to a boil.
- ❖ Add the kale and cook for 2 minutes.
- ❖ Drain the kale and set it aside.
- ❖ Turn the heat down to medium and place the empty pot back on the burner.
- ❖ Add the oil and onion. Saute for 3 to 4 minutes.
- ❖ Combine the garlic into the oil mixture and saute for another minute.
- ❖ Add the capers, olives, and red pepper.
- ❖ Cook the ingredients for another minute while stirring.
- ❖ Pour in the sugar and stir while you toss in the kale. Mix all the ingredients thoroughly and ensure the kale is thoroughly coated.
- ❖ Cover the pot and set the timer for 8 minutes.
- ❖ Turn off the heat and add in the tuna, pepper, beans, salt, and any other herbs that will make this one of the best Mediterranean-Style dishes you've ever made.

Nutrition: calories: 265, fats: 12 grams, carbohydrates: 26 grams, protein: 16 grams.

359) POMODORO SOUP

Cooking Time: 30 Minutes   **Servings:** 8

Ingredients:

- ✓ 4 tbsp olive oil
- ✓ 2 medium yellow onions, thinly sliced
- ✓ 1 tsp salt (extra for taste if needed)
- ✓ 2 tsp curry powder
- ✓ 1 tsp red curry powder
- ✓ 1 tsp ground coriander
- ✓ 1 tsp ground cumin
- ✓ ¼-½ tsp red pepper flakes
- ✓ 1 15-ounce can diced tomatoes, undrained
- ✓ 1 28-ounce can diced or plum tomatoes, undrained
- ✓ 5½ cups water (vegetable broth or chicken broth also usable)
- ✓ 1 14-ounce can coconut milk optional add-ins: cooked brown rice, lemon wedges, fresh thyme, etc.

Directions:

- ❖ Heat oil in a medium-sized pot over medium heat.
- ❖ Add onions and salt and cook for about 10-1minutes until browned.
- ❖ Stir in curry powder, coriander, red pepper flakes, cumin, and cook for seconds, being sure to keep stirring well.
- ❖ Add tomatoes and water (or broth if you prefer).
- ❖ Simmer the mixture for 1minutes.
- ❖ Take an immersion blender and puree the mixture until a soupy consistency is achieved.
- ❖ Enjoy as it is, or add some extra add-ins for a more flavorful experience

Nutrition: Calories: 217, Total Fat: 19.3 g, Saturated Fat: 11.5 g, Cholesterol: 0 mg, Sodium: 40 mg, Total Carbohydrate: 12.1 g, Dietary Fiber: 3.g, Total Sugars: 7.1 g, Protein: 3 g, Vitamin D: 0 mcg, Calcium: 58 mg, Iron: 2 mg, Potassium: 570 mg

360) ONION CHEESE SOUP

Cooking Time: 25 Minutes   **Servings:** 4

Ingredients:

- ✓ 2 large onions, finely sliced
- ✓ 2 cups vegetable stock
- ✓ 1 tsp brown sugar
- ✓ 1 cup red wine
- ✓ 1 measure of brandy
- ✓ 1 tsp herbs de Provence
- ✓ 4 slices stale bread
- ✓ 4 ounces grated strong cheese
- ✓ 1-ounce grated parmesan
- ✓ 1 tbsp plain flour
- ✓ 2 tbsp olive oil
- ✓ 1-ounce butter
- ✓ salt
- ✓ pepper

Directions:

- ❖ Heat oil and butter in a pan over medium-high heat.
- ❖ Add onions and brown sugar.
- ❖ Cook until the onions are golden brown.
- ❖ Pour brandy and flambé, making sure to keep stirring until the flames are out.
- ❖ Add plain flour and herbs de Provence and keep stirring well.
- ❖ Slowly add the stock and red wine.
- ❖ Season well and simmer for 20 minutes, making sure to add water if the soup becomes too thick.
- ❖ Ladle the soup into jars.
- ❖ Before serving, place rounds of stale bread on top.
- ❖ Add strong cheese.
- ❖ Garnish with some parmesan.
- ❖ Place the bowls under a hot grill or in an oven until the cheese has melted.

Nutrition: Calories: 403, Total Fat: 22.4 g, Saturated Fat: 10.9 g, Cholesterol: 41 mg, Sodium: 886 mg, Total Carbohydrate: 24.9 g, Dietary Fiber: 3.6 g, Total Sugars: 7 g, Protein: 16.2 g, Vitamin D: 4 mcg, Calcium: 371 mg, Iron: 1 mg, Potassium: 242 mg

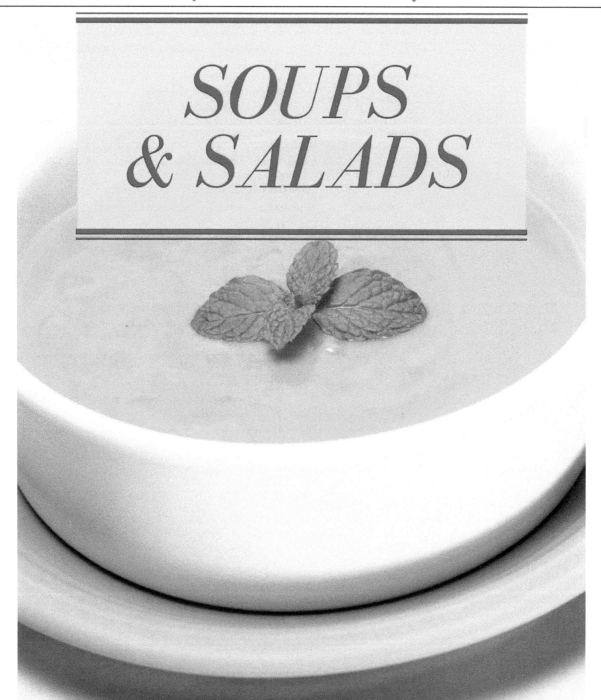

SOUPS & SALADS

361) TURKEY MEATBALL WITH DITALINI SOUP

Cooking Time: 40 Minutes   **Servings:** 4

Ingredients:

- ✓ meatballs:
- ✓ 1 pound 93% lean ground turkey
- ✓ 1/3 cup seasoned breadcrumbs
- ✓ 3 tbsp grated Pecorino Romano cheese
- ✓ 1 large egg, beaten
- ✓ 1 clove crushed garlic
- ✓ 1 tbsp fresh minced parsley
- ✓ 1/2 tsp kosher salt
- ✓ Soup:
- ✓ cooking spray
- ✓ 1 tsp olive oil
- ✓ 1/2 cup chopped onion
- ✓ 1/2 cup chopped celery
- ✓ 1/2 cup chopped carrot
- ✓ 3 cloves minced garlic
- ✓ 1 can (28 ounces diced San Marzano tomatoes
- ✓ 4 cups reduced sodium chicken broth
- ✓ 4 torn basil leaves
- ✓ 2 bay leaves
- ✓ 1 cup ditalini pasta
- ✓ 1 cup zucchini, diced small
- ✓ Parmesan rind, optional
- ✓ Grated parmesan cheese, optional for serving

Directions:

- ❖ Thoroughly combine turkey with egg, garlic, parsley, salt, pecorino and breadcrumbs in a bowl.
- ❖ Make 30 equal sized meatballs out of this mixture.
- ❖ Preheat olive oil in the insert of the Instant Pot on Sauté mode.
- ❖ Sear the meatballs in the heated oil in batches, until brown.
- ❖ Set the meatballs aside in a plate.
- ❖ Add more oil to the insert of the Instant Pot.
- ❖ Stir in carrots, garlic, celery, and onion. Sauté for 4 minutes.
- ❖ Add basil, bay leaves, tomatoes, and Parmesan rind.
- ❖ Return the seared meatballs to the pot along with the broth.
- ❖ Secure and sear the Instant Pot lid and select Manual mode for 15 minutes at high pressure.
- ❖ Once done, release the pressure completely then remove the lid.
- ❖ Add zucchini and pasta, cook it for 4 minutes on Sauté mode.
- ❖ Garnish with cheese and basil.
- ❖ Serve.

Nutrition: Calories: 261;Carbohydrate: 11.2g;Protein: 36.6g;Fat: 7g;Sugar: 3g;Sodium: 198g

362) LOVELY MINT AVOCADO CHILLED SOUP

Cooking Time: 5 Minutes   **Servings:** 2

Ingredients:

- ✓ 1 cup coconut milk, chilled
- ✓ 1 medium ripe avocado
- ✓ 1 tbsp lime juice
- ✓ Salt, to taste
- ✓ 20 fresh mint leaves

Directions:

- ❖ Put all the ingredients into an immersion blender and blend until a thick mixture is formed.
- ❖ Allow to cool in the fridge for about 10 minutes and serve chilled.

Nutrition: Calories: 286;Carbs: 12.6g;Fats: 26.9g;Proteins: 4.2g;Sodium: 70mg;Sugar: 4.6g

363) CLASSIC SPLIT PEA SOUP

Cooking Time: 30 Minutes   **Servings:** 6

Ingredients:

- ✓ 3 tbsp butter
- ✓ 1 onion diced
- ✓ 2 ribs celery diced
- ✓ 2 carrots diced
- ✓ 6 oz. diced ham
- ✓ 1 lb. dry split peas sorted and rinsed
- ✓ 6 cups chicken stock
- ✓ 2 bay leaves
- ✓ kosher salt and black pepper

Directions:

- ❖ Set your Instant Pot on Sauté mode and melt butter in it.
- ❖ Stir in celery, onion, carrots, salt, and pepper.
- ❖ Sauté them for 5 minutes then stir in split peas, ham bone, chicken stock, and bay leaves.
- ❖ Seal and lock the Instant Pot lid then select Manual mode for 15 minutes at high pressure.
- ❖ Once done, release the pressure completely then remove the lid.
- ❖ Remove the ham bone and separate meat from the bone.
- ❖ Shred or dice the meat and return it to the soup.
- ❖ Adjust seasoning as needed then serve warm.
- ❖ Enjoy.

Nutrition: Calories: 190;Carbohydrate: 30.5g;Protein: 8g;Fat: 3.5g;Sugar: 4.2g;Sodium: 461mg

364) SPECIAL BUTTERNUT SQUASH SOUP

Cooking Time: 40 Minutes   **Servings: 4**

Ingredients:

- ✓ 1 tbsp olive oil
- ✓ 1 medium yellow onion chopped
- ✓ 1 large carrot chopped
- ✓ 1 celery rib chopped
- ✓ 3 cloves of garlic minced
- ✓ 2 lbs. butternut squash, peeled chopped
- ✓ 2 cups vegetable broth
- ✓ 1 green apple peeled, cored, and chopped
- ✓ 1/4 tsp ground cinnamon
- ✓ 1 sprig fresh thyme
- ✓ 1 sprig fresh rosemary
- ✓ 1 tsp kosher salt
- ✓ 1/2 tsp black pepper
- ✓ Pinch of nutmeg optional

Directions:

- ❖ Preheat olive oil in the insert of the Instant Pot on Sauté mode.
- ❖ Add celery, carrots, and garlic, sauté for 5 minutes.
- ❖ Stir in squash, broth, cinnamon, apple nutmeg, rosemary, thyme, salt, and pepper.
- ❖ Mix well gently then seal and secure the lid.
- ❖ Select Manual mode to cook for 10 minutes at high pressure.
- ❖ Once done, release the pressure completely then remove the lid.
- ❖ Puree the soup using an immersion blender.
- ❖ Serve warm.

Nutrition: Calories: 282;Carbohydrate: 50g;Protein: 13g;Fat: 4.7g;Sugar: 12.8g;Sodium: 213mg

365) LOVELY CREAMY CILANTRO LIME COLESLAW

Cooking Time: 10 Minutes   **Servings: 2**

Ingredients:

- ✓ ¾ avocado
- ✓ 1 lime, juiced
- ✓ 1/8 cup water
- ✓ Cilantro, to garnish
- ✓ 6 oz coleslaw, bagged
- ✓ 1/8 cup cilantro leaves
- ✓ 1 garlic clove
- ✓ ¼ tsp salt

Directions:

- ❖ Put garlic and cilantro in a food processor and process until chopped.
- ❖ Add lime juice, avocado and water and pulse until creamy.
- ❖ Put coleslaw in a large bowl and stir in the avocado mixture.
- ❖ Refrigerate for a few hours before serving.

Nutrition: Calories: 240;Carbs: 17.4g;Fats: 19.6g;Proteins: 2.8g;Sodium: 0mg;Sugar: 0.5g

366) CLASSIC SNAP PEA SALAD

Cooking Time: 15 Minutes   **Servings: 2**

Ingredients:

- ✓ 1/8 cup lemon juice
- ✓ ½ clove garlic, crushed
- ✓ 4 ounces cauliflower riced
- ✓ 1/8 cup olive oil
- ✓ ¼ tsp coarse grain Dijon mustard
- ✓ ½ tsp granulated stevia
- ✓ ¼ cup sugar snap peas, ends removed and each pod cut into three pieces
- ✓ 1/8 cup chives
- ✓ 1/8 cup red onions, minced
- ✓ Sea salt and black pepper, to taste
- ✓ ¼ cup almonds, sliced

Directions:

- ❖ Pour water in a pot fitted with a steamer basket and bring water to a boil.
- ❖ Place riced cauliflower in the steamer basket and season with sea salt.
- ❖ Cover the pot and steam for about 10 minutes until tender.
- ❖ Drain the cauliflower and dish out in a bowl to refrigerate for about 1 hour.
- ❖ Meanwhile, make a dressing by mixing olive oil, lemon juice, garlic, mustard, stevia, salt and black pepper in a bowl.
- ❖ Mix together chilled cauliflower, peas, chives, almonds and red onions in another bowl.
- ❖ Pour the dressing over this mixture and serve.

Nutrition: Calories: 203;Carbs: 7.6g;Fats: 18g;Proteins: 4.2g;Sodium: 28mg;Sugar: 2.9g

367) SPINACH AND BACON SALAD

Cooking Time: 15 Minutes   **Servings: 4**

Ingredients:

- ✓ 2 eggs, boiled, halved, and sliced
- ✓ 10 oz. organic baby spinach, rinsed, and dried
- ✓ 8 pieces thick bacon, cooked and sliced
- ✓ ½ cup plain mayonnaise
- ✓ ½ medium red onion, thinly sliced

Directions:

- ❖ Mix together the mayonnaise and spinach in a large bowl.
- ❖ Stir in the rest of the ingredients and combine well.
- ❖ Dish out in a glass bowl and serve well.

Nutrition: Calories: 373;Carbs: ;Fats: 34.5g;Proteins: 11g;Sodium: 707mg;Sugar: 1.1g

Sauces and Dressings Recipes

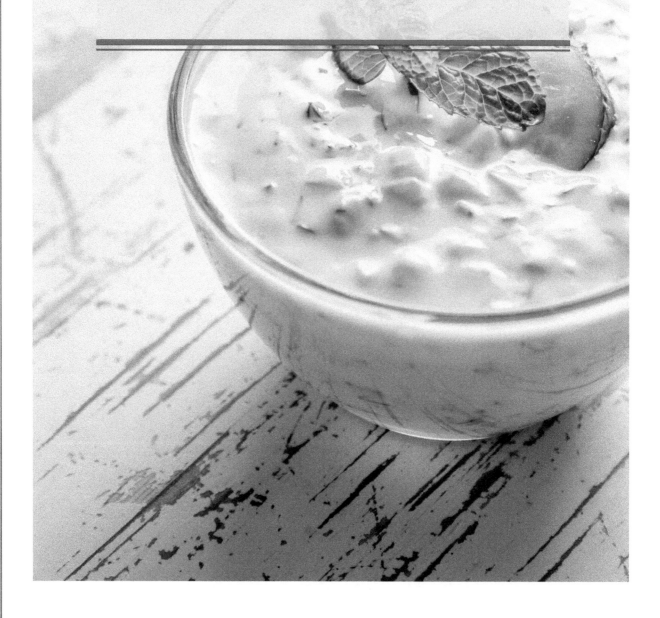

SAUCES & DRESSINGS

368) GREEK-STYLE CHICKEN AND POTATOES

Preparation Time: 10 minutes   **Cooking Time:** 50 minutes   **Servings:** 4

Ingredients:

- ✓ 4 lb chicken thighs 2 tbsp oregano
- ✓ 1 tbsp salt
- ✓ 1 tsp black pepper
- ✓ 2/3 cup chicken stock
- ✓ One pinch of cayenne pepper

- ✓ 1 tsp rosemary
- ✓ ½ cup lemon juice
- ✓ Six minced garlic cloves
- ✓ ½ cup olive oil
- ✓ Three sliced russet potatoes
- ✓ 1 tbsp chopped oregano

Directions:

- ❖ Add lemon juice, oregano, oil, cayenne pepper, salt, garlic, rosemary, black pepper potatoes, and chicken in a bowl. Mix them to coat everything well.
- ❖ Place chicken in a roasting tray.
- ❖ Spread potato pieces, 2/3 cup of stock, and marinade over chicken pieces.
- ❖ Bake in a preheated oven at 425 degrees for 20 minutes.
- ❖ Change the sides of the chicken and bake for 20 more minutes.
- ❖ Bake until chicken is done and shift chicken in serving dish.
- ❖ Mix potatoes with remaining juice and broil for three minutes.
- ❖ Shift the potatoes in the serving dish beside the chicken.
- ❖ Concentrate chicken stock left in a roasting tray on the stove over medium flame.

Nutrition: Calories: 138 kcal Fat: 74.5 g Protein: 80.4 g Carbs: 34.4 g Fiber: 3 g

369) ITALIAN BAKED FISH

Preparation Time: 5 minutes   **Cooking Time:** 30 minutes   **Servings:** 6

Ingredients:

- ✓ 1/3 cup olive oil
- ✓ Two diced tomatoes 1.5 chopped red onion
- ✓ Ten chopped garlic cloves
- ✓ 1 tsp Spanish paprika 2 tsp coriander
- ✓ 1 tsp cumin
- ✓ 1.5 tbsp capers
- ✓ ½ tsp cayenne pepper

- ✓ Salt to taste
- ✓ 1/3 cup raisins
- ✓ 1 tbsp of lemon juice
- ✓ Black pepper to taste
- ✓ Parsley for garnishing
- ✓ Zest of one lemon
- ✓ 1.5 lb white fish fillet
- ✓ Mint for garnishing

Directions:

- ❖ Cook onions in heated olive oil in a saucepan for three minutes.
- ❖ Stir in tomatoes, salt, capers, garlic, raisins, and spices and let them boil.
- ❖ Reduce the flame to low and simmer for 15 minutes.
- ❖ Rub fish with pepper and salt and set aside.
- ❖ Transfer half of the cooked tomato mixture to the baking pan, followed by fish, lemon juice, zest, and leftover tomato mixture.
- ❖ Bake in a preheated oven at 400 degrees for 18 minutes.
- ❖ Sprinkle mint and parsley and serve.

Nutrition: Calories: 308 kcal Fat: 17.4 g Protein: 27 g Carbs: 13.3 g Fiber: 2 g

370) GREEK TZATZIKI SAUCE AND DIP

Preparation Time: 10 minutes   **Cooking Time:** 0 minute   **Servings:** 4

Ingredients:

- ✓ ½ halved cucumber
- ✓ 3/4 cup Yogurt
- ✓ Two minced garlic cloves 2 tbsp red wine vinegar

- ✓ 1 tbsp minced dill
- ✓ One pinch of kosher salt
- ✓ One pinch of black pepper

Directions:

- ❖ Place dried shredded cucumber in a bowl.
- ❖ Mix garlic, vinegar, salt, yogurt, dill, and pepper in cucumber and mix well.
- ❖ Cover the bowl and place it in the refrigerator. The Tzatziki sauce is ready.
- ❖ Can store up to three days.

Nutrition: Calories: 30 kcal Fat: 1 g Protein: 4 g Carbs: 3 g Fiber: 1 g

371) ITALIAN PESTO AND GARLIC SHRIMP BRUSCHETTA

Preparation Time: 10 minutes   **Cooking Time:** 15 minutes   **Servings:** 12

Ingredients:

- ✓ 8 oz shrimp
- ✓ Black pepper to taste
- ✓ 2 tbsp butter
- ✓ 4 tbsp olive oil
- ✓ 20 basil leaves One bread

- ✓ Four minced garlic cloves 3 oz pesto
- ✓ 2 oz capers 3 oz sun-dried tomatoes
- ✓ 1 oz feta cheese
- ✓ kosher salt to taste
- ✓ Glaze Balsamic for garnishing

Directions:

- ❖ Sprinkle salt and pepper over shrimps in a bowl. Set aside for ten minutes.
- ❖ Add olive oil and butter of about 2 tbsp each in the pan and cook for 2 minutes over medium flame.
- ❖ Stir in garlic and sauté for one more minute.
- ❖ Mix shrimps and cook for four minutes.
- ❖ Remove from flame and let it set.
- ❖ Slice the bread and place in a baking tray and drizzle oil and toast in the oven for five minutes.
- ❖ Spread pesto sauce over each bread slice followed by sun-dried tomatoes, shrimp, caper, cheese, basil, and balsamic glaze and serve.

Nutrition: Calories: 168 kcal Fat: 7 g Protein: 5 g Carbs: 19 g Fiber: 1 g

372)   EASY PAN-SEARED CITRUS SHRIMP

Preparation Time: 5 minutes   **Cooking Time:** 10 minutes   **Servings:** 6

Ingredients:

- ✓ 1 tbsp olive oil
- ✓ 6 tbsp cup lemon juice
- ✓ 1 cup of orange juice
- ✓ One sliced orange
- ✓ Five minced garlic cloves
- ✓ 1 tbsp chopped parsley
- ✓ 1 tbsp chopped red onion
- ✓ One pinch of red pepper flakes
- ✓ Kosher salt to taste
- ✓ Black pepper to taste 3 lb shrimp
- ✓ One wedge cut lemon

Directions:

- ❖ Mix parsley, pepper flakes, orange juice, oil, garlic, lemon juice, and onions in a bowl.
- ❖ Transfer the onion mixture to skillet and cook over medium flame for eight minutes.
- ❖ Add salt, pepper, and shrimps in a skillet and cook for five minutes or until shrimps are done.
- ❖ Garnish with parsley and lemon slices and serve.

Nutrition: Calories: 291 kcal Fat: 6 g Protein: 47 g Carbs: 11 g Fiber: 1 g

373)   SIMPLE CUCUMBER AND TOMATO SALAD

Preparation Time: 10 minutes   **Cooking Time:** 0 minute   **Servings:** 4

Ingredients:

- ✓ One sliced English cucumber
- ✓ ½ sliced red onion
- ✓ Three diced tomatoes
- ✓ 2 tbsp olive oil
- ✓ Salt to taste
- ✓ 1 tbsp red wine vinegar
- ✓ Black pepper to taste

Directions:

- ❖ In a large mixing bowl, mix all the ingredients and place in the refrigerator for 20 minutes.
- ❖ Serve and enjoy it.

Nutrition: Calories: 104 kcal Fat: 8 g Protein: 2 g Carbs: 7 g Fiber: 2 g

374)   EASY CITRUS AVOCADO DIP

Preparation Time: 15 minutes   **Cooking Time:** 0 minute   **Servings:** 8

Ingredients:

- ✓ Two diced oranges
- ✓ ½ cup chopped onions
- ✓ ½ cup chopped mint
- ✓ ½ cup chopped cilantro
- ✓ Olive oil as required
- ✓ Two sliced avocados
- ✓ ½ cup chopped walnuts
- ✓ Black pepper to taste
- ✓ Cayenne as required
- ✓ Salt to taste
- ✓ 1 tbsp of lime juice
- ✓ ¾ tsp sumac
- ✓ 1.75 oz shredded feta cheese

Directions:

- ❖ In a bowl, combine all the ingredients and mix well.
- ❖ Serve and enjoy it.

Nutrition: Calories: 147 kcal Fat: 10.3 g Protein: 2.8 g Carbs: 14.6 g Fiber: 2.1 g

375)   TOMATOES ROAST WITH THYME AND FETA

Preparation Time: 5 minutes   **Cooking Time:** 20 minutes   **Servings:** 4

Ingredients:

- ✓ ½ tsp dried thyme
- ✓ 16 oz cherry tomatoes
- ✓ Black pepper to taste
- ✓ 3 tbsp olive oil
- ✓ Salt to taste
- ✓ 6 tbsp feta cheese

Directions:

- ❖ In a baking tray, put tomatoes.
- ❖ Pour olive oil and drizzle pepper, thyme leaves, and salt over tomatoes and mix well.
- ❖ Bake in a preheated oven at 450 degrees for 15 minutes.
- ❖ Drizzle cheese and broil for five minutes and serve when the cheese melts.

Nutrition: Calories: 195 kcal Fat: 7.3 g Protein: 2 g Carbs: 3.1 g Fiber: 1.1 g

376) GREEK-STYLE CHICKEN AND POTATOES

Preparation Time: 10 minutes   **Cooking Time:** 50 minutes   **Servings: 4**

Ingredients:

- ✓ 4 lb chicken thighs 2 tbsp oregano
- ✓ 1 tbsp salt
- ✓ 1 tsp black pepper
- ✓ 2/3 cup chicken stock
- ✓ One pinch of cayenne pepper

- ✓ 1 tsp rosemary
- ✓ ½ cup lemon juice
- ✓ Six minced garlic cloves
- ✓ ½ cup olive oil
- ✓ Three sliced russet potatoes
- ✓ 1 tbsp chopped oregano

Directions:

- ❖ Add lemon juice, oregano, oil, cayenne pepper, salt, garlic, rosemary, black pepper potatoes, and chicken in a bowl. Mix them to coat everything well.
- ❖ Place chicken in a roasting tray.
- ❖ Spread potato pieces, 2/3 cup of stock, and marinade over chicken pieces.
- ❖ Bake in a preheated oven at 425 degrees for 20 minutes.
- ❖ Change the sides of the chicken and bake for 20 more minutes.
- ❖ Bake until chicken is done and shift chicken in serving dish.
- ❖ Mix potatoes with remaining juice and broil for three minutes.
- ❖ Shift the potatoes in the serving dish beside the chicken.
- ❖ Concentrate chicken stock left in a roasting tray on the stove over medium flame.

Nutrition: Calories: 138 kcal Fat: 74.5 g Protein: 80.4 g Carbs: 34.4 g Fiber: 3 g

377) ITALIAN BAKED FISH

Preparation Time: 5 minutes   **Cooking Time:** 30 minutes   **Servings: 6**

Ingredients:

- ✓ 1/3 cup olive oil
- ✓ Two diced tomatoes 1.5 chopped red onion
- ✓ Ten chopped garlic cloves
- ✓ 1 tsp Spanish paprika 2 tsp coriander
- ✓ 1 tsp cumin
- ✓ 1.5 tbsp capers
- ✓ ½ tsp cayenne pepper

- ✓ Salt to taste
- ✓ 1/3 cup raisins
- ✓ 1 tbsp of lemon juice
- ✓ Black pepper to taste
- ✓ Parsley for garnishing
- ✓ Zest of one lemon
- ✓ 1.5 lb white fish fillet
- ✓ Mint for garnishing

Directions:

- ❖ Cook onions in heated olive oil in a saucepan for three minutes.
- ❖ Stir in tomatoes, salt, capers, garlic, raisins, and spices and let them boil.
- ❖ Reduce the flame to low and simmer for 15 minutes.
- ❖ Rub fish with pepper and salt and set aside.
- ❖ Transfer half of the cooked tomato mixture to the baking pan, followed by fish, lemon juice, zest, and leftover tomato mixture.
- ❖ Bake in a preheated oven at 400 degrees for 18 minutes.
- ❖ Sprinkle mint and parsley and serve.

Nutrition: Calories: 308 kcal Fat: 17.4 g Protein: 27 g Carbs: 13.3 g Fiber: 2 g

378) GREEK TZATZIKI SAUCE AND DIP

Preparation Time: 10 minutes   **Cooking Time:** 0 minute   **Servings: 4**

Ingredients:

- ✓ ½ halved cucumber
- ✓ 3/4 cup Yogurt
- ✓ Two minced garlic cloves 2 tbsp red wine vinegar

- ✓ 1 tbsp minced dill
- ✓ One pinch of kosher salt
- ✓ One pinch of black pepper

Directions:

- ❖ Place dried shredded cucumber in a bowl.
- ❖ Mix garlic, vinegar, salt, yogurt, dill, and pepper in cucumber and mix well.
- ❖ Cover the bowl and place it in the refrigerator. The Tzatziki sauce is ready.
- ❖ Can store up to three days.

Nutrition: Calories: 30 kcal Fat: 1 g Protein: 4 g Carbs: 3 g Fiber: 1 g

379) ITALIAN PESTO AND GARLIC SHRIMP BRUSCHETTA

Preparation Time: 10 minutes   **Cooking Time:** 15 minutes   **Servings: 12**

Ingredients:

- ✓ 8 oz shrimp
- ✓ Black pepper to taste
- ✓ 2 tbsp butter
- ✓ 4 tbsp olive oil
- ✓ 20 basil leaves One bread

- ✓ Four minced garlic cloves 3 oz pesto
- ✓ 2 oz capers 3 oz sun-dried tomatoes
- ✓ 1 oz feta cheese
- ✓ kosher salt to taste
- ✓ Glaze Balsamic for garnishing

Directions:

- ❖ Sprinkle salt and pepper over shrimps in a bowl. Set aside for ten minutes.
- ❖ Add olive oil and butter of about 2 tbsp each in the pan and cook for 2 minutes over medium flame.
- ❖ Stir in garlic and sauté for one more minute.
- ❖ Mix shrimps and cook for four minutes.
- ❖ Remove from flame and let it set.
- ❖ Slice the bread and place in a baking tray and drizzle oil and toast in the oven for five minutes.
- ❖ Spread pesto sauce over each bread slice followed by sun-dried tomatoes, shrimp, caper, cheese, basil, and balsamic glaze and serve.

Nutrition: Calories: 168 kcal Fat: 7 g Protein: 5 g Carbs: 19 g Fiber: 1 g

380) EASY PAN-SEARED CITRUS SHRIMP

Preparation Time: 5 minutes   **Cooking Time:** 10 minutes   **Servings: 6**

Ingredients:

- ✓ 1 tbsp olive oil
- ✓ 6 tbsp cup lemon juice
- ✓ 1 cup of orange juice
- ✓ One sliced orange
- ✓ Five minced garlic cloves

- ✓ 1 tbsp chopped parsley
- ✓ 1 tbsp chopped red onion
- ✓ One pinch of red pepper flakes
- ✓ Kosher salt to taste
- ✓ Black pepper to taste 3 lb shrimp
- ✓ One wedge cut lemon

Directions:

- ❖ Mix parsley, pepper flakes, orange juice, oil, garlic, lemon juice, and onions in a bowl.
- ❖ Transfer the onion mixture to skillet and cook over medium flame for eight minutes.
- ❖ Add salt, pepper, and shrimps in a skillet and cook for five minutes or until shrimps are done.
- ❖ Garnish with parsley and lemon slices and serve.

Nutrition: Calories: 291 kcal Fat: 6 g Protein: 47 g Carbs: 11 g Fiber: 1 g

381) SIMPLE CUCUMBER AND TOMATO SALAD

Preparation Time: 10 minutes   **Cooking Time:** 0 minute   **Servings: 4**

Ingredients:

- ✓ One sliced English cucumber
- ✓ ½ sliced red onion
- ✓ Three diced tomatoes

- ✓ 2 tbsp olive oil
- ✓ Salt to taste
- ✓ 1 tbsp red wine vinegar
- ✓ Black pepper to taste

Directions:

- ❖ In a large mixing bowl, mix all the ingredients and place in the refrigerator for 20 minutes.
- ❖ Serve and enjoy it.

Nutrition: Calories: 104 kcal Fat: 8 g Protein: 2 g Carbs: 7 g Fiber: 2 g

382) EASY CITRUS AVOCADO DIP

Preparation Time: 15 minutes   **Cooking Time:** 0 minute   **Servings: 8**

Ingredients:

- ✓ Two diced oranges
- ✓ ½ cup chopped onions
- ✓ ½ cup chopped mint
- ✓ ½ cup chopped cilantro
- ✓ Olive oil as required
- ✓ Two sliced avocados

- ✓ ½ cup chopped walnuts
- ✓ Black pepper to taste
- ✓ Cayenne as required
- ✓ Salt to taste
- ✓ 1 tbsp of lime juice
- ✓ ¾ tsp sumac
- ✓ 1.75 oz shredded feta cheese

Directions:

- ❖ In a bowl, combine all the ingredients and mix well.
- ❖ Serve and enjoy it.

Nutrition: Calories: 147 kcal Fat: 10.3 g Protein: 2.8 g Carbs: 14.6 g Fiber: 2.1 g

383) TOMATOES ROAST WITH THYME AND FETA

Preparation Time: 5 minutes   **Cooking Time:** 20 minutes   **Servings: 4**

Ingredients:

- ✓ ½ tsp dried thyme
- ✓ 16 oz cherry tomatoes
- ✓ Black pepper to taste

- ✓ 3 tbsp olive oil
- ✓ Salt to taste
- ✓ 6 tbsp feta cheese

Directions:

- ❖ In a baking tray, put tomatoes.
- ❖ Pour olive oil and drizzle pepper, thyme leaves, and salt over tomatoes and mix well.
- ❖ Bake in a preheated oven at 450 degrees for 15 minutes.
- ❖ Drizzle cheese and broil for five minutes and serve when the cheese melts.

Nutrition: Calories: 195 kcal Fat: 7.3 g Protein: 2 g Carbs: 3.1 g Fiber: 1.1 g

Desserts & Snacks Recipes

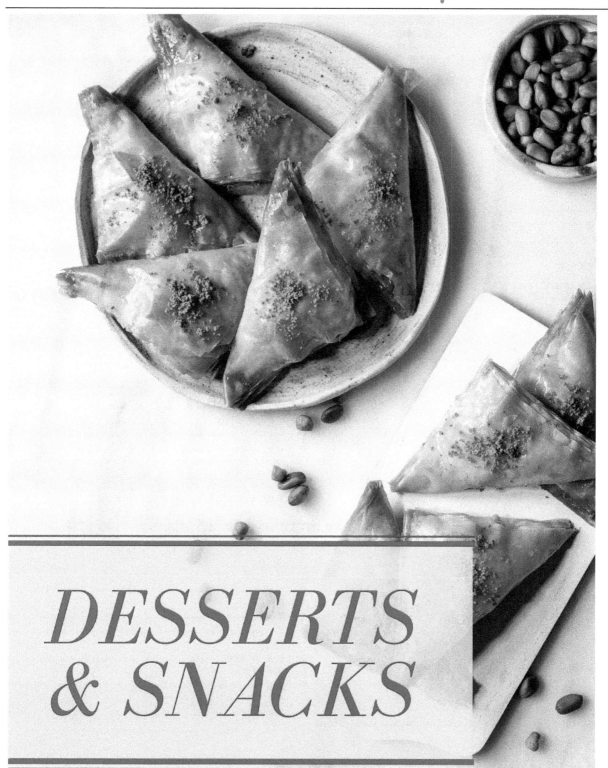

DESSERTS & SNACKS

384) SPECIAL CHUNKY MONKEY TRAIL MIX

Cooking Time: 1 Hour 30 Minutes   **Servings:** 6

Ingredients:

- ✓ 1 cup cashews, halved
- ✓ 2 cups raw walnuts, chopped or halved
- ✓ ⅓ cup coconut sugar
- ✓ ½ cup of chocolate chips
- ✓ 1 tsp vanilla extract
- ✓ 1 cup coconut flakes, unsweetened and make sure you have big flakes and not shredded
- ✓ 6 ounces dried banana slices
- ✓ 1 ½ tsp coconut oil at room temperature

Directions:

- ❖ Turn your crockpot to high and add the cashews, walnuts, vanilla, coconut oil, and sugar. Combine until the ingredients are well mixed and then cook for 45 minutes.
- ❖ Reduce the temperature on your crockpot to low.
- ❖ Continue to cook the mixture for another 20 minutes.
- ❖ Place a piece of parchment paper on your counter.
- ❖ Once the mix is done cooking, remove it from the crockpot and set on top of the parchment paper.
- ❖ Let the mixture sit and cool for 20 minutes.
- ❖ Pour the contents into a bowl and add the dried bananas and chocolate chips. Gently mix the ingredients together. You can store the mixture in Ziplock bags for a quick and easy snack.

Nutrition: calories: 250, fats: 6 grams, carbohydrates: 1grams, protein: 4 grams

385) DELICIOUS FIG-PECAN ENERGY BITES

Cooking Time: 20 Minutes   **Servings:** 6

Ingredients:

- ✓ ½ cup chopped pecans
- ✓ 2 tbsp honey
- ✓ ¾ cup dried figs, about 6 to 8, diced
- ✓ 2 tbsp wheat flaxseed
- ✓ ¼ cup quick oats
- ✓ 2 tbsp regular or powdered peanut butter

Directions:

- ❖ Combine the figs, quick oats, pecans, peanut butter, and flaxseed into a bowl. Stir the ingredients well.
- ❖ Drizzle honey onto the ingredients and mix everything with a wooden spoon. Do your best to press all the ingredients into the honey as you are stirring. If you start to struggle because the mixture is too sticky, set it in the freezer for 3 to 5 minutes.
- ❖ Divide the mixture into four sections.
- ❖ Take a wet rag and get your hands damp. You don't want them too wet or they won't work well with the mixture.
- ❖ Divide each of the four sections into 3 separate sections.
- ❖ Take one of the three sections and roll them up. Repeat with each section so you have a dozen energy bites once you are done.
- ❖ If you want to firm them up, you can place them into the freezer for a few minutes. Otherwise, you can enjoy them as soon as they are little energy balls.
- ❖ To store them, you'll want to keep them in a sealed container and set them in the fridge. They can be stored for about a week.

Nutrition: calories: 157, fats: 6 grams, carbohydrates: 26 grams, protein: 3 grams

386) MEDITERRANEAN STYLE BAKED APPLES

Cooking Time: 25 Minutes   **Servings:** 4

Ingredients:

- ✓ ½ lemon, squeezed for juice
- ✓ 1 ½ pounds of peeled and sliced apples
- ✓ ¼ tsp cinnamon

Directions:

- ❖ Set the temperature of your oven to 350 degrees Fahrenheit so it can preheat.
- ❖ Take a piece of parchment paper and lay on top of a baking pan.
- ❖ Combine your lemon juice, cinnamon, and apples into a medium bowl and mix well.
- ❖ Pour the apples onto the baking pan and arrange them so they are not doubled up.
- ❖ Place the pan in the oven and set your timer to 2minutes. The apples should be tender but not mushy.
- ❖ Remove from the oven, plate and enjoy!

Nutrition: calories: 90, fats: 0.3 grams, carbohydrates: 24 grams, protein: 0.5 grams

387) LOVELY STRAWBERRY POPSICLE

Cooking Time: 10 Minutes   **Servings: 5**

Ingredients:

- ✓ ½ cup almond milk
- ✓ 1 ½ cups fresh strawberries

Directions:

- ❖ Using a blender or hand mixer, combine the almond milk and strawberries thoroughly in a bowl.
- ❖ Using popsicle molds, pour the mixture into the molds and place the sticks into the mixture.
- ❖ Set in the freezer for at least 4 hours.
- ❖ Serve and enjoy—especially on a hot day!

Nutrition: calories: 3 fats: 0.5 grams, carbohydrates: 7 grams, protein: 0.6 grams.

388) SPECIAL FROZEN BLUEBERRY YOGURT

Cooking Time: 30 Minutes   **Servings: 6**

Ingredients:

- ✓ ⅔ cup honey
- ✓ 2 cups chilled yogurt
- ✓ 1 pint fresh blueberries
- ✓ 1 juiced and zested lime or lemon. You can even substitute an orange if your tastes prefer.

Directions:

- ❖ With a saucepan on your burner set to medium heat, add the honey, juiced fruit, zest, and blueberries.
- ❖ Stir the mixture continuously as it begins to simmer for 15 minutes.
- ❖ When the liquid is nearly gone, pour the contents into a bowl and place in the fridge for several minutes. You will want to stir the ingredients and check to see if they are chilled.
- ❖ Once the fruit is chilled, combine with the yogurt.
- ❖ Mix until the ingredients are well incorporated and enjoy.

Nutrition: calories: 233, fats: 3 grams, carbohydrates: 52 grams, protein: 3.5 grams

389) Cherry Brownies and Walnuts

Cooking Time: 25 To 30 Minutes   **Servings: 9**

Ingredients:

- ✓ 9 fresh cherries that are stemmed and pitted or 9 frozen cherries
- ✓ ½ cup sugar or sweetener substitute
- ✓ ¼ cup extra virgin olive oil
- ✓ 1 tsp vanilla extract
- ✓ ¼ tsp sea salt
- ✓ ½ cup whole-wheat pastry flour
- ✓ ¼ tsp baking powder
- ✓ ⅓ cup walnuts, chopped
- ✓ 2 eggs
- ✓ ½ cup plain Greek yogurt
- ✓ ⅓ cup cocoa powder, unsweetened

Directions:

- ❖ Make sure one of the metal racks in your oven is set in the middle.
- ❖ Turn the temperature on your oven to 375 degrees Fahrenheit.
- ❖ Using cooking spray, grease a 9-inch square pan.
- ❖ Take a large bowl and add the oil and sugar or sweetener substitute. Whisk the ingredients well.
- ❖ Add the eggs and use a mixer to beat the ingredients together.
- ❖ Pour in the yogurt and continue to beat the mixture until it is smooth.
- ❖ Take a medium bowl and combine the cocoa powder, flour, sea salt, and baking powder by whisking them together.
- ❖ Combine the powdered ingredients into the wet ingredients and use your electronic mixer to incorporate the ingredients together thoroughly.
- ❖ Add in the walnuts and stir.
- ❖ Pour the mixture into the pan.
- ❖ Sprinkle the cherries on top and push them into the batter. You can use any design, but it is best to make three rows and three columns with the cherries. This ensures that each piece of the brownie will have one cherry.
- ❖ Put the batter into the oven and turn your timer to 20 minutes.
- ❖ Check that the brownies are done using the toothpick test before removing them from the oven. Push the toothpick into the middle of the brownies and once it comes out clean, remove the brownies.
- ❖ Let the brownies cool for 5 to 10 minutes before cutting and serving.

Nutrition: calories: 225, fats: 10 grams, carbohydrates: 30 grams, protein: 5 grams

390) SPECIAL FRUIT DIP

Cooking Time: 10 To 15 Minutes   **Servings: 10**

Ingredients:

- ¼ cup coconut milk, full-fat is best
- ¼ cup vanilla yogurt
- ⅓ cup marshmallow creme
- 1 cup cream cheese, set at room temperature
- 2 tbsp maraschino cherry juice

Directions:

- ❖ In a large bowl, add the coconut milk, vanilla yogurt, marshmallow creme, cream cheese, and cherry juice.
- ❖ Using an electric mixer, set to low speed and blend the ingredients together until the fruit dip is smooth.
- ❖ Serve the dip with some of your favorite fruits and enjoy!

Nutrition: calories: 110, fats: 11 grams, carbohydrates: 3 grams, protein: 3 grams

391) Delicious Almond Shortbread Cookies

Cooking Time: 25 Minutes   **Servings: 16**

Ingredients:

- ½ cup coconut oil
- 1 tsp vanilla extract
- 2 egg yolks
- 1 tbsp brandy
- 1 cup powdered sugar
- 1 cup finely ground almonds
- 3 ½ cups cake flour
- ½ cup almond butter
- 1 tbsp water or rose flower water

Directions:

- ❖ In a large bowl, combine the coconut oil, powdered sugar, and butter. If the butter is not soft, you want to wait until it softens up. Use an electric mixer to beat the ingredients together at high speed.
- ❖ In a small bowl, add the egg yolks, brandy, water, and vanilla extract. Whisk well.
- ❖ Fold the egg yolk mixture into the large bowl.
- ❖ Add the flour and almonds. Fold and mix with a wooden spoon.
- ❖ Place the mixture into the fridge for at least 1 hour and 30 minutes.
- ❖ Preheat your oven to 325 degrees Fahrenheit.
- ❖ Take the mixture, which now looks like dough, and divide it into 1-inch balls.
- ❖ With a piece of parchment paper on a baking sheet, arrange the cookies and flatten them with a fork or your fingers.
- ❖ Place the cookies in the oven for 13 minutes, but watch them so they don't burn.
- ❖ Transfer the cookies onto a rack to cool for a couple of minutes before enjoying!

Nutrition: calories: 250, fats: 14 grams, carbohydrates: 30 grams, protein: 3 grams

392) CLASSIC CHOCOLATE FRUIT KEBABS

Cooking Time: 30 Minutes   **Servings: 6**

Ingredients:

- 24 blueberries
- 12 strawberries with the green leafy top part removed
- 12 green or red grapes, seedless
- 12 pitted cherries
- 8 ounces chocolate

Directions:

- ❖ Line a baking sheet with a piece of parchment paper and place 6, -inch long wooden skewers on top of the paper.
- ❖ Start by threading a piece of fruit onto the skewers. You can create and follow any pattern that you like with the ingredients. An example pattern is 1 strawberry, 1 cherry, blueberries, 2 grapes. Repeat the pattern until all of the fruit is on the skewers.
- ❖ In a saucepan on medium heat, melt the chocolate. Stir continuously until the chocolate has melted completely.
- ❖ Carefully scoop the chocolate into a plastic sandwich bag and twist the bag closed starting right above the chocolate.
- ❖ Snip the corner of the bag with scissors.
- ❖ Drizzle the chocolate onto the kebabs by squeezing it out of the bag.
- ❖ Put the baking pan into the freezer for 20 minutes.
- ❖ Serve and enjoy!

Nutrition: calories: 254, fats: 15 grams, carbohydrates: 28 grams, protein: 4 grams

393)

394) MEDITERRANEAN-STYLE BLACKBERRY ICE CREAM

Cooking Time: 15 Minutes   **Servings:** 6

Ingredients:

- 3 egg yolks
- 1 container of Greek yogurt
- 1 pound mashed blackberries
- ½ tsp vanilla essence
- 1 tsp arrowroot powder
- ¼ tsp ground cloves
- 5 ounces sugar or sweetener substitute
- 1 pound heavy cream

Directions:

- In a small bowl, add the arrowroot powder and egg yolks. Whisk or beat them with an electronic mixture until they are well combined.
- Set a saucepan on top of your stove and turn your heat to medium.
- Add the heavy cream and bring it to a boil.
- Turn off the heat and add the egg mixture into the cream through folding.
- Turn the heat back on to medium and pour in the sugar. Cook the mixture for 10 minutes or until it starts to thicken.
- Remove the mixture from heat and place it in the fridge so it can completely cool. This should take about one hour.
- Once the mixture is cooled, add in the Greek yogurt, ground cloves, blackberries, and vanilla by folding in the ingredients.
- Transfer the ice cream into a container and place it in the freezer for at least two hours.
- Serve and enjoy!

Nutrition: calories: 402, fats: 20 grams, carbohydrates: 52 grams, protein: 8 grams

395) CLASSIC STUFFED FIGS

Cooking Time: 20 Minutes   **Servings:** 6

Ingredients:

- 10 halved fresh figs
- 20 chopped almonds
- 4 ounces goat cheese, divided
- 2 tbsp of raw honey

Directions:

- Turn your oven to broiler mode and set it to a high temperature.
- Place your figs, cut side up, on a baking sheet. If you like to place a piece of parchment paper on top you can do this, but it is not necessary.
- Sprinkle each fig with half of the goat cheese.
- Add a tbsp of chopped almonds to each fig.
- Broil the figs for 3 to 4 minutes.
- Take them out of the oven and let them cool for 5 to 7 minutes.
- Sprinkle with the remaining goat cheese and honey.

396) PEACHES AND BLUE CHEESE CREAM

Cooking Time: 20 Hours 10 Minutes   **Servings:** 4

- ¼ tsp cardamom pods
- ⅔ cup red wine
- 2 tbsp honey, raw or your preferred variety
- 1 vanilla bean
- 1 tsp allspice berries
- 4 tbsp dried cherries

Directions:

- Set a saucepan on top of your stove range and add the cinnamon stick, cloves, orange juice, cardamom, vanilla, allspice, red wine, and orange zest. Whisk the ingredients well. Add your peaches to the mixture and poach them for hours or until they become soft.
- Take a spoon to remove the peaches and boil the rest of the liquid to make the syrup. You want the liquid to reduce itself by at least half.
- While the liquid is boiling, combine the dried cherries, blue cheese, and honey into a bowl. Once your peaches are cooled, slice them into halves.
- Top each peach with the blue cheese mixture and then drizzle the liquid onto the top. Serve and enjoy!

Nutrition: calories: 211, fats: 24 grams, carbohydrates: 15 grams, protein: 6 grams

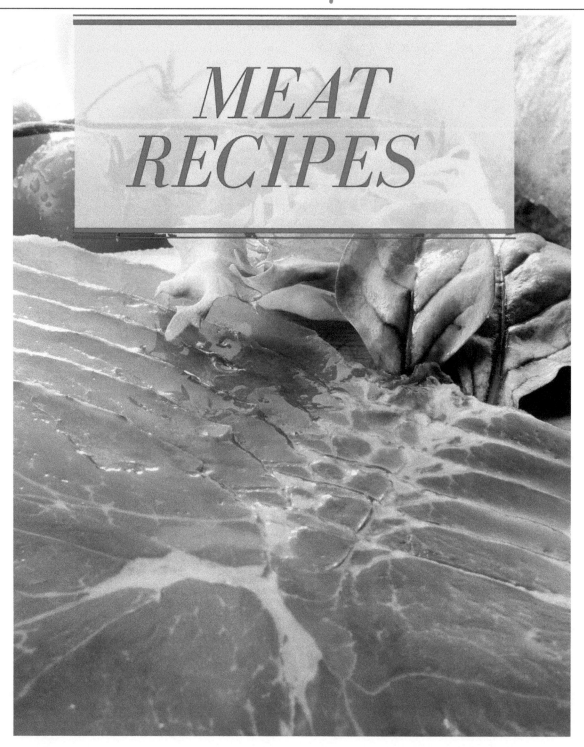

397) SPECIAL GROUND PORK SKILLET

Cooking Time: 25 Minutes   **Servings: 4**

Ingredients:

- ✓ 1 ½ pounds ground pork
- ✓ 2 tbsp olive oil
- ✓ 1 bunch kale, trimmed and roughly chopped
- ✓ 1 cup onions, sliced
- ✓ 1/4 tsp black pepper, or more to taste
- ✓ 1/4 cup tomato puree
- ✓ 1 bell pepper, chopped
- ✓ 1 tsp sea salt
- ✓ 1 cup chicken bone broth
- ✓ 1/4 cup port wine
- ✓ 2 cloves garlic, pressed
- ✓ 1 chili pepper, sliced

Directions:

- ❖ Heat tbsp of the olive oil in a cast-iron skillet over a moderately high heat. Now, sauté the onion, garlic, and peppers until they are tender and fragrant; reserve.
- ❖ Heat the remaining tbsp of olive oil; once hot, cook the ground pork and approximately 5 minutes until no longer pink.
- ❖ Add in the other ingredients and continue to cook for 15 to 17 minutes or until cooked through.
- ❖ Storing
- ❖ Place the ground pork mixture in airtight containers or Ziploc bags; keep in your refrigerator for up to 3 to 4 days.
- ❖ For freezing, place the ground pork mixture in airtight containers or heavy-duty freezer bags. Freeze up to 2 to 3 months. Defrost in the refrigerator. Bon appétit!

Nutrition: 349 Calories; 13g Fat; 4.4g Carbs; 45.3g Protein; 1.2g Fiber

398) LOVELY CHEESY GREEK-STYLE PORK

Cooking Time: 20 Minutes   **Servings: 6**

Ingredients:

- ✓ 1 tbsp sesame oil
- ✓ 1 ½ pounds pork shoulder, cut into strips
- ✓ Himalayan salt and freshly ground black pepper, to taste
- ✓ 1/2 tsp cayenne pepper
- ✓ 1/2 cup shallots, roughly chopped
- ✓ 2 bell peppers, sliced
- ✓ 1/4 cup cream of onion soup
- ✓ 1/2 tsp Sriracha sauce
- ✓ 1 tbsp tahini (sesame butter
- ✓ 1 tbsp soy sauce
- ✓ 4 ounces gouda cheese, cut into small pieces

Directions:

- ❖ Heat he sesame oil in a wok over a moderately high flame.
- ❖ Stir-fry the pork strips for 3 to 4 minutes or until just browned on all sides. Add in the spices, shallots and bell peppers and continue to cook for a further 4 minutes.
- ❖ Stir in the cream of onion soup, Sriracha, sesame butter, and soy sauce; continue to cook for to 4 minutes more.
- ❖ Top with the cheese and continue to cook until the cheese has melted.
- ❖ Storing
- ❖ Place your stir-fry in six airtight containers or Ziploc bags; keep in your refrigerator for 3 to 4 days.
- ❖ For freezing, wrap tightly with heavy-duty aluminum foil or freezer wrap. It will maintain the best quality for 2 to 3 months. Defrost in the refrigerator and reheat in your wok.

Nutrition: 424 Calories; 29.4g Fat; 3. Carbs; 34.2g Protein; 0.6g Fiber

399) SPECIAL PORK IN BLUE CHEESE SAUCE

Cooking Time: 30 Minutes   **Servings: 6**

Ingredients:

- ✓ 2 pounds pork center cut loin roast, boneless and cut into 6 pieces
- ✓ 1 tbsp coconut aminos
- ✓ 6 ounces blue cheese
- ✓ 1/3 cup heavy cream
- ✓ 1/3 cup port wine
- ✓ 1/3 cup roasted vegetable broth, preferably homemade
- ✓ 1 tsp dried hot chile flakes
- ✓ 1 tsp dried rosemary
- ✓ 1 tbsp lard
- ✓ 1 shallot, chopped
- ✓ 2 garlic cloves, chopped
- ✓ Salt and freshly cracked black peppercorns, to taste

Directions:

- ❖ Rub each piece of the pork with salt, black peppercorns, and rosemary.
- ❖ Melt the lard in a saucepan over a moderately high flame. Sear the pork on all sides about 15 minutes; set aside.
- ❖ Cook the shallot and garlic until they've softened. Add in port wine to scrape up any brown bits from the bottom.
- ❖ Reduce the heat to medium-low and add in the remaining ingredients; continue to simmer until the sauce has thickened and reduced.
- ❖ Storing
- ❖ Divide the pork and sauce into six portions; place each portion in a separate airtight container or Ziploc bag; keep in your refrigerator for 3 to 4 days.
- ❖ Freeze the pork and sauce in airtight containers or heavy-duty freezer bags. Freeze up to 4 months. Defrost in the refrigerator. Bon appétit!

Nutrition: 34Calories; 18.9g Fat; 1.9g Carbs; 40.3g Protein; 0.3g Fiber

400) MISSISSIPPI-STYLE PULLED PORK

Cooking Time: 6 Hours   **Servings: 4**

Ingredients:

- ✓ 1 ½ pounds pork shoulder
- ✓ 1 tbsp liquid smoke sauce
- ✓ 1 tsp chipotle powder
- ✓ Au Jus gravy seasoning packet
- ✓ 2 onions, cut into wedges
- ✓ Kosher salt and freshly ground black pepper, taste

Directions:

- ❖ Mix the liquid smoke sauce, chipotle powder, Au Jus gravy seasoning packet, salt and pepper. Rub the spice mixture into the pork on all sides.
- ❖ Wrap in plastic wrap and let it marinate in your refrigerator for 3 hours.
- ❖ Prepare your grill for indirect heat. Place the pork butt roast on the grate over a drip pan and top with onions; cover the grill and cook for about 6 hours.
- ❖ Transfer the pork to a cutting board. Now, shred the meat into bite-sized pieces using two forks.
- ❖ Storing
- ❖ Divide the pork between four airtight containers or Ziploc bags; keep in your refrigerator for up to 3 to 5 days.
- ❖ For freezing, place the pork in airtight containers or heavy-duty freezer bags. Freeze up to 4 months. Defrost in the refrigerator. Bon appétit!

Nutrition: 350 Calories; 11g Fat; 5g Carbs; 53.6g Protein; 2.2g Fiber

401) SPICY WITH CHEESY TURKEY DIP

Cooking Time: 25 Minutes   **Servings: 4**

Ingredients:

- ✓ 1 Fresno chili pepper, deveined and minced
- ✓ 1 ½ cups Ricotta cheese, creamed, 4% fat, softened
- ✓ 1/4 cup sour cream
- ✓ 1 tbsp butter, room temperature
- ✓ 1 shallot, chopped
- ✓ 1 tsp garlic, pressed
- ✓ 1 pound ground turkey
- ✓ 1/2 cup goat cheese, shredded
- ✓ Salt and black pepper, to taste
- ✓ 1 ½ cups Gruyère, shredded

Directions:

- ❖ Melt the butter in a frying pan over a moderately high flame. Now, sauté the onion and garlic until they have softened.
- ❖ Stir in the ground turkey and continue to cook until it is no longer pink.
- ❖ Transfer the sautéed mixture to a lightly greased baking dish. Add in Ricotta, sour cream, goat cheese, salt, pepper, and chili pepper.
- ❖ Top with the shredded Gruyère cheese. Bake in the preheated oven at 350 degrees F for about 20 minutes or until hot and bubbly in top.
- ❖ Storing
- ❖ Place your dip in an airtight container; keep in your refrigerator for up 3 to 4 days. Enjoy!

Nutrition: 284 Calories; 19g Fat; 3.2g Carbs; 26. Protein; 1.6g Fiber

402) TURKEY CHORIZO AND BOK CHOY

Cooking Time: 50 Minutes   **Servings: 4**

Ingredients:

- ✓ 4 mild turkey Chorizo, sliced
- ✓ 1/2 cup full-fat milk
- ✓ 6 ounces Gruyère cheese, preferably freshly grated
- ✓ 1 yellow onion, chopped
- ✓ Coarse salt and ground black pepper, to taste
- ✓ 1 pound Bok choy, tough stem ends trimmed
- ✓ 1 cup cream of mushroom soup
- ✓ 1 tbsp lard, room temperature

Directions:

- ❖ Melt the lard in a nonstick skillet over a moderate flame; cook the Chorizo sausage for about 5 minutes, stirring occasionally to ensure even cooking; reserve.
- ❖ Add in the onion, salt, pepper, Bok choy, and cream of mushroom soup. Continue to cook for 4 minutes longer or until the vegetables have softened.
- ❖ Spoon the mixture into a lightly oiled casserole dish. Top with the reserved Chorizo.
- ❖ In a mixing bowl, thoroughly combine the milk and cheese. Pour the cheese mixture over the sausage.
- ❖ Cover with foil and bake at 36degrees F for about 35 minutes.
- ❖ Storing
- ❖ Cut your casserole into four portions. Place each portion in an airtight container; keep in your refrigerator for 3 to 4 days.
- ❖ For freezing, wrap your portions tightly with heavy-duty aluminum foil or freezer wrap. Freeze up to 1 to 2 months. Defrost in the refrigerator. Enjoy!

Nutrition: 18Calories; 12g Fat; 2.6g Carbs; 9.4g Protein; 1g Fiber

403)   CLASSIC SPICY CHICKEN BREASTS

Cooking Time: 30 Minutes   **Servings: 6**

Ingredients:

- ✓ 1 ½ pounds chicken breasts
- ✓ 1 bell pepper, deveined and chopped
- ✓ 1 leek, chopped
- ✓ 1 tomato, pureed
- ✓ 2 tbsp coriander
- ✓ 2 garlic cloves, minced
- ✓ 1 tsp cayenne pepper
- ✓ 1 tsp dry thyme
- ✓ 1/4 cup coconut aminos
- ✓ Sea salt and ground black pepper, to taste

Directions:

- ❖ Rub each chicken breasts with the garlic, cayenne pepper, thyme, salt and black pepper. Cook the chicken in a saucepan over medium-high heat.
- ❖ Sear for about 5 minutes until golden brown on all sides.
- ❖ Fold in the tomato puree and coconut aminos and bring it to a boil. Add in the pepper, leek, and coriander.
- ❖ Reduce the heat to simmer. Continue to cook, partially covered, for about 20 minutes.
- ❖ Storing
- ❖ Place the chicken breasts in airtight containers or Ziploc bags; keep in your refrigerator for 3 to 4 days.
- ❖ For freezing, place the chicken breasts in airtight containers or heavy-duty freezer bags. It will maintain the best quality for about 4 months. Defrost in the refrigerator. Bon appétit!

Nutrition: 239 Calories; 6g Fat; 5.5g Carbs; 34.3g Protein; 1g Fiber

404)   DELICIOUS SAUCY BOSTON BUTT

Cooking Time: 1 Hour 20 Minutes   **Servings: 8**

Ingredients:

- ✓ 1 tbsp lard, room temperature
- ✓ 2 pounds Boston butt, cubed
- ✓ Salt and freshly ground pepper
- ✓ 1/2 tsp mustard powder
- ✓ A bunch of spring onions, chopped
- ✓ 2 garlic cloves, minced
- ✓ 1/2 tbsp ground cardamom
- ✓ 2 tomatoes, pureed
- ✓ 1 bell pepper, deveined and chopped
- ✓ 1 jalapeno pepper, deveined and finely chopped
- ✓ 1/2 cup unsweetened coconut milk
- ✓ 2 cups chicken bone broth

Directions:

- ❖ In a wok, melt the lard over moderate heat. Season the pork belly with salt, pepper and mustard powder.
- ❖ Sear the pork for 8 to 10 minutes, stirring periodically to ensure even cooking; set aside, keeping it warm.
- ❖ In the same wok, sauté the spring onions, garlic, and cardamom. Spoon the sautéed vegetables along with the reserved pork into the slow cooker.
- ❖ Add in the remaining ingredients, cover with the lid and cook for 1 hour 10 minutes over low heat.
- ❖ Storing
- ❖ Divide the pork and vegetables between airtight containers or Ziploc bags; keep in your refrigerator for up to 3 to 5 days.
- ❖ For freezing, place the pork and vegetables in airtight containers or heavy-duty freezer bags. Freeze up to 4 months. Defrost in the refrigerator. Bon appétit!

Nutrition: 369 Calories; 20.2g Fat; 2.9g Carbs; 41.3g Protein; 0.7g Fiber

405)   OLD-FASHIONED HUNGARIAN GOULASH

Cooking Time: 9 Hours 10 Minutes   **Servings: 4**

Ingredients:

- ✓ 1 ½ pounds pork butt, chopped
- ✓ 1 tsp sweet Hungarian paprika
- ✓ 2 Hungarian hot peppers, deveined and minced
- ✓ 1 cup leeks, chopped
- ✓ 1 ½ tbsp lard
- ✓ 1 tsp caraway seeds, ground
- ✓ 4 cups vegetable broth
- ✓ 2 garlic cloves, crushed
- ✓ 1 tsp cayenne pepper
- ✓ 2 cups tomato sauce with herbs
- ✓ 1 ½ pounds pork butt, chopped
- ✓ 1 tsp sweet Hungarian paprika
- ✓ 2 Hungarian hot peppers, deveined and minced
- ✓ 1 cup leeks, chopped
- ✓ 1 ½ tbsp lard
- ✓ 1 tsp caraway seeds, ground
- ✓ 4 cups vegetable broth
- ✓ 2 garlic cloves, crushed
- ✓ 1 tsp cayenne pepper
- ✓ 2 cups tomato sauce with herbs

Directions:

- ❖ Melt the lard in a heavy-bottomed pot over medium-high heat. Sear the pork for 5 to 6 minutes until just browned on all sides; set aside.
- ❖ Add in the leeks and garlic; continue to cook until they have softened.
- ❖ Place the reserved pork along with the sautéed mixture in your crock pot. Add in the other ingredients and stir to combine.
- ❖ Cover with the lid and slow cook for 9 hours on the lowest setting.
- ❖ Storing
- ❖ Spoon your goulash into four airtight containers or Ziploc bags; keep in your refrigerator for up to 3 to 4 days.
- ❖ For freezing, place the goulash in airtight containers. Freeze up to 4 to 6 months. Defrost in the refrigerator. Enjoy!

Nutrition: 456 Calories; 27g Fat; 6.7g Carbs; 32g Protein; 3.4g Fiber

406) FLATBREAD AND CHICKEN LIVER PÂTÉ

Cooking Time: 2 Hours 15 Minutes   **Servings:** 4

Ingredients:

- ✓ 1 yellow onion, finely chopped
- ✓ 10 ounces chicken livers
- ✓ 1/2 tsp Mediterranean seasoning blend
- ✓ 4 tbsp olive oil
- ✓ 1 garlic clove, minced

- ✓ For Flatbread:
- ✓ 1 cup lukewarm water
- ✓ 1/2 stick butter
- ✓ 1/2 cup flax meal
- ✓ 1 ½ tbsp psyllium husks
- ✓ 1 ¼ cups almond flour

Directions:

- ❖ Pulse the chicken livers along with the seasoning blend, olive oil, onion and garlic in your food processor; reserve.
- ❖ Mix the dry ingredients for the flatbread. Mix in all the wet ingredients. Whisk to combine well.
- ❖ Let it stand at room temperature for 2 hours. Divide the dough into 8 balls and roll them out on a flat surface.
- ❖ In a lightly greased pan, cook your flatbread for 1 minute on each side or until golden.
- ❖ Storing
- ❖ Wrap the chicken liver pate in foil before packing it into airtight containers; keep in your refrigerator for up to 7 days.
- ❖ For freezing, place the chicken liver pate in airtight containers or heavy-duty freezer bags. Freeze up to 2 months. Defrost overnight in the refrigerator.
- ❖ As for the keto flatbread, wrap them in foil before packing them into airtight containers; keep in your refrigerator for up to 4 days.
- ❖ Bon appétit!

Nutrition: 395 Calories; 30.2g Fat; 3.6g Carbs; 17.9g Protein; 0.5g Fiber

407) SATURDAY CHICKEN WITH CAULIFLOWER SALAD

Cooking Time: 20 Minutes   **Servings:** 2

Ingredients:

- ✓ 1 tsp hot paprika
- ✓ 2 tbsp fresh basil, snipped
- ✓ 1/2 cup mayonnaise
- ✓ 1 tsp mustard
- ✓ 2 tsp butter
- ✓ 2 chicken wings

- ✓ 1/2 cup cheddar cheese, shredded
- ✓ Sea salt and ground black pepper, to taste
- ✓ 2 tbsp dry sherry
- ✓ 1 shallot, finely minced
- ✓ 1/2 head of cauliflower

Directions:

- ❖ Boil the cauliflower in a pot of salted water until it has softened; cut into small florets and place in a salad bowl.
- ❖ Melt the butter in a saucepan over medium-high heat. Cook the chicken for about 8 minutes or until the skin is crisp and browned. Season with hot paprika salt, and black pepper.
- ❖ Whisk the mayonnaise, mustard, dry sherry, and shallot and dress your salad. Top with cheddar cheese and fresh basil.
- ❖ Storing
- ❖ Place the chicken wings in airtight containers or Ziploc bags; keep in your refrigerator for up 3 to 4 days.
- ❖ Keep the cauliflower salad in your refrigerator for up 3 days.
- ❖ For freezing, place the chicken wings in airtight containers or heavy-duty freezer bags. Freeze up to 3 months. Once thawed in the refrigerator, reheat in a saucepan until thoroughly warmed.

Nutrition: 444 Calories; 36g Fat; 5.7g Carbs; 20.6g Protein; 4.3g Fiber

408) SPECIAL KANSAS-STYLE MEATLOAF

Cooking Time: 1 Hour 10 Minutes   **Servings:** 8

Ingredients:

- ✓ 2 pounds ground pork
- ✓ 2 eggs, beaten
- ✓ 1/2 cup onions, chopped
- ✓ 1/2 cup marinara sauce, bottled
- ✓ 8 ounces Colby cheese, shredded
- ✓ 1 tsp granulated garlic

- ✓ Sea salt and freshly ground black pepper, to taste
- ✓ 1 tsp lime zest
- ✓ 1 tsp mustard seeds
- ✓ 1/2 cup tomato puree
- ✓ 1 tbsp Erythritol

Directions:

- ❖ Mix the ground pork with the eggs, onions, marinara salsa, cheese, granulated garlic, salt, pepper, lime zest, and mustard seeds; mix to combine.
- ❖ Press the mixture into a lightly-greased loaf pan. Mix the tomato paste with the Erythritol and spread the mixture over the top of your meatloaf.
- ❖ Bake in the preheated oven at 5 degrees F for about 1 hour 10 minutes, rotating the pan halfway through the cook time. Storing Wrap your meatloaf tightly with heavy-duty aluminum foil or plastic wrap. Then, keep in your refrigerator for up to 3 to 4 days.
- ❖ For freezing, wrap your meatloaf tightly to prevent freezer burn. Freeze up to 3 to 4 months. Defrost in the refrigerator. Bon appétit!

Nutrition: 318 Calories; 14. Fat; 6.2g Carbs; 39.3g Protein; 0.3g Fiber

409) ORIGINAL TURKEY KEBABS

Cooking Time: 30 Minutes   **Servings:** 6

Ingredients:

- ✓ 1 ½ pounds turkey breast, cubed
- ✓ 3 Spanish peppers, sliced
- ✓ 2 zucchinis, cut into thick slices
- ✓ 1 onion, cut into wedges
- ✓ 2 tbsp olive oil, room temperature
- ✓ 1 tbsp dry ranch seasoning

Directions:

- ❖ Thread the turkey pieces and vegetables onto bamboo skewers. Sprinkle the skewers with dry ranch seasoning and olive oil.
- ❖ Grill your kebabs for about 10 minutes, turning them periodically to ensure even cooking.
- ❖ Storing
- ❖ Wrap your kebabs in foil before packing them into airtight containers; keep in your refrigerator for up to 3 to days.
- ❖ For freezing, place your kebabs in airtight containers or heavy-duty freezer bags. Freeze up to 2-3 months. Defrost in the refrigerator. Bon appétit!

Nutrition: 2 Calories; 13.8g Fat; 6.7g Carbs; 25.8g Protein; 1.2g Fiber

410) ORIGINAL MEXICAN-STYLE TURKEY BACON BITES

Cooking Time: 5 Minutes   **Servings:** 4

Ingredients:

- ✓ 4 ounces turkey bacon, chopped
- ✓ 4 ounces Neufchatel cheese
- ✓ 1 tbsp butter, cold
- ✓ 1 jalapeno pepper, deveined and minced
- ✓ 1 tsp Mexican oregano
- ✓ 2 tbsp scallions, finely chopped

Directions:

- ❖ Thoroughly combine all ingredients in a mixing bowl.
- ❖ Roll the mixture into 8 balls.
- ❖ Storing
- ❖ Divide the turkey bacon bites between two airtight containers or Ziploc bags; keep in your refrigerator for up 3 to days.

Nutrition: 19Calories; 16.7g Fat; 2.2g Carbs; 8.8g Protein; 0.3g Fiber

411) ORIGINAL MUFFINS WITH GROUND PORK

Cooking Time: 25 Minutes   **Servings:** 6

Ingredients:

- ✓ 1 stick butter
- ✓ 3 large eggs, lightly beaten
- ✓ 2 tbsp full-fat milk
- ✓ 1/2 tsp ground cardamom
- ✓ 3 ½ cups almond flour
- ✓ 2 tbsp flaxseed meal
- ✓ 1 tsp baking powder
- ✓ 2 cups ground pork
- ✓ Salt and pepper, to your liking
- ✓ 1/2 tsp dried basil

Directions:

- ❖ In the preheated frying pan, cook the ground pork until the juices run clear, approximately 5 minutes.
- ❖ Add in the remaining ingredients and stir until well combined.
- ❖ Spoon the mixture into lightly greased muffin cups. Bake in the preheated oven at 5 degrees F for about 17 minutes.
- ❖ Allow your muffins to cool down before unmolding and storing.
- ❖ Storing
- ❖ Place your muffins in the airtight containers or Ziploc bags; keep in the refrigerator for a week.
- ❖ For freezing, divide your muffins among Ziploc bags and freeze up to 3 months. Defrost in your microwave for a couple of minutes. Bon appétit!

Nutrition: 330 Calories; 30.3g Fat; 2.3g Carbs; 19g Protein; 1.2g Fiber

412) Authentic Pork Chops With Herbs

Cooking Time: 20 Minutes   **Servings:** 4

Ingredients:

- ✓ 1 tbsp butter
- ✓ 1 pound pork chops
- ✓ 2 rosemary sprigs, minced
- ✓ 1 tsp dried marjoram
- ✓ 1 tsp dried parsley
- ✓ A bunch of spring onions, roughly chopped
- ✓ 1 thyme sprig, minced
- ✓ 1/2 tsp granulated garlic
- ✓ 1/2 tsp paprika, crushed
- ✓ Coarse salt and ground black pepper, to taste

Directions:

- ❖ Season the pork chops with the granulated garlic, paprika, salt, and black pepper.
- ❖ Melt the butter in a frying pan over a moderate flame. Cook the pork chops for 6 to 8 minutes, turning them occasionally to ensure even cooking.
- ❖ Add in the remaining ingredients and cook an additional 4 minutes.
- ❖ Storing
- ❖ Divide the pork chops into four portions; place each portion in a separate airtight container or Ziploc bag; keep in your refrigerator for 3 to 4 days.
- ❖ Freeze the pork chops in airtight containers or heavy-duty freezer bags. Freeze up to 4 months. Defrost in the refrigerator. Bon appétit!

413) TYPICAL MEDITERRANEAN-STYLE CHEESY PORK LOIN

Cooking Time: 25 Minutes   **Servings: 4**

Ingredients:

- ✓ 1 pound pork loin, cut into 1-inch-thick pieces
- ✓ 1 tsp Mediterranean seasoning mix
- ✓ Salt and pepper, to taste
- ✓ 1 onion, sliced
- ✓ 1 tsp fresh garlic, smashed
- ✓ 2 tbsp black olives, pitted and sliced
- ✓ 2 tbsp balsamic vinegar
- ✓ 1/2 cup Romano cheese, grated
- ✓ 2 tbsp butter, room temperature
- ✓ 1 tbsp curry paste
- ✓ 1 cup roasted vegetable broth
- ✓ 1 tbsp oyster sauce

Directions:

- ❖ In a frying pan, melt the butter over a moderately high heat. Once hot, cook the pork until browned on all sides; season with salt and black pepper and set aside.
- ❖ In the pan drippings, cook the onion and garlic for 4 to 5 minutes or until they've softened.
- ❖ Add in the Mediterranean seasoning mix, curry paste, and vegetable broth. Continue to cook until the sauce has thickened and reduced slightly or about 10 minutes. Add in the remaining ingredients along with the reserved pork.
- ❖ Top with cheese and cook for 10 minutes longer or until cooked through.
- ❖ Storing
- ❖ Divide the pork loin between four airtight containers; keep in your refrigerator for 3 to 5 days.
- ❖ For freezing, place the pork loin in airtight containers or heavy-duty freezer bags. Freeze up to 4 to 6 months. Defrost in the refrigerator. Enjoy!

Nutrition: 476 Calories; 35.3g Fat; 6.2g Carbs; 31.1g Protein; 1.4g Fiber

414) OVEN-ROASTED SPARE RIBS

Cooking Time: 3 Hour 40 Minutes   **Servings: 6**

Ingredients:

- ✓ 2 pounds spare ribs
- ✓ 1 garlic clove, minced
- ✓ 1 tsp dried marjoram
- ✓ 1 lime, halved
- ✓ Salt and ground black pepper, to taste

Directions:

- ❖ Toss all ingredients in a ceramic dish.
- ❖ Cover and let it refrigerate for 5 to 6 hours.
- ❖ Roast the foil-wrapped ribs in the preheated oven at 275 degrees F degrees for about hours 30 minutes.
- ❖ Storing
- ❖ Divide the ribs into six portions. Place each portion of ribs in an airtight container; keep in your refrigerator for 3 to 5 days.
- ❖ For freezing, place the ribs in airtight containers or heavy-duty freezer bags. Freeze up to 4 to months. Defrost in the refrigerator and reheat in the preheated oven. Bon appétit!

Nutrition: 385 Calories; 29g Fat; 1.8g Carbs; 28.3g Protein; 0.1g Fiber

415) HEALTHY PARMESAN CHICKEN SALAD

Cooking Time: 20 Minutes   **Servings: 6**

Ingredients:

- ✓ 2 romaine hearts, leaves separated
- ✓ Flaky sea salt and ground black pepper, to taste
- ✓ 1/4 tsp chili pepper flakes
- ✓ 1 tsp dried basil
- ✓ 1/4 cup Parmesan, finely grated
- ✓ 2 chicken breasts
- ✓ 2 Lebanese cucumbers, sliced
- ✓ For the dressing:
- ✓ 2 large egg yolks
- ✓ 1 tsp Dijon mustard
- ✓ 1 tbsp fresh lemon juice
- ✓ 1/4 cup olive oil
- ✓ 2 garlic cloves, minced

Directions:

- ❖ In a grilling pan, cook the chicken breast until no longer pink or until a meat thermometer registers 5 degrees F. Slice the chicken into strips.
- ❖ Storing
- ❖ Place the chicken breasts in airtight containers or Ziploc bags; keep in your refrigerator for to 4 days.
- ❖ For freezing, place the chicken breasts in airtight containers or heavy-duty freezer bags. It will maintain the best quality for about months. Defrost in the refrigerator.
- ❖ Toss the chicken with the other ingredients. Prepare the dressing by whisking all the ingredients.
- ❖ Dress the salad and enjoy! Keep the salad in your refrigerator for 3 to 5 days.

Nutrition: 183 Calories; 12.5g Fat; 1. Carbs; 16.3g Protein; 0.9g Fiber

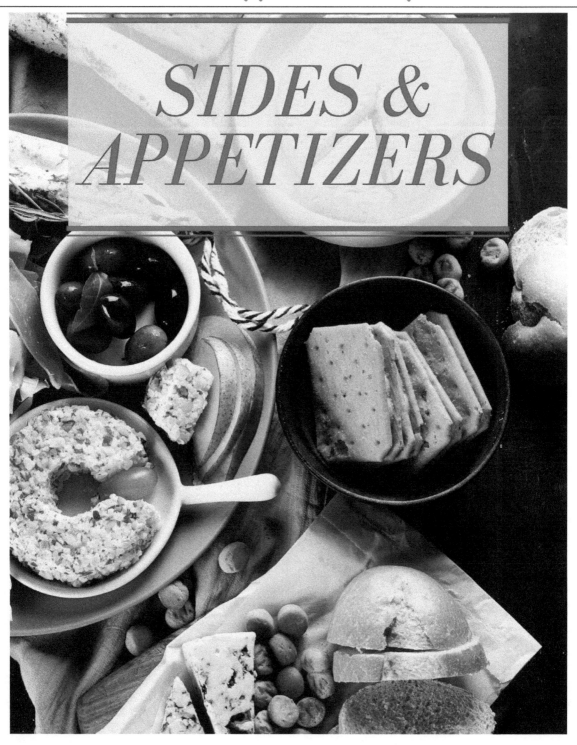

SIDES &
APPETIZERS

416) TUSCAN BAKED MUSHROOMS

Cooking Time: 20 Minutes   **Servings: 2**

Ingredients:

- ½ pound mushrooms (sliced)
- 2 tbsp olive oil (onion and garlic flavored)
- 1 can tomatoes
- 1 cup Parmesan cheese
- ½ tsp oregano
- 1 tbsp basil
- sea salt or plain salt
- freshly ground black pepper

Directions:

- Heat the olive oil in the pan and add the mushrooms, salt, and pepper. Cook for about 2 minutes.
- Then, transfer the mushrooms into a baking dish.
- Now, in a separate bowl mix the tomatoes, basil, oregano, salt, and pepper, and layer it on the mushrooms. Top it with Parmesan cheese.
- Finally, bake the dish at 0 degrees F for about 18-22 minutes or until done.
- Serve warm.

Nutrition: Calories: 358, Total Fat: 27 g, Saturated Fat: 10.2 g, Cholesterol: 40 mg, Sodium: 535 mg, Total Carbohydrate: 13 g, Dietary Fiber: 3.5 g, Total Sugars: 6.7 g, Protein: 23.2 g, Vitamin D: 408 mcg, Calcium: 526 mg, Iron: 4 mg, Potassium: 797 mg

417) TYPICAL MINT TABBOULEH

Cooking Time: 15 Minutes   **Servings: 6**

Ingredients:

- ¼ cup fine bulgur
- 1/3 cup water, boiling
- 3 tbsp lemon juice
- ¼ tsp honey
- 1 1/3 cups pistachios, finely chopped
- 1 cup curly parsley, finely chopped
- 1 small cucumber, finely chopped
- 1 medium tomato, finely chopped
- 4 green onions, finely chopped
- 1/3 cup fresh mint, finely chopped
- 3 tbsp olive oil

Directions:

- Take a large bowl and add bulgur and 3 cup of boiling water.
- Allow it to stand for about 5 minutes.
- Stir in honey and lemon juice and allow it to stand for 5 minutes more.
- Fluff up the bulgur with a fork and stir in the rest of the Ingredients.
- Season with salt and pepper.
- Enjoy!

Nutrition: Calories: 15 Total Fat: 13.5 g, Saturated Fat: 1.8 g, Cholesterol: 0 mg, Sodium: 78 mg, Total Carbohydrate: 9.2 g, Dietary Fiber: 2.8 g, Total Sugars: 2.9 g, Protein: 3.8 g, Vitamin D: 0 mcg, Calcium: 46 mg, Iron: 2 mg, Potassium: 359 mg

418) Italian Scallops Pea Fettuccine

Cooking Time: 15 Minutes   **Servings: 5**

Ingredients:

- 8 ounces whole-wheat fettuccine (pasta, macaroni)
- 1 pound large sea scallops
- ¼ tsp salt, divided
- 1 tbsp extra virgin olive oil
- 1 8-ounce bottle of clam juice
- 1 cup low-fat milk
- ¼ tsp ground white pepper
- 3 cups frozen peas, thawed
- ¾ cup finely shredded Romano cheese, divided
- 1/3 cup fresh chives, chopped
- ½ tsp freshly grated lemon zest
- 1 tsp lemon juice

Directions:

- Boil water in a large pot and cook fettuccine according to package instructions.
- Drain well and put it to the side.
- Heat oil in a large, non-stick skillet over medium-high heat.
- Pat the scallops dry and sprinkle them with 1/8 tsp of salt.
- Add the scallops to the skillet and cook for about 2-3 minutes per side until golden brown. Remove scallops from pan.
- Add clam juice to the pan you removed the scallops from.
- In another bowl, whisk in milk, white pepper, flour, and remaining 1/8 tsp of salt.
- Once the mixture is smooth, whisk into the pan with the clam juice.
- Bring the entire mix to a simmer and keep stirring for about 1-2 minutes until the sauce is thick.
- Return the scallops to the pan and add peas. Bring it to a simmer.
- Stir in fettuccine, chives, ½ a cup of Romano cheese, lemon zest, and lemon juice.
- Mix well until thoroughly combined.
- Cool and spread over containers.
- Before eating, serve with remaining cheese sprinkled on top.
- Enjoy!

Nutrition: Calories: 388, Total Fat: 9.2 g, Saturated Fat: 3.7 g, Cholesterol: 33 mg, Sodium: 645 mg, Total Carbohydrate: 50.1 g, Dietary Fiber: 10.4 g, Total Sugars: 8.7 g, Protein: 24.9 g, Vitamin D: 25 mcg, Calcium: 293 mg, Iron: 4 mg, Potassium: 247 mg

419) **CLASSIC BASIL PASTA**

Cooking Time: 40 Minutes   **Servings: 4**

Ingredients:

- ✓ 2 red peppers, de-seeded and cut into chunks
- ✓ 2 red onions cut into wedges
- ✓ 2 mild red chilies, de-seeded and diced
- ✓ 3 garlic cloves, coarsely chopped
- ✓ 1 tsp golden caster sugar
- ✓ 2 tbsp olive oil, plus extra for serving

- ✓ 2 pounds small ripe tomatoes, quartered
- ✓ 12 ounces pasta
- ✓ a handful of basil leaves, torn
- ✓ 2 tbsp grated parmesan
- ✓ salt
- ✓ pepper

Directions:

- ❖ Preheat oven to 390 degrees F.
- ❖ On a large roasting pan, spread peppers, red onion, garlic, and chilies.
- ❖ Sprinkle sugar on top.
- ❖ Drizzle olive oil and season with salt and pepper.
- ❖ Roast the veggies for 1minutes.
- ❖ Add tomatoes and roast for another 15 minutes.
- ❖ In a large pot, cook your pasta in salted boiling water according to instructions.
- ❖ Once ready, drain pasta.
- ❖ Remove the veggies from the oven and carefully add pasta.
- ❖ Toss everything well and let it cool.
- ❖ Spread over the containers.
- ❖ Before eating, place torn basil leaves on top, and sprinkle with parmesan.
- ❖ Enjoy!

Nutrition: Calories: 384, Total Fat: 10.8 g, Saturated Fat: 2.3 g, Cholesterol: 67 mg, Sodium: 133 mg, Total Carbohydrate: 59.4 g, Dietary Fiber: 2.3 g, Total Sugars: 5.7 g, Protein: 1 g, Vitamin D: 0 mcg, Calcium: 105 mg, Iron: 4 mg, Potassium: 422 mg

420) **Veggie Mediterranean-style Pasta**

Cooking Time: 2 Hours   **Servings: 4**

Ingredients:

- ✓ 1 tbsp olive oil
- ✓ 1 small onion, finely chopped
- ✓ 2 small garlic cloves, finely chopped
- ✓ 2 14-ounce cans diced tomatoes
- ✓ 1 tbsp sun-dried tomato paste
- ✓ 1 bay leaf
- ✓ 1 tsp dried thyme
- ✓ 1 tsp dried basil
- ✓ 1 tsp oregano
- ✓ 1 tsp dried parsley
- ✓ bread of your choice

- ✓ ½ tsp salt
- ✓ ½ tsp brown sugar
- ✓ freshly ground black pepper
- ✓ 1 piece aubergine
- ✓ 2 pieces courgettes
- ✓ 2 pieces red peppers, de-seeded
- ✓ 2 garlic cloves, peeled
- ✓ 2-3 tbsp olive oil
- ✓ 12 small vine-ripened tomatoes
- ✓ 16 ounces of pasta of your preferred shape, such as Gigli, conchiglie, etc.
- ✓ 3½ ounces parmesan cheese

Directions:

- ❖ Heat oil in a pan over medium heat.
- ❖ Add onions and fry them until tender.
- ❖ Add garlic and stir-fry for 1 minute.
- ❖ Add the remaining Ingredients: listed under the sauce and bring to a boil.
- ❖ Reduce the heat, cover, and simmer for 60 minutes.
- ❖ Season with black pepper and salt as needed. Set aside.
- ❖ Preheat oven to 350 degrees F.
- ❖ Chop up courgettes, aubergine and red peppers into 1-inch pieces.
- ❖ Place them on a roasting pan along with whole garlic cloves.
- ❖ Drizzle with olive oil and season with salt and black pepper.
- ❖ Mix the veggies well and roast in the oven for 45 minutes until they are tender.
- ❖ Add tomatoes just before 20 minutes to end time.
- ❖ Cook your pasta according to package instructions.
- ❖ Drain well and stir into the sauce.
- ❖ Divide the pasta sauce between 4 containers and top with vegetables.
- ❖ Grate some parmesan cheese on top and serve with bread.
- ❖ Enjoy!

Nutrition: Calories: 211, Total Fat: 14.9 g, Saturated Fat: 2.1 g, Cholesterol: 0 mg, Sodium: 317 mg, Total Carbohydrate: 20.1 g, Dietary Fiber: 5.7 g, Total Sugars: 11.7 g, Protein: 4.2 g, Vitamin D: 0 mcg, Calcium: 66 mg, Iron: 2 mg, Potassium: 955 mg

421) ORIGINAL RED ONION KALE PASTA

Cooking Time: 25 Minutes   **Servings:** 4

Ingredients:

- ✓ 2½ cups vegetable broth
- ✓ ¾ cup dry lentils
- ✓ ½ tsp of salt
- ✓ 1 bay leaf
- ✓ ¼ cup olive oil
- ✓ 1 large red onion, chopped
- ✓ 1 tsp fresh thyme, chopped
- ✓ ½ tsp fresh oregano, chopped
- ✓ 1 tsp salt, divided
- ✓ ½ tsp black pepper
- ✓ 8 ounces vegan sausage, sliced into ¼-inch slices
- ✓ 1 bunch kale, stems removed and coarsely chopped
- ✓ 1 pack rotini

Directions:

- ❖ Add vegetable broth, ½ tsp of salt, bay leaf, and lentils to a saucepan over high heat and bring to a boil.
- ❖ Reduce the heat to medium-low and allow to cook for about minutes until tender.
- ❖ Discard the bay leaf.
- ❖ Take another skillet and heat olive oil over medium-high heat.
- ❖ Stir in thyme, onions, oregano, ½ a tsp of salt, and pepper; cook for 1 minute.
- ❖ Add sausage and reduce heat to medium-low.
- ❖ Cook for 10 minutes until the onions are tender.
- ❖ Bring water to a boil in a large pot, and then add rotini pasta and kale.
- ❖ Cook for about 8 minutes until al dente.
- ❖ Remove a bit of the cooking water and put it to the side.
- ❖ Drain the pasta and kale and return to the pot.
- ❖ Stir in both the lentils mixture and the onions mixture.
- ❖ Add the reserved cooking liquid to add just a bit of moistness.
- ❖ Spread over containers.

Nutrition: Calories: 508, Total Fat: 17 g, Saturated Fat: 3 g, Cholesterol: 0 mg, Sodium: 2431 mg, Total Carbohydrate: 59.3 g, Dietary Fiber: 6 g, Total Sugars: 4.8 g, Protein: 30.9 g, Vitamin D: 0 mcg, Calcium: 256 mg, Iron: 8 mg, Potassium: 1686 mg

422) Special Braised Artichokes

Cooking Time: 30 Minutes   **Servings:** 6

Ingredients:

- ✓ 6 tbsp olive oil
- ✓ 2 pounds baby artichokes, trimmed
- ✓ ½ cup lemon juice
- ✓ 4 garlic cloves, thinly sliced
- ✓ ½ tsp salt
- ✓ 1½ pounds tomatoes, seeded and diced
- ✓ ½ cup almonds, toasted and sliced

Directions:

- ❖ Heat oil in a skillet over medium heat.
- ❖ Add artichokes, garlic, and lemon juice, and allow the garlic to sizzle.
- ❖ Season with salt.
- ❖ Reduce heat to medium-low, cover, and simmer for about 15 minutes.
- ❖ Uncover, add tomatoes, and simmer for another 10 minutes until the tomato liquid has mostly evaporated.
- ❖ Season with more salt and pepper.
- ❖ Sprinkle with toasted almonds.
- ❖ Enjoy!

Nutrition: Calories: 265, Total Fat: 1g, Saturated Fat: 2.6 g, Cholesterol: 0 mg, Sodium: 265 mg, Total Carbohydrate: 23 g, Dietary Fiber: 8.1 g, Total Sugars: 12.4 g, Protein: 7 g, Vitamin D: 0 mcg, Calcium: 81 mg, Iron: 2 mg, Potassium: 1077 mg

423) DELICIOUS FRIED GREEN BEANS

Cooking Time: 15 Minutes   **Servings:** 2

Ingredients:

- ✓ ½ pound green beans, trimmed
- ✓ 1 egg
- ✓ 2 tbsp olive oil
- ✓ 1¼ tbsp almond flour
- ✓ 2 tbsp parmesan cheese
- ✓ ½ tsp garlic powder
- ✓ sea salt or plain salt
- ✓ freshly ground black pepper

Directions:

- ❖ Start by beating the egg and olive oil in a bowl.
- ❖ Then, mix the remaining Ingredients: in a separate bowl and set aside.
- ❖ Now, dip the green beans in the egg mixture and then coat with the dry mix.
- ❖ Finally, grease a baking pan, then transfer the beans to the pan and bake at 5 degrees F for about 12-15 minutes or until crisp.
- ❖ Serve warm.

Nutrition: Calories: 334, Total Fat: 23 g, Saturated Fat: 8.3 g, Cholesterol: 109 mg, Sodium: 397 mg, Total Carbohydrate: 10.9 g, Dietary Fiber: 4.3 g, Total Sugars: 1.9 g, Protein: 18.1 g, Vitamin D: 8 mcg, Calcium: 398 mg, Iron: 2 mg, Potassium: 274 mg

424)   ARTICHOKE OLIVE PASTA

Cooking Time: 25 Minutes   **Servings: 4**

Ingredients:

- ✓ salt
- ✓ pepper
- ✓ 2 tbsp olive oil, divided
- ✓ 2 garlic cloves, thinly sliced
- ✓ 1 can artichoke hearts, drained, rinsed, and quartered lengthwise
- ✓ 1-pint grape tomatoes, halved lengthwise, divided
- ✓ ½ cup fresh basil leaves, torn apart
- ✓ 12 ounces whole-wheat spaghetti
- ✓ ½ medium onion, thinly sliced
- ✓ ½ cup dry white wine
- ✓ 1/3 cup pitted Kalamata olives, quartered lengthwise
- ✓ ¼ cup grated Parmesan cheese, plus extra for serving

Directions:

- ❖ Fill a large pot with salted water.
- ❖ Pour the water to a boil and cook your pasta according to package instructions until al dente.
- ❖ Drain the pasta and reserve 1 cup of the cooking water.
- ❖ Return the pasta to the pot and set aside.
- ❖ Heat 1 tbsp of olive oil in a large skillet over medium-high heat.
- ❖ Add onion and garlic, season with pepper and salt, and cook well for about 3-4 minutes until nicely browned.
- ❖ Add wine and cook for 2 minutes until evaporated.
- ❖ Stir in artichokes and keep cooking 2-3 minutes until brown.
- ❖ Add olives and half of your tomatoes.
- ❖ Cook well for 1-2 minutes until the tomatoes start to break down.
- ❖ Add pasta to the skillet.
- ❖ Stir in the rest of the tomatoes, cheese, basil, and remaining oil.
- ❖ Thin the mixture with the reserved pasta water if needed.
- ❖ Place in containers and sprinkle with extra cheese.
- ❖ Enjoy!

Nutrition: 340, Total Fat: 11.9 g, Saturated Fat: 3.3 g, Cholesterol: 10 mg, Sodium: 278 mg, Total Carbohydrate: 35.8 g, Dietary Fiber: 7.8 g, Total Sugars: 4.8 g, Protein: 11.6 g, Vitamin D: 0 mcg, Calcium: 193 mg, Iron: 3 mg, Potassium: 524 mg

425)   MEDITERRANEAN OLIVE TUNA PASTA

Cooking Time: 20 Minutes   **Servings: 4**

Ingredients:

- ✓ 8 ounces of tuna steak, cut into 3 pieces
- ✓ ¼ cup green olives, chopped
- ✓ 3 cloves garlic, minced
- ✓ 2 cups grape tomatoes, halved
- ✓ ½ cup white wine
- ✓ 2 tbsp lemon juice
- ✓ 6 ounces pasta - whole wheat gobetti, rotini, or penne
- ✓ 1 10-ounce package frozen artichoke hearts, thawed and squeezed dry
- ✓ 4 tbsp extra-virgin olive oil, divided
- ✓ 2 tsp fresh grated lemon zest
- ✓ 2 tsp fresh rosemary, chopped, divided
- ✓ ½ tsp salt, divided
- ✓ ¼ tsp fresh ground pepper
- ✓ ¼ cup fresh basil, chopped

Directions:

- ❖ Preheat grill to medium-high heat.
- ❖ Take a large pot of water and put it on to boil.
- ❖ Place the tuna pieces in a bowl and add 1 tbsp of oil, 1 tsp of rosemary, lemon zest, a ¼ tsp of salt, and pepper.
- ❖ Grill the tuna for about 3 minutes per side.
- ❖ Transfer tuna to a plate and allow it to cool.
- ❖ Place the pasta in boiling water and cook according to package instructions.
- ❖ Drain the pasta.
- ❖ Flake the tuna into bite-sized pieces.
- ❖ In a large skillet, heat remaining oil over medium heat.
- ❖ Add artichoke hearts, garlic, olives, and remaining rosemary.
- ❖ Cook for about 3-4 minutes until slightly browned.
- ❖ Add tomatoes, wine, and bring the mixture to a boil.
- ❖ Cook for about 3 minutes until the tomatoes are broken down.
- ❖ Stir in pasta, lemon juice, tuna, and remaining salt.
- ❖ Cook for 1-2 minutes until nicely heated.
- ❖ Spread over the containers.
- ❖ Before eating, garnish with some basil and enjoy!

Nutrition: 455, Total Fat: 21.2 g, Saturated Fat: 3.5 g, Cholesterol: 59 mg, Sodium: 685 mg, Total Carbohydrate: 38.4 g, Dietary Fiber: 6.1 g, Total Sugars: 3.5 g, Protein: 25.5 g, Vitamin D: 0 mcg, Calcium: 100 mg, Iron: 5 mg, Potassium: 800 mg

AUTHOR BIBLIOGRAPHY

THE MEDITERRANEAN DIET:

Cookbook for Beginners: Master Guidance, and More than 100 Recipes to Get You Started.

THE MEDITERRANEAN DIET FOR BEGINNERS:

The Complete Guide with More than 100 Delicious Recipes, and

Tips for Success!

THE MEDITERRANEAN DIET COOKBOOK:

A Guide for Beginners: Discover 100+ Delicious Recipes for Healthy Eating. Enjoy your Food Every Day!!!

THE MEDITERRANEAN DIET COPLETE GUIDE FOR BEGINNER:

2 Books in 1: The Ultimate Guide for Beginners: Discover 200+ Delicious Recipes and Start to Lose Weight for a Healthy Eating! Enjoy your Food

Every Day!!!

THE MEDITERRANEAN DIET FOR VEGETARIANS:

Complete Guide and More than 100 Delicious Mediterranean recipes suitable for Vegetarians

THE MEDITERRANEAN & KETO DIET:

The Guide on the Combination of the Mediterranean Diet and the Keto Diet to boost your weight loss and Get Fit and Healthy! Cookbook for

Beginners: Master Guidance, and More than 150 Recipes to Get You Started! 4-week Meal Plan Included

THE MEDITERRANEAN DIET SPECIAL EDITION:

4 Books in 1: A Simple Guide to Start the Mediterranean Diet suitable for Vegetarian and Athlete with more 400+ Recipes! 4-Week Keto Meal

Plan Included! Start to be Healthy and Fit!

THE MEDITERRANEAN DIET RECIPE BOOK:

2 Books in 1: 200 + Easy Recipes to Start a Heathy Lifestyle!!! Taste the Mediterranean Meals Flavors and Follow the Guide for Beginners Inside!

THE MEDITERRANEAN DIET FOR ATHLETE:

200+ Delicious Recipes for Healthy Eating. Enjoy your Food Every Day!!! Expert Tips to Improve your Health, Performance and Energy!

THE MEDITERRANEAN DIET FOR ABSOLUTE BEGINNERS:

3 Books in 1: The Ultimate and Complete Guide for Beginners: Discover 300+ Healthy, Delicious, and Easy to Follow Recipes to Enjoy your Food

Every Day and a New Lifestyle!!!

THE MEDITERRANEAN DIET FOR ONE:

Mediterranean diet to lose weight, burn fat and reset your metabolism! Quick & Easy Recipes to Change your Lifestyle!

THE MEDITERRANEAN DIET FOR TWO:

2 Books in 1: Easy, Healthy and Delicious Recipes That Will Make Your Life Way Easier! Quick, and Delicious Mediterranean Recipes That a Busy Person Can Cook to Kick-Start a Healthy Lifestyle!

THE MEDITERRANEAN DIET SIMPLE GUIDE:

2 Books in 1: The Complete Beginner Guide With 250+ Delicious and Easy-To-Make Low Calories Recipes to Boost Your Metabolism and Weight Loss!

THE MEDITERRANEAN HEALTHY DIET:

3 Books in 1: The Complete Guide, with 350+ Unique and Delicious Recipes to Get the Most out of Your Mediterranean-Style Cooking State-of-The-Art!

THE MEDITERRANEAN DIET COMPLETE COLLECTION:

4 Books in 1: The Master Mediterranean Guide to Lose Weight. Everything you Need to Get Started! A Fresh Guide to 455+ Vibrant Dishes Using Greens, Vegetables, Grains, Proteins, and More!

THE MEDITERRANEAN DIET FOR MEN:

120 + Easy Recipes to Start a Heathy Lifestyle!!! Taste the Mediterranean Meals Food Flavors Like a Restaurant!

THE MEDITERRANEAN DIET FOR MEN OVER 50:

2 Books in 1: 240+ Unique and Delicious Recipes to Get the Most out of Your Mediterranean-Style Cooking! Italian, Spanish, and Greek Food Meals!

THE MEDITERRANEAN DIET FOR FITNESS:

2 Books in 1: 240+ Recipes All Mediterranean with High-Protein! Beginners Guide to Increase Muscle Mass with Healthy and Whole-Food Italian, Spanish, and Greek Recipes to Fuel Your Workouts!

THE MEDITERRANEAN DIET QUICK AND EASY:

2 Books in 1: 240+ New Delicious Natural Mediterranean Food Quick & Easy-to-Follow Recipe to Taste!

THE MEDITERRANEAN DIET FOR LOSE WEIGHT:

2 Books in 1: Recipe Book for Beginners: 240+ Mediterranean Meals to Energize Your Body and Get to Know About How this Diet Can Help to Weight Loss!

THE MEDITERRANEAN DIET FOR HEALTHY BODY ENERGY:

2 Books in 1: Discover 240+ Healthy and Natural, Food-based Delicious, and Easy to Follow Recipes to Enjoy your Food Every Day and a New Lifestyle!!! Meat, Seafood, and Vegetarian Food

THE MEDITERRANEAN DIET FOR BEGINNERS' CHEF:

3 Books in 1: Cook Like in Restaurant! 340+ New Mediterranean Recipes Idea to Transform your Home into a Restaurant! Italian, Spanish, and Greek Food Recipes All with Natural Foods (Meat, Seafood, and Vegetables)!

THE MEDITERRANEAN DIET FOR FAMILY:

3 Books in 1: All You Need to Know About the Mediterranean Cooking + More Than 350+ Delicious Italian, Spanish, and Greek Style Recipes for Weight Loss and Live Healthy!

THE MEDITERRANEAN RESTAURANT COLLECTION:

4 Books in 1: A Game-Changing Approach to Peak Performance! 450+ Recipes All Mediterranean with High-Protein! Natural Food to Live a Healthy Lifestyle and Lose- Weight! Cook Like in Restaurant!

CONCLUSIONS

The Mediterranean diet emphasizes fresh foods such as fruits and vegetables in combination with whole grains. It is low in red meat and high in fish, poultry, nuts, and beans. This diet has many different types of food groups to help you bring variety into your day: bread (whole grain), beans/lentils/nuts/seeds, berries/vegetables, dairy (low fat), olive oil, refrigerated or uncooked fish/meat (preferably fatty fish), unlimited wine and alcohol (usually no more than one glass per day), cheese (low fat), fruit (fresh), eggplant, potatoes (unpeeled), cabbage (raw), and pasta (whole grain). Add other vegetables to meals, such as tomatoes. Don't overcook the meat. All meats should be grilled or broiled over a low flame that does not brown the meat to reduce cancer risk. It is best to use steaks instead of hamburgers or ground beef. Make sure poultry is white meat from chicken or turkey, not dark meat, including liver or bones. Use lean cuts of beef/pork such as round steak or tenderloin instead of fattier cuts such as sirloin or rib-eye steaks. Fish should be firm-fleshed and skin-on and fried in relatively light oil such as olive oil instead of butter or margarine, as this can increase the number of calories you eat per serving. Always use white meat turkey instead of dark meat breast for recipes that call for one type of meat since white meat has less fat: per serving than dark meat chicken breast. All fruits should be eaten raw to provide taste plus their vitamin content, including vitamin C plus others. Mediterranean health is a healthy lifestyle that includes eating lots of fresh fruits, lots of vegetables, whole grains, healthy fats, moderate amounts of alcohol, seafood, poultry, and engaging in physical activity. The Mediterranean diet is a healthy eating pattern recommended for people living in northern climates who are at low risk of developing cardiovascular disease or diabetes. It is called the Mediterranean diet because it originated in Italy, Spain, Greece, Turkey, and the Mediterranean Sea's southern countries. These countries (and others in the region) share many cultural and culinary similarities.

The Mediterranean diet, often called the Mediterranean lifestyle, has been getting a lot of hype lately. More and more people are trying to eat healthier or simply starting to think about what they eat. Mediterranean diets, sometimes called the traditional Mediterranean diet or traditional lifestyle was initially designed for those who worked on farms. They contain foods that lead to healthy hearts and muscular bodies. Many call the Mediterranean diet a "bikini-body diet." As surprising as it may be, there is not much difference between the Mediterranean diet and the Atkins diet. All three focus on eating healthy foods. The Mediterranean diet is based on the fact that food often contains more than one nutrient. Most fruits and vegetables have some fat: or sugar in them. The idea is to eat various foods from all parts of the world, which includes different types of meats, cheeses, grains, legumes, nuts, and other foods. In addition to being a great way to eat well naturally, the Mediterranean diet is good for your health. It has been shown to help with weight loss and cardiovascular disease prevention. It also promotes weight maintenance after weight loss. Studies have shown that it can reduce cholesterol levels in obese people and reduce blood pressure in people with hypertension. People with high cholesterol can have their grades lowered by following a Mediterranean diet. Studies have also shown that it can help fight cancer naturally, causing tumors to shrink faster than other dietary regimens.

Alexander Sandler

Lightning Source UK Ltd.
Milton Keynes UK
UKHW050734070621
385067UK00002B/108